MUSCLEMAG INTERNATIONAL'S

BODYFitness
FOR WOMEN

Your Way To Physical Perfection
By Gerard Thorne & Phil Embleton

Published by MuscleMag International
6465 Airport Road
Mississauga, Ontario
Canada L4V 1E4

Designed by Jackie Kydyk
Edited by Mandy Morgan
Printed in Canada

10 9 8 7 6 5 4 3 2 1 Pbk.

Canadian Cataloguing in Publication Data

Thorne, Gerard, 1963–
   Bodyfitness for women: your way to physical perfection

Includes index.
ISBN 1-55210-014-6

   1. Bodybuilding for women. I. Embleton, Phil J.,
1963– II. Title.

GV546.6. W64T48 1999   646.7'5'082   C99-900013-6

Distributed in Canada by
CANBOOK Distribution Services
1220 Nicholson Road
Newmarket, Ontario
L3Y 7V1
800-399-6858

Distributed in the States by
BookWorld Services
1933 Whitfield Park Loop
Sarasota, FL 34243
800-444-2524

BODYFITNESS FOR WOMEN

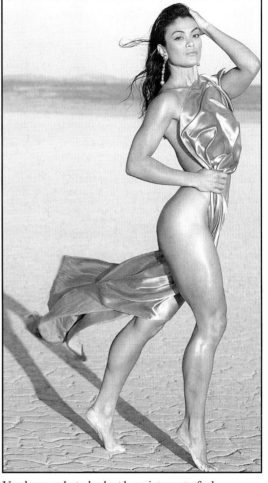

...Chain'd to a rock she stood; young Perseus stay'd
his rapid flight, to view the beauteous maid.
So sweet her frame, so exquisitely fine,
She seem'd a statue by a hand divine,
Had not the wind her waving tresses show'd,
And down her cheeks the melting sorrows flow'd.
Her faultless form the hero's bosom fires;
The more he looks, the more he still admires...

Ovid,
from the classic poem, *Metamorphoses*

The transience of human beauty has challenged writers and artists since the dawn of civilization. Poets use words to capture a moment in time. Painters and now photographers use their talents to share a mortal image, to preserve its enjoyment and inspiration for those not yet born.

My task as both a writer and photographer has been to communicate the beauty of the pursuit and achievement of physical fitness. But talent and technology can only do so much. Every artist dreams of finding a special model, an individual who is able to embody everything the artist wants to say. The model who, almost on a telepathic level, communicates with the artist in such a way that the vision captured is exactly what the artist wanted to express.

For me, that individual was Debbie Dobbins. You have only to look at her pictures to feel the positive energy she radiated. I couldn't have taken a bad picture of Debbie if I'd tried. We lost Debbie in a tragic house fire in 1993. When you lose someone close to you, you grieve. But not so much for what you had, but for what could have been. I believe Debbie would have been a champion fitness contestant, a contributing writer to *Oxygen*, a media star; anything she wanted to be. We would have had great photoshoots, and she would have been one of the best friends MuscleMag, and I, ever had.

How fair is youth that flies so fast!
Then be happy, you who may; what's
to come is still unsure.

Lorenzo De Medici
(Lorenzo the Magnificent),
1449-1492

Before her death, I never contemplated the existence of angels. Now I know there's one in our midst. Debbie Dobbins, on behalf of all your friends here at MuscleMag, we dedicate this book to your memory and to your life, which was too short for one so talented and inspirational.

Robert Kennedy,
and the staff of MuscleMag International

ACKNOWLEDGMENTS

As with our previous publications, we have to thank numerous individuals for their help in creating this book. To our ladies at the St. John's YM/YWCA, Laura Dwyer, Melanie Hiscock, Annette Powell, and Laura McHugh. Thanks for giving two guys the female perspective on things!

Once again, thanks to Rick Martin at the St. John's YM/YWCA, for his valuable input. And Rick, congratulations on finally getting your name in print!

To Mrs. Bertha Thorne, never has one secretary done so much for absolutely nothing! One day, we will express our thanks monetarily. We've been saying that since 1991, but we're optimists.

To Mrs. Irina Embleton, registered massage therapist and aesthetician, of Radiant Reflections Salon, and Mrs. Jacqueline Molyneaux-Petrie, owner/operator of Whispers Salon, both of Charlottetown, Prince Edward Island. Thanks, without your knowledge of haircare and cosmetics we would have been lost!

To Mrs. Nicola Embleton-Lake, your ability to make any computer progam user friendly has saved us weeks of production time. Congratulations on the completion of your Masters in Architecture!

To Jackie Kydyk, Mandy Morgan, and the staff at MuscleMag International, thanks once again for your expertise in putting another book together.

Finally, to the person who started it all over 25 years ago, Robert Kennedy, thanks for yet another opportunity to add to MuscleMag's growing line of publications.

Gerard Thorne and Phil Embleton

Contents

CONTENTS

CONTENTS

CONTENTS

CONTENTS

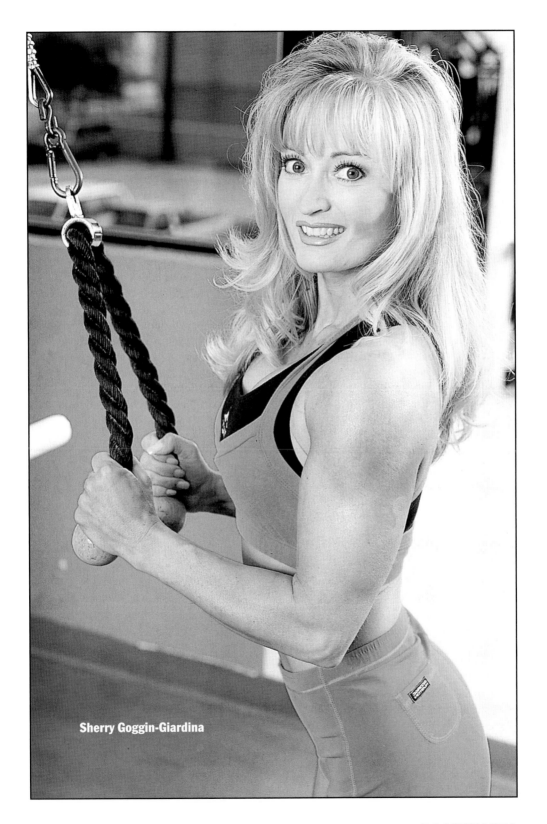

Sherry Goggin-Giardina

CONTENTS

Foreword

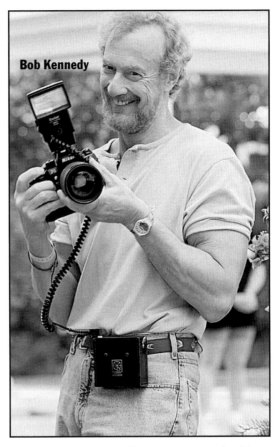

Bob Kennedy

The first fitness athlete I ever met never competed. As I was taking my first painful steps into adolescence, I met Eva, a Swedish girl of 16, who was staying with a local family and studying English. I first saw her at the local park. It wasn't her long mane of golden white hair, her penetrating blue eyes, or her long, firm body that grabbed my attention, it was what she was doing. Pullups. I watched and counted, slack-jawed as she reached thirty! Then she dropped down, and without missing a beat, began doing pushups, followed by several laps around a nearby field. Then she walked up to me smiling, and asked me in her broken, heavily accented English, if I could hold her feet while she did some situps. How could I refuse? Beads of sweat were rolling down her face (mine too), as she strained to raise her body repeatedly. After 4 sets of 50, she said I could let go, and said thank you. She then asked me if I wanted to jog with her cross-country. My adrenaline was already flowing, and in no time we were flying across the fields and hills that surround my little village. We ran for at least an hour when I signaled her to stop. I sat on the ground, loudly gasping for air, and I blurted out, "Why do you do this?" She replied with a smile, "Because I can."

That summer we ran together. Almost every day after her lessons, we'd meet at the park, rain or shine. I started her on lifting weights, and she was soon making remarkable progress. The day before she left for Sweden we ran one last time. Then she kissed me goodbye.

No, I never saw her again. But she taught me that the female body was every bit as strong and competitive as my own. As I later became involved in bodybuilding and fitness, I would often reflect on that summer, and how Eva would forever symbolize, at least for me, what a fitness contestant should strive for; to be her personal best. Which brings me to this book, *BodyFitness For Women*. It is a companion for all who wish to take that personal journey into fitness. Inside this book you'll find all the techniques and tricks to take you to the winning edge, both in life and onstage.

With the explosion in popularity of fitness competitions, it became clear to the staff at MuscleMag International that we needed to address the void in sound advice available to competitors. Through our women's fitness magazine, *Oxygen*, and now *BodyFitness For Women*, we provide women readers with the latest in fitness information.

Why would you want to test your body to the limit? Because you can!

Robert Kennedy,
editor and publisher of
MuscleMag International* and *Oxygen

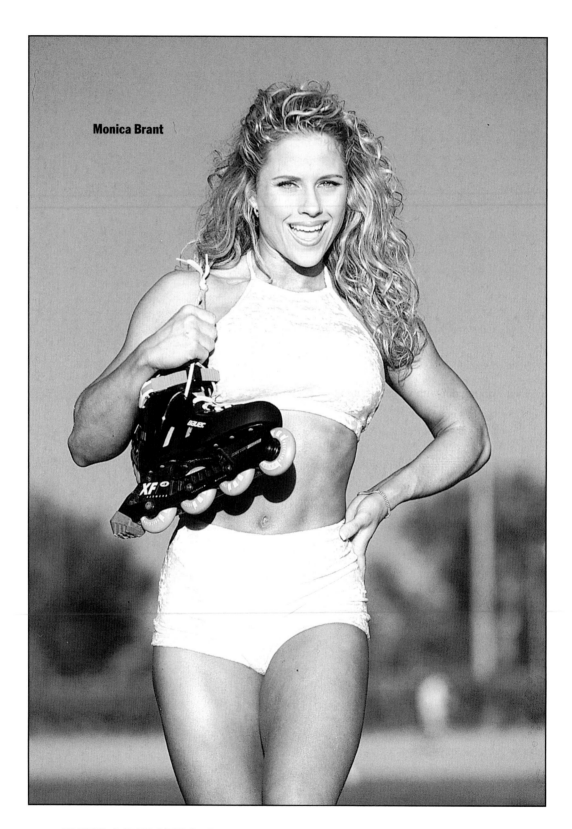

Monica Brant

Introduction

Congratulations! You've just taken the first step toward a healthier you. You're now one of millions about to reap the benefits of strength training. No longer are gyms the exclusive domain of the male segment of society. You might be surprised to know that, in many gyms, female memberships outnumber male memberships.

WHY STRENGTH TRAIN?

Twenty years ago most women not only avoided working out with weights but in many cases were advised not to. Thankfully, a combination of positive media coverage and medical advice has changed such archaic views.

There are a number of reasons why women should train with weights. Perhaps the most obvious is the strength aspect. An aerobic workout is great for the cardiovascular system, but it does very little to strengthen the body's muscles and connective tissues. While you may move the body faster during an aerobics workout, the amount of stress placed on the muscles – your bodyweight – remains the same. Even then it's only your lower-body muscles that receive the most benefit. The upper body is virtually neglected

during a typical aerobics workout. And while some instructors have added light handweights to their classes, it's really only the heart and lungs that benefit from such exercise. Jumping, running, and dancing are a great way to work the cardiovascular system but they do very little to stimulate the musculoskeletal system. Only a regular weight-training program using free weights and machines can adequately stimulate the body's muscles.

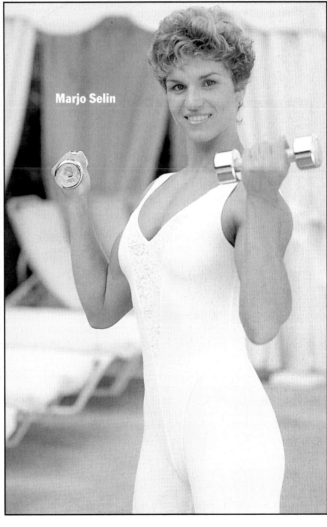

Marjo Selin

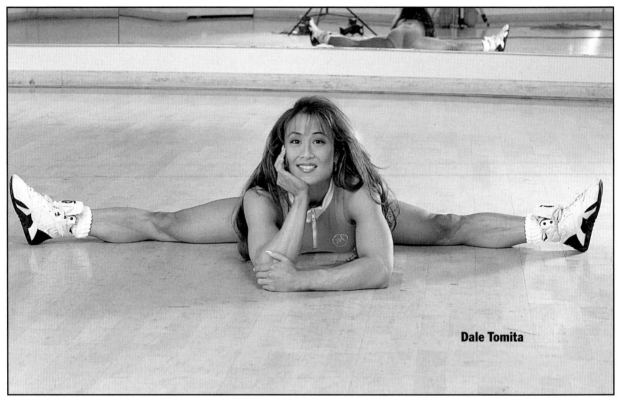

Dale Tomita

A second benefit to weight training is toning. We should add that toning is a very misunderstood word. Toning does not mean to shape and define a muscle. Shape is determined by genetics, and while you can tailor a program to emphasize different parts of a muscle giving the illusion of changing its shape, the muscles' final appearance is predetermined. As for definition – meaning how prominent the muscle fibers stand out – this is primarily controlled by bodyfat percentage. The less fat, the more the striations and fibers become visible. You can't spot reduce by weight training (train one muscle group of the body and only lose fat from that area). The best example of this is the abdominals. No amount of crunches or leg raises will shrink the fat and define the waist (although abdominal exercises will strengthen and tone the muscles – two very worthwhile benefits).

Misconceptions about weight training are still very common. Some people assume resistance training is only beneficial for bulking men with low IQ's. The truth is actually the opposite.

Will Brink, regular *MuscleMag* **columnist**

Despite what many body shaping programs tell you, toning means to firm and strengthen a muscle. By increasing the resistance placed on a muscle in the form of weight, the muscle fibers increase slightly, producing a stronger, harder muscle – collectively called tonus. By using weights to tone the muscles throughout the body you can make great changes to your physique. And it doesn't take years to accomplish either. A couple of months on a quality exercise program, combined with a proper diet, and people may not recognize you!

A third benefit to weight training involves its effects on the body's metabolism. Aerobic exercise burns more calories per unit of time than strength training, but the effects are short-lived. After you stop running or jumping, the body's metabolic rate returns to normal. The effects of weight training on the other hand last long after you leave the gym. A stronger, well-toned muscle system will burn more calories at rest than a nontoned muscle system. In simple terms, being in shape helps keep you in shape by burning more calories.

The fourth reason to strength train is one of the least known but most important. As the human body ages, one of the negative effects is the loss of calcium from the body's skeleton. And while both sexes experience this phenomena, the effect is much more pronounced in post-menopausal women. The condition is called osteoporosis and it is believed, among other things, to be caused by the decline in estrogen levels that accompany menopause. Estrogen not only causes the bones to absorb calcium but also helps prevent existing calcium from being lost. Easily broken hips, often suffered by elderly women, are the end result of such calcium loss. While most are aware that weight training strengthens muscles, many are surprised to learn that strength training also stimulates the bones to hold and absorb calcium. Studies with elderly women have found weight training returns bone calcium levels to near pre-menopausal levels. And while weight training doesn't prevent osteoporosis, it does appear to offer a partial treatment.

Fear not! Except for a truly select number of genetically gifted women, large muscles are unlikely. It takes a certain way of eating and working out in a very disciplined, intense fashion that constantly pushes for muscle growth.

Kathleen Engel, *Oxygen* contributor

Younger women reading the previous may gloss over these findings, subscribing to the old adage "I'll cross that bridge when I come to it." This is the wrong attitude to take as studies suggest weight training may also help reduce the onset of osteoporosis. It seems that strengthening the muscles and bones with resistance exercise acts as a sort of preventative medicine.[1] Strength training may not be the fountain of youth but it helps insure your golden years are healthy and rewarding.

A fifth benefit to strength training has psychological undertones. Many therapists now incorporate regular exercise,

I usually tell people that looking masculine is not going to happen unless they're a genetic freak or they're chemically enhancing their bodies to grow masculine-looking muscles.

Marla Duncan, *Oxygen* columnist

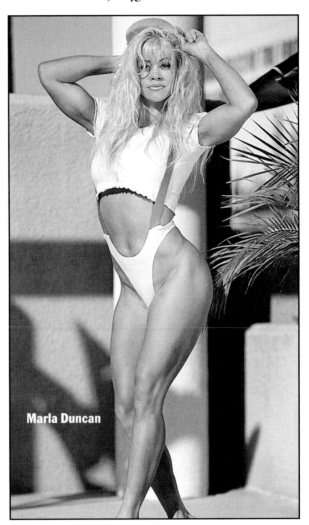

Marla Duncan

including strength training, as a form of recreational therapy. Improving health and appearance is a great way to boost self-esteem and self-image. This is especially true of older women who may feel "left out" of social activities because of age-related declines in physical health. Both physical and psychological health are heavily dependent on one another.

MYTHS EXPOSED

Despite the valid reasons outlined in the previous section, we're sure many readers are still sceptical about weight training. This may be the result of a list of misconceptions. How often have gym instructors heard the lines "I don't want to look like a man," or "I don't want to gain any muscle mass, just tone up!" Let us reassure you that a couple of months of weight training won't have you stunt doubling for Arnold Schwarzenegger. Look at it

Bodyweight is a poor indicator of fitness level.
– Debi Lee Stern

another way, millions of guys are trying to do just that – gain pounds of muscle mass – yet have to struggle for every ounce! It's virtually impossible for women to gain an appreciable amount of muscle mass. The key word here is appreciable. True, women can and will gain some muscle tissue by following a quality weight-training program, but nothing comparable to men. Female biochemistry won't allow it. No doubt many readers may respond by asking "but what about the women bodybuilders I see on TV?" Yes it's true these women are more muscular than the average female. But keep in mind many have resorted to anabolic steroids and other bodybuilding drugs to achieve such a condition. They have masculinized their body chemistry in favor of building large defined muscles. Few women can do this naturally. You can, however, build a great-looking physique that's both healthy and feminine in appearance.

DIETING ALONE WON'T DO IT

Another myth that gets tossed around these days is that dieting alone is a great way to lose weight. Restricting calories will help you lose a few pounds, but as many readers can attest to, it's not long before you gain most of the weight back. In many cases there's a rebound effect and our unfortunate dieter gains the weight back, as well as a few extra pounds. The reason is that the body assumes it's in a period of famine or starvation and begins to store every calorie consumed. It's not long before people become frustrated and blow their diets. The combination of extra calories plus the body's revved up storage mechanisms results in more calories being turned into fat. Another crash diet and the cycle continues.

Besides the physiological aspect, dieting can be the source of much mental anguish. Few individuals can

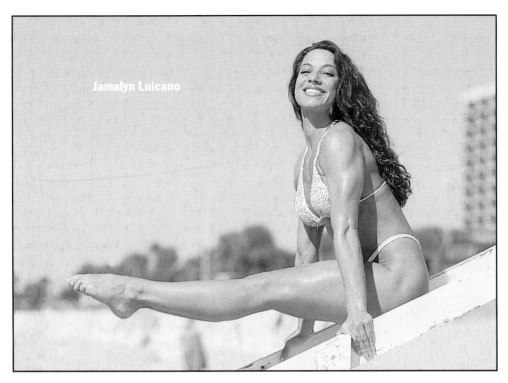

Jamalyn Luicano

handle cutting their calorie intake by half or even a third. Yet this is what many people do in trying to lose weight. A week or two of such restraint is all most can handle, and you guessed it, another post-diet binge.

A third problem with strict diets is their effect on muscle mass. This is especially important for competitive bodybuilders. As soon as the body's fat reserves drop below a certain point, the body begins to use muscle tissue as a fuel source. Unless the individual follows good eating habits, hard-earned muscle mass will be lost. Even though many readers won't be competing in bodybuilding contests, any habit that forces the body to consume muscle tissue should be avoided at all costs.

WHO CARES WHAT YOU WEIGH?

A fourth myth that most women get consumed by is what the authors call "the folly of the scales." If there's one thing you take from this chapter it's that bodyweight is a poor indicator of fitness level. Two women with the same frame and bodyweight may be at opposite ends of the fitness spectrum. It all depends on what the weight is composed of. Muscle is healthy living tissue. On the other hand, fat remains inactive until it's needed as a source of energy. And as most individuals consume more energy in the form of food than they need, the stored fat deposits never get called to active duty. They keep growing. Fat not only gets stored on the outside but on the inside as well. By the time fat shows up around the hips and midsection it's already in and around the body's major organs.

If you lose fat and gain muscle, the scales might not change drastically, but you will be losing inches. This is exactly why most people should throw their scales out the window.

Will Brink, *MuscleMag* columnist and published author

You don't always have to lose bodyweight to improve health. Granted, if you're carrying 30 to 40 extra pounds of fat, yes it would be a good idea to get rid of it. But an increase or decrease on the scales does not necessarily mean a corresponding increase or

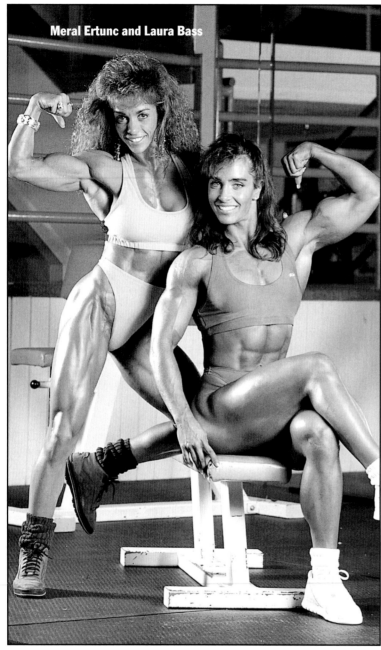

Meral Ertunc and Laura Bass

WHAT HAPPENS IF I STOP?

Before we start offering advice on training we should put another myth to rest. Many individuals are afraid that once they reach a certain level of fitness they're condemned to intense exercising for life. How often have you heard someone say "But if I stop it will all turn to fat!" The problem with such a statement is that it defies the laws of bio-chemistry. Muscle cannot turn into fat. The two are distinct entities. True, some athletes who stop train-ing become fat, but their muscles did not turn to fat. More than likely the increased appetite they devel-oped while training remained after they stopped working out. The excess calories, once burned as energy, are now being stored around the midsection. The previously toned muscles will also lose some of their firmness and give the appearance of being fat.

Your muscles won't turn to fat if you stop working out. This raises the question, Why stop work-ing out? Most individuals who make strength training a regular part of their lives never stop training entirely. A short vacation here, a few weeks off there, but they rarely quit training cold turkey. Maintaining a physique is much easier than getting there in the first place. Two to three days a week for about 45 to 60 minutes is all it takes. And something tells us

decrease in fitness level. You can make a drastic change in your physique without gaining or losing a pound. A couple of months of exercise could help shed 10 pounds of fat, and help you gain 10 pounds of muscle. And as muscle is more compact than fat, you will no doubt be "smaller" in all the right places. Yet step on the scale and nothing has changed.

that once the weight-training bug bites, your problem won't be finding the time to train. You'll become one of millions who hate to miss a workout!

Reference
1. W. Katz and C. Sherman, "Osteoporosis: The Role of Exercise in Optimal Management," *Physician and Sports Medicine*, 26:2 (1998), 33-41.

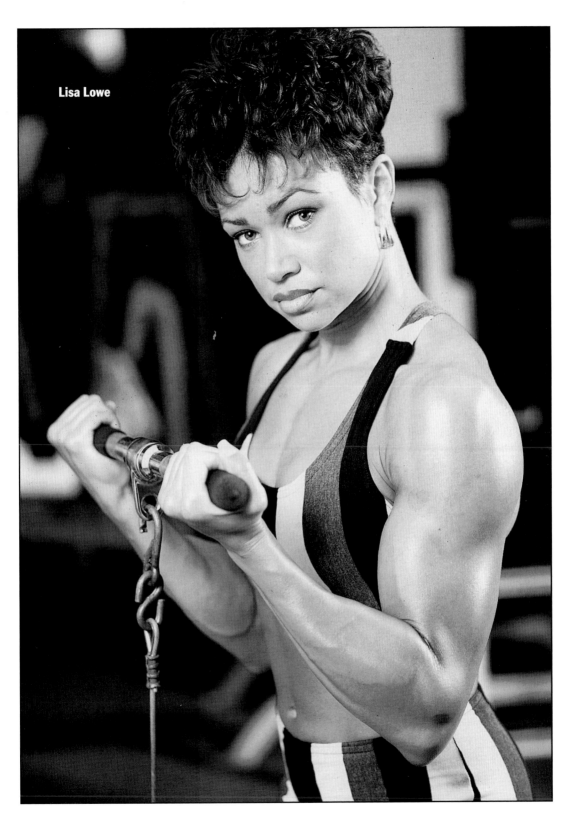

Lisa Lowe

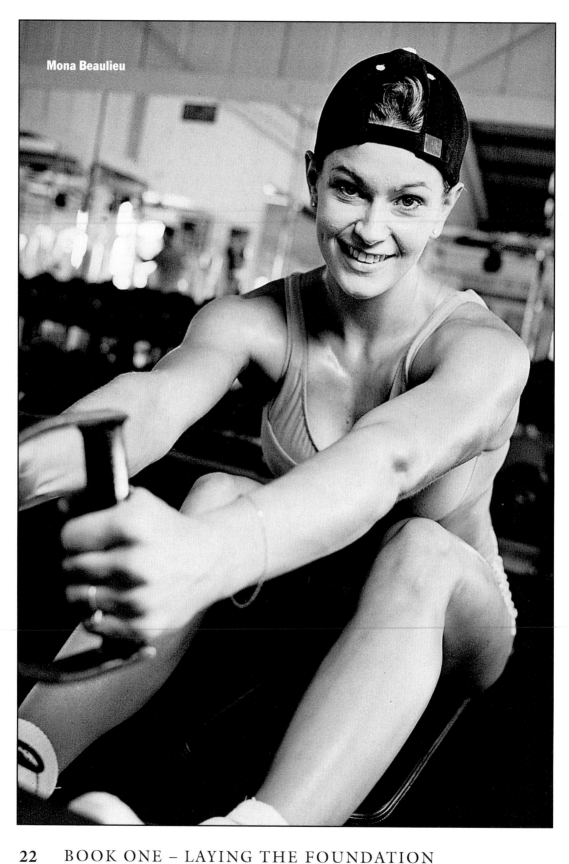
Mona Beaulieu

Book One

Laying the Foundation

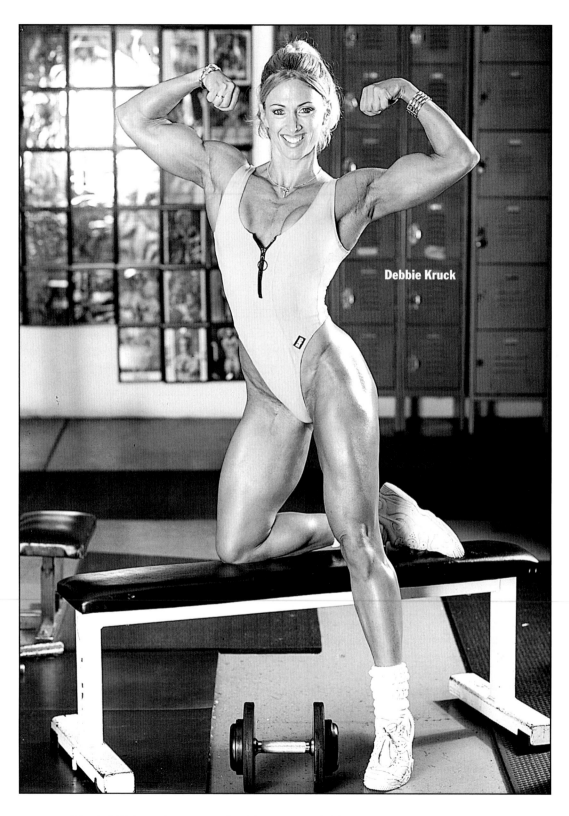

Debbie Kruck

Chapter 1

Getting Started

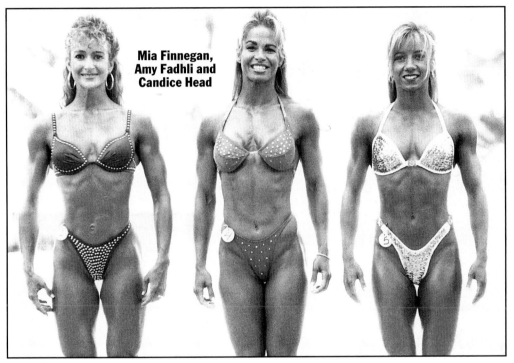

Mia Finnegan, Amy Fadhli and Candice Head

It may have taken you five years to put on those excess pounds, but it may only take you a year to get back into super shape.

Nina Simone, *Oxygen* contributor

WHERE TO WORK OUT

You have two choices when it comes to working out. You can set up a mini gym in your basement or you can join a commercial gym. Both have advantages and disadvantages.

HOME SWEET HOME

In terms of cost and convenience nothing beats training at home. For the investment of a few hundred dollars you can set up an ideal training facility in your basement. All you need is a couple of benches, dumbells, and an adjustable barbell set. If you have the extra cash you can even add one of those small compact multi-stations that are sold in most department and sports stores.

The advantages to working out at home are numerous. For starters you don't have a monthly or yearly membership to worry about. Once you spend the first few dollars everything is free from then on. Another point concerns parking. Peak times at the more popular gyms can be a lesson in survival. If you're lucky you'll get a parking spot in the first few minutes but in many cases you'll be waiting a while. Worse case scenario sees you parking a block or two away. And we don't need to remind you what this could mean in a large city. Training at home, however, means parking your car in the driveway or garage. No fighting for that last parking space.

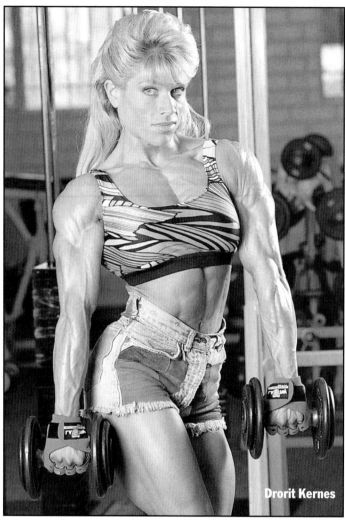
Drorit Kernes

point where you'll outgrow your meager provisions. Dumbells and barbells are a great way to start training, and you'll make use of them throughout your training career, but they have their limits.

Another disadvantage is the atmosphere. Unless you enjoy doing things alone, training by yourself can be boring. There's nothing like being surrounded by other people doing the same thing to get the motivational spirits flowing.

Closely related to the previous is the issue of safety. On numerous occasions weight lifters have been found dead in their basements after becoming trapped under a barbell. This is unlikely at a gym because within a matter of seconds someone would rush to your aid.

Perhaps the biggest disadvantage to working out at home is ironically an advantage. Following the old adage "never procrastinate today if you can do it tomorrow," many individuals give up training at home because it's so convenient to put it off. They assume that since the equipment is in the basement they can always do it later. Unfortunately, later never comes. Eventually your investment becomes another piece of equipment gathering dust in the basement. If you have to drive to the gym however, it forces you to work out (hopefully the word "force" will quickly disappear from your vocabulary). Let's face it, what else are you going to do there! All of the previous leads us to the second place you can workout – the commercial gym.

Another advantage to working out at home concerns hygiene. While better gyms keep their facilities clean, let's face it, if you have hundreds, or even thousands of individuals using a facility, you will be exposed to a wide range of germs and diseases. Without sounding paranoid, having to use a piece of equipment immediately after someone has perspired all over it – whether he or she cleaned it or not – is not very appealing. You don't have to worry about other people's germs when working out at home.

ON THE OTHER HAND...

The biggest drawback to home training is equipment variety. Unless you've got the room and the finances, you'll quickly reach the

THE GYM

You can get a great workout at home, but most individuals opt for the many advantages offered by commercial training establishments. The first walk through the door of any large gym should be enough to convince you of the many positive attributes of such facilities. The most obvious is the variety of equipment available. No home gym can compare to a modern commercial gym when it comes to training apparatus. There will be complete lines of state-of-the-art training machines. Every sort of rack, barbell, and bench imaginable, will be found throughout the premises. While purists will tell you much of the equipment is not needed, most experts agree that to optimize your training nothing beats variety.

Another advantage to training at a gym is the atmosphere. Being in among dozens of other people doing the same thing is a sure way to get motivated. You may have arrived at the gym tired from a hard day at the office but chances are someone's humorous statement will make you forget all that and it's down to some serious training. Besides the general atmosphere created by crowds there's a practical consideration as well. Books and magazines are a great way to learn new things, but it's always nice to get the information firsthand. You can't beat the pool of knowledge available at large gyms. Better-run facilities have highly knowledgeable instructors on hand to answer all your questions. Also, the sheer number of members you will come in contact with means you'll be surrounded by individuals with years of strength-training experience. The solution to your problem may be one question away.

I used to move heavy weights in the beginning. The guy I was training with had me do everything heavy to build a base. He didn't really make it clear to me that applying different training methods would impact how I looked, so I'd go into the gym, day in, day out, and press heavy weight.

**Monica Brant,
1998 Ms. Fitness Olympia**

Although the advantages to training at gyms far outweigh the disadvantages, there are a few drawbacks. For starters you have the cost to consider. Although it varies, gym memberships generally range from a low of about $300 to $1000 or more per year. While we consider this a great value for your dollar, for some this is beyond their budget. We should add that most gyms have monthly payment plans so you don't have to lay out all

Yes, joining a gym is the best way because you are hands-on right in the middle of the activity.

**Robert Kennedy,
Oxygen founder
and publisher**

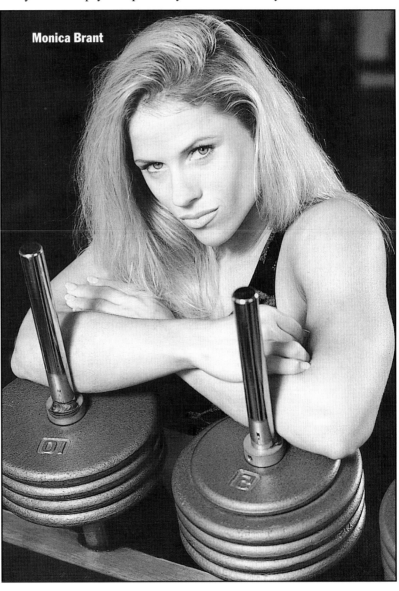

Monica Brant

the cash at once. Some allow you to pay month by month. Others will accept post-dated cheques; and still others will charge your credit-card account on a predetermined schedule.

Another disadvantage to gyms is their hours of operation. Training at home means 24 hours of availability. Most gyms accommodate the bulk of their membership by being open a couple of hours before and after standard working hours. This translates to about 7 in the morning to 10 or 11 at night. If you live in a large city, you can probably find a 24-hour gym, but be prepared to be flexible with your workout hours.

Closely related to the previous are the peak times experienced by most gyms. As

If by now we've convinced you to join a gym, the next section is a must read – especially if you live in an area where there is a wide selection of training establishments.

CHOOSING A GYM

Picking a gym is much like buying a house or car – you don't jump at the first one that comes along. You have to shop around. To make things easier we're going to classify gyms into three basic categories. Each have their merits and hopefully our tidbits will make things easier when you finally decide to go gym hunting.

At one end of the spectrum we have what can be called health spas. These facilities tend to cater to upscale clients, particularly

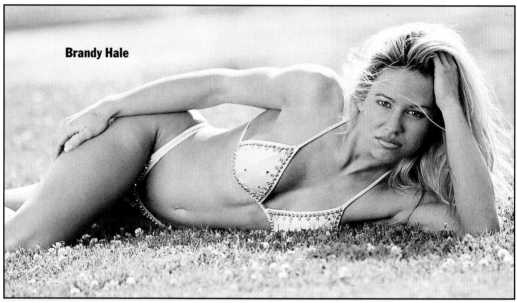

Brandy Hale

most people get off work between 5 and 6 pm, and prefer to be home by 9 or 10 at night, the hours between these times are by far the busiest. Some gyms have a mini peak around 3:30 when the high school students show up, but by and large, 5 to 9 pm is the busiest time period. If your job or daily schedule allows you to work out before or after these hours, we strongly suggest doing so. It's one thing to have people around for inspiration and safety, but another thing to have to wait five to 10 minutes for each piece of equipment.

Like most women, when I became interested in fitness, I was out-and-out afraid to go to the gym. I stayed in the women's section of the workout area, sort of hiding and learning until I had the confidence to really integrate myself into the mainstream workout crowd.

Brandy Hale, fitness model and competitor

business executives. For serious weight trainers health spas are a poor place to work out. Serious types are not generally welcome. That extra rep on the bench press or slight

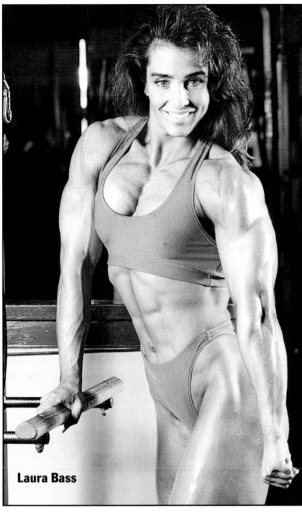

Laura Bass

hardcore bodybuilding gyms. You won't find much chrome equipment in here, nor business people utilizing them. Hardcore gyms are loaded with the very best in strength-training equipment – endless supplies of barbells, dumbells, and machines. The one fault of hardcore gyms is that they tend to be weak in the cardio aspect. And while the focus of this book is strength training, you should also make cardio training a regular part of your exercise routine. With the emphasis on total health these days, most of the better hardcore gyms have enhanced their range of cardio equipment.

Another potential drawback to hardcore gyms is their atmosphere. We say potential as it all depends on what you're looking for. In a word, hardcore gyms are intense. You won't find many slackers in here. Where spas try to shun serious weight trainers, hardcore gyms may intimidate executive types! Many members are competitive bodybuilders or other athletes. You have to see their training intensity to believe it. If you don't

groan on the squat may get you banned! Tongue-in-cheek aside, health spas devote most of their resources to cardio equipment, saunas, and whirlpools than serious weight-training equipment. You may find a few chrome-plated strength-training machines, but don't expect to find much in the way of barbells and dumbells. Such ungainly instruments don't fit the average spa's idea of proper exercising. In addition, spas are the most expensive of the three types of gyms. A couple thousands of dollars a year is the norm for such establishments. By now you can guess our feelings about health spas. Unless you have no choice, our advice is to seek out one of the next two types of gyms.

At the other end of the spectrum we have a different beast all together. They go by many names but all can be classified as

mind the occasional grunt or groan, give a hardcore gym a try. Motivation and intensity seems to saturate the atmosphere of these places. Given the variety of equipment available, hardcore gyms are reasonably priced averaging $400 to $600 per year. Some of the biggest names in the hardcore gym business are Gold's, World Gym, and Powerhouse Gyms.

If you consider yourself average or middle of the road, the third category of gyms is probably the one most suited to your needs. Called multipurpose fitness facilities, they try to cater to just about everyone in society. Where the other two are like medical specialists, multipurpose gyms are like the family physician – they offer a little of everything. These establishments usually contain a larger weight training and cardio area, a pool, a gym,

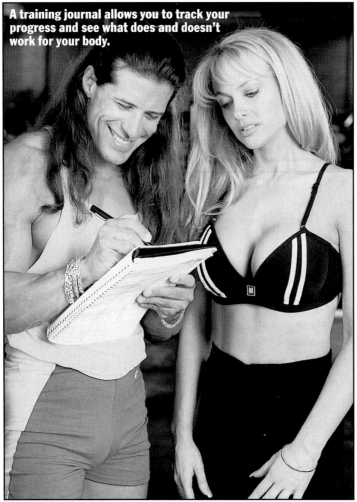

A training journal allows you to track your progress and see what does and doesn't work for your body.

then closes; or worse, has a grand opening, offering lifetime memberships and then mysteriously disappears. A couple of gym chains back in the 1960s and 1970s were notorious for this.

Following the previous advice may take a bit of time, but it will be worth it in the end, providing you with years of productive workouts.

KEEPING A TRAINING JOURNAL

Although not a necessity, you probably should get in the habit of keeping a training diary. Not only is it a great way to see progress, but it serves as a motivational tool. You can record just about anything you want in the journal. The following are a few suggestions:

1) Cardio activity – keep track of such variables as form, number of calories burned, intensity level, and time.

2) Weight-training – record such important items as numbers of sets, reps, exercises, and weight used. You may also want to record the time it takes to complete the workout.

3) Nutritional information – although you can record every morsel of food eaten, it's easier to keep track of the approximate number of calories eaten and the amounts of the three main food groups – fats, carbohydrates, and protein.

4) Optional information – you may want to record your weight (weekly or monthly, not daily!) as well as measurements, and energy levels.

WHAT TO WEAR

Although it's not a high school prom you're going to, it does make a difference what you wear when working out. Too many clothes and you'll dehydrate, too little and the more sweat you transfer to the equipment. Our advice is to dress both casually and practically. During the summer, T-shirts or tanktops and shorts are comfortable. For our northern readers winter training may mean altering

and possibly an indoor track. Most also have saunas, whirlpools, and large shower and change areas. Dollar for dollar you can't beat the price either, with a yearly membership averaging $500.

If you live in a larger metropolitan center, you'll have the chance to check out each type of gym for yourself. As you evaluate your choices take into account such factors as cost, location, hours of operation, and above all, reputation. If you have close friends who work out don't hesitate to get their advice. Those who work out regularly often have an insight into the reputations of the various gyms in town. You don't want to join some fly-by-night organization that gives you three months of a year membership and your wardrobe. Try a sweatsuit. This is enough to stay warm without going overboard. You can even get trendy if you want. In fact, your gym may have the equivalent of a golf pro shop. For $40 to $50 you may be able to outfit yourself right then and there.

Before moving onto the next topic we should say a word about one of the most popular types of training attire – spandex. First used by competitive athletes – especially for reducing wind resistance in races – spandex is worn by everyone these days. It is very light, durable, allows the skin to breath (allows sweat to evaporate), and hugs the body like a second skin. If spandex has a disadvantage it is that it can't hide anything. A few excess pounds can easily be covered with baggy sweat clothes, but no such luck with spandex. Everything is on display. A few use this as an incentive to work out harder, but if you are self-conscious about your physical appearance, we suggest leaving spandex for a few months down the road. Consider spandex your graduation present and stick with the sweat clothes or shorts and T-shirts. If there's any doubt as to what to wear, a couple of days at the gym will give you a pretty good idea of your possible choices.

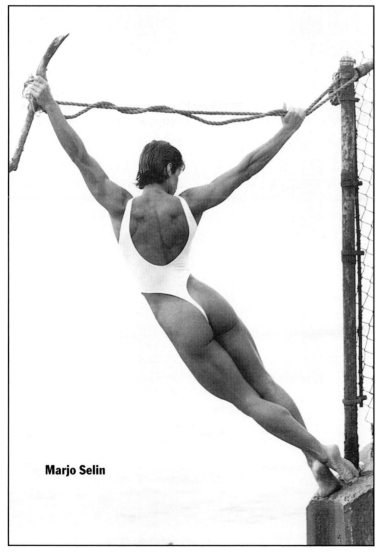

Marjo Selin

WHEN TO TRAIN

When is the optimal time to train? Biologists tell us that the human body reaches peak efficiency about four to six hours after awakening. But the human body is very adaptive and quickly becomes accustomed to training at a certain time each day.

You should train at a time that is most convenient for you. Based on your workout schedule, find a time when you feel ready to work out. Whether it's before you go to work, during early morning hours, or after you're finished for the day, it's up to you.

**Marjo Selin,
former *MuscleMag* columnist**

Some individuals prefer to train at 4 or 5 am, while others get the most out of late evening workouts. As Marjo Selin states in the above quote, train when it's most convenient for you. The bottom line is not so much when you train but that you do train.

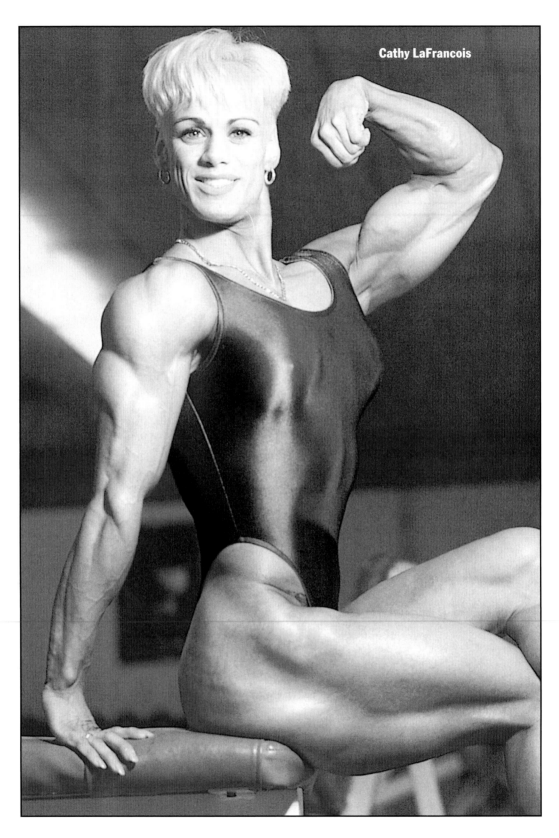

Cathy LaFrancois

Chapter 2
Vocab 101

Now that you've bought your workout clothes and selected a gym, it's time to get started. Before doing so, however, there's a few additional pieces of information that must be discussed. Weight training is like most athletic endeavours; done properly it provides years of fun and enjoyment; done improperly and it becomes an orthopaedic surgeon's best friend! The following suggestions will help insure that your workouts are effective and injury free. And while a few are not safety issues, they are part of the etiquette rules of most gyms.

Choose an initial routine that won't be so demanding or draining that you won't stick with it. It should be something that fits easily into your schedule and an activity you look forward to doing.

Karen Voight, fitness pioneer

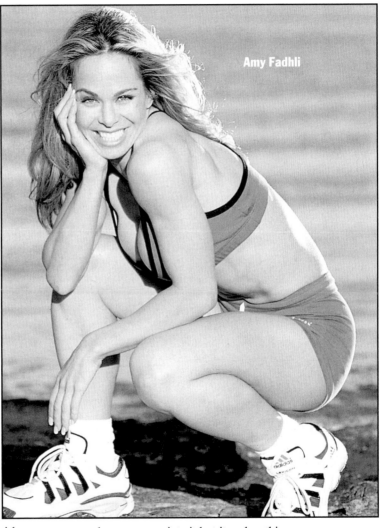

Amy Fadhli

EIGHT TIPS FOR SAFE, EFFECTIVE WORKOUTS

1) Keep long hair tied back. As most of the machines have many moving parts – pulley wheels, cables, weight stacks – we strongly suggest tying long hair out of harm's reach. Numerous patrons have received a nasty fright after getting their hair tangled around a cable pulley wheel. Losing a few strands of hair could be the least of your worries. Under the right (or wrong depending on your view) circumstances you could twist your neck.

2) Put your weights away. Nothing irks gym staff and members like individuals who chronically leave their weights on the floor. It may be one of those days you're in a rush, or have something important on your mind, but try to get in the habit from day one of putting your weights away. Not only will the gym employees appreciate it but it makes things a whole lot safer for everyone.

3) Do not perform maximum single-repetition sets. This usually applies to the male ego, nevertheless, a few women may want to see how much they can lift. By a one-rep max we mean the heaviest weight you can lift for one

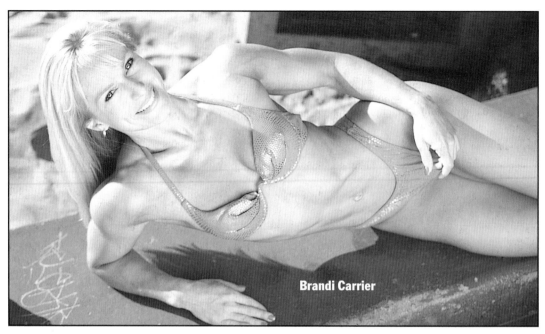
Brandi Carrier

complete rep. With the possible exception of power lifters, one-rep maxes add little to weight training as a form of physical fitness. Not only are they relatively ineffective but they're downright dangerous.

4) Do not hog the equipment. Nothing disrupts the flow of members' workouts like an equipment hog. While cardiovascular training necessitates staying on the same piece of equipment for 25 to 30 minutes, the same does not hold true for weight training. At the most you should be on a piece of weight-training equipment for five to six minutes. And even then we suggest letting others work in with you. Few gyms tolerate members who monopolize the same machine for endless numbers of sets.

5) Don't drop your weights. This is another rule that most gyms enforce. Dropping weights damages the floor, the weights themselves, and could potentially injure another member. When you're finished your set simply lower the weights to the floor. If there's any doubt, enlist the aid of a rack or another gym member.

6) No spitting in the fountain. As disgusting as this sounds most gyms have a couple of chronics who continuously do this. Under the best of circumstances water fountains can be the source of much germ transmission. Spitting does not help matters. If you must spit go to the bathroom. To protect yourself from others invest a few dollars in a water bottle.

7) Wear proper attire. Although we touched on this before, it's an issue that needs repeating. Most gyms have dress codes. This usually means a minimum of a halter top and pair of shorts. This keeps everything legally covered and at the same time helps cut down on the amount of sweat transferred to gym equipment.

8) Always use collars. No matter how strict your technique, odds are that one side of the bar will be lower than the other, causing the plates to slide off. To save the floor, plates, and possibly your feet, lock the weights in place using collars.

BASIC TERMINOLOGY

Weight training is similar to other athletic endeavours in that it has its own vocabulary. Although there are differences, for practical purposes we are going to use the terms weight training, strength training, bodybuilding, and weightlifting interchangeably throughout the book. The following terms can be considered the foundation of any strength-training program. As time moves on you'll be using weight-training terms such as sets, reps, and spotting, like a golfer talks about putts, birdies, and bogeys.

THE WARMUP

For those who do their cardio training earlier in the day, or after weight training, a warmup is an absolute must before hitting the weights. Even with proper exercise technique, it's dangerous to start stressing the muscles without warming them and elevating your body temperature and heart rate.

I do two warmups before training. First I warm up the entire body by spending 15 minutes on the stationary bike, stairclimber, or treadmill. The second kind of warmup is what I call a "microwarmup" for the more delicate joints like the elbows and knees.

Robert Kennedy,
MuscleMag International
founder and best-selling author

Warmups fall into two categories, overall body preparation, and individual muscle preparation. Hop on a piece of cardio equipment for five to 10 minutes of light-intensity exercise. Doing so elevates heart rate, blood flow, and conditions the overall body for the more intense exercise to follow.

The second type of warmup involves doing a few light sets for the individual muscles being worked. For example, if you were using 100 pounds on the bench press you wouldn't start with that weight. Instead, take 30 to 40 pounds and do 15 to 20 reps. For the next set put about 75 to 80 pounds on the bar and perform 12 to 15 reps. Then on the third set you can put on 100 pounds and start your heavy training. In other words, go from light to moderate, to heavy. For previously injured areas or muscles that are more prone to injury, (for example, the shoulders), it's probably a good idea

to do a few extra light sets to be on the safe side. By getting as much blood into the area as possible, you are not only increasing the muscle's exercising efficiency, but also decreasing your chance of injury.

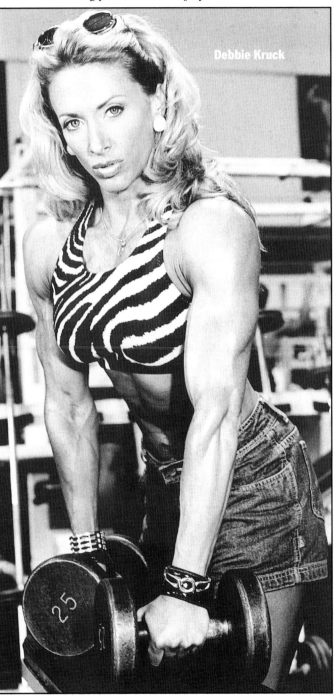

Debbie Kruck

REPS

Perhaps the most basic term to weight training is rep. The word rep is actually an abbreviation of the word repetition. It refers to the execution of one complete movement of an exercise. For example, curling a barbell from the hips to the chest and then back down is one rep. Both the raising and lowering are part of the same rep. Many beginners take the easy way out and call the raising portion one rep and the lowering another rep. Raising the bar in a curling exer-

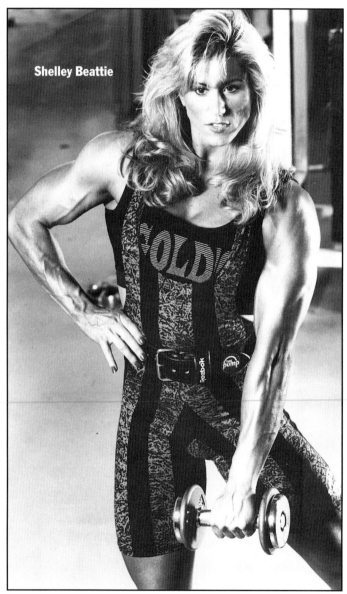

Shelley Beattie

cise is called the positive portion of the movement, and lowering is called the negative. Kinesiologists use the terms concentric for raising and eccentric for lowering.

HOW MANY REPS?

Like the controversy surrounding machines and free weights, few topics garner as much debate as rep numbers. While we'll give general recommendations, keep in mind everyone is unique. It may take months if not years for you to find the rep range that works best for you.

Rep ranges can be subdivided into three broad categories. At one end we have the toning range consisting of reps in the 12 to 15 range. For those going for sheer strength, increase the weight and drop the reps into the three to five range. Those going for muscle size will respond best to reps in the six to 10 range.

It would be nice if things were this simple, but they're not. Many individuals find they need to do reps in the 12 to 15 range to increase muscle size, while others respond best to reps in the three to five powerlifting range. The above numbers are meant as a guide to get you started. As time goes by we encourage you to experiment with different rep ranges. In this manner you will discover what works best for your body.

The programs outlined in this text mainly use rep ranges in the 12 to 15 range. This is because the majority of women who work out are primarily interested in muscle tone, not sheer strength and size. For those seeking these traits it's only a matter of dropping the rep range and increasing the weight. The exercises stay the same.

REP TEMPO

Twenty years ago the standard rep took about two to three seconds to complete – about two seconds up and one second down. Recent research suggests the negative part of the exercise is as important if not more important than the positive portion. The traditional two- to three-second rep is fast being replaced by reps lasting four to five seconds. And instead of the

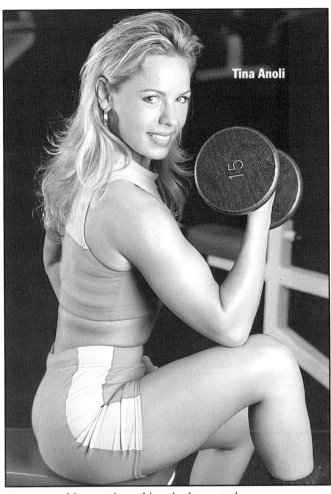

Tina Anoli

ment where the exercise changes direction. For example, numerous weight trainers have ripped bicep tendons from bouncing the bar at the bottom of the preacher curl. We cannot emphasize the importance of performing your reps in a slow and controlled manner.

SETS

Sets are nothing more than groups of reps. Perform 12 reps of a given exercise, wait a minute and perform 12 more reps and you would have performed two sets of the exercise. While you have performed 24 reps total, you do them in two groups of 12. Don't try to speed things up and perform 24 or 36 (three sets of 12) reps all at once. Let's face it, if you can do 24 or 36 reps in a set you are using an almost useless amount of weight. The standard number of sets per exercise is three.

HOW MUCH WEIGHT?

Now that you've got the sets and reps straight, the next order of business is for you to choose the correct weight to use for your exercises. Notice we said you choose the weight. While the routines later in the book will be laid out with exercises, reps, sets, etc., the one thing we can't do is tell you how much to lift. There's no magic formula to calculate workout poundages. About all we can do is offer a few tips as a rough guide.

In a 12-rep set you should start feeling the "burn" in the target muscle around the seventh to eighth rep. You then have to work for the last four to five reps. The key word is work not strain. If you can't complete the desired number of reps, the weight is too heavy. But there's also another side to the story. If after completing 12 reps you say to yourself "I could have done three or four more with that weight," the weight is too light. Please don't worry if this description seems vague. In a couple of weeks you will be picking and choosing weights with ease.

positive portion taking the longest, the negative part now receives the greatest emphasis.

The main disadvantage of fast reps is physics. The faster a weight is moved, the more momentum that is generated, which means less effort is required to keep the weight moving. Slow the movement down, however, and less momentum is generated and hence the muscles have to work harder to keep the weight moving. A slow four- to five-second rep scheme will necessitate using less weight but in a more efficient manner.

Besides effectiveness there's the issue of safety to consider. A fast moving weight places much more negative stress on the joints and connective tissues than a weight moved in a slow and controlled manner. This is especially true at the bottom of the move-

You simply need to replace the fat on your rump with muscle tissue, which will take some serious glute training and a regular maintenance program. Most women are so afraid to put any poundage into their leg programs that they're never able to replace the fat on that area with muscle.

Marla Duncan, *Oxygen* **columnist**

"THE PUMP"

Few topics are as unique to weightlifting as "the pump," defined as the engorging of a muscle with blood in response to exercise. Many weight trainers rate their workouts by the degree of muscle pump they achieve; however, even within individuals there's variation. One day the muscles pump by merely looking at a weight, while on other days nothing seems to get the job done. Weight trainers in tune with their bodies train until the muscles fully pump up, and then stop at the first sign of losing the desired feeling.

Is the pump necessary for muscle growth? Although the evidence is mixed, the reports seem to suggest it helps. Certainly a well-pumped muscle is indicative of good blood flow to the muscle – to bring in nutrients and remove fatigue toxins. Also, a fast-pumping muscle means there's a good neuromuscular pathway.

If you have trouble pumping the muscles on a regular basis, we suggest reassessing your training and diet. A constant lack of a pump is often a sign of overtraining or improper technique. Try reducing the number of sets but concentrating more during each rep. Muscles with low-glycogen (sugar) levels are also much harder to pump. Check your diet to see that you are consuming adequate amounts of complex carbohydrates.

SPOTTING

Spotting is another term that you'll hear frequently while working out. It's a technique that you can do for someone else or have him or her do for you. Spotting is gym jargon for

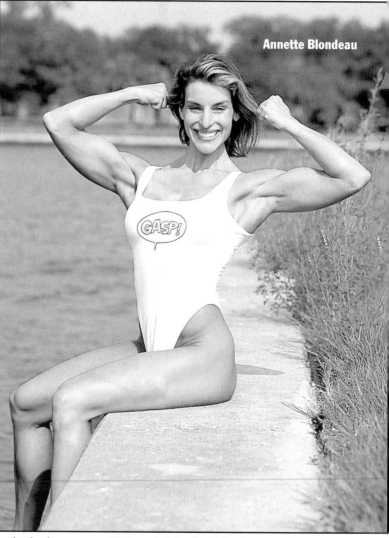

Annette Blondeau

GASP!

offering a helping hand. Let's say you're doing barbell bench presses and want to do 12 reps but realize after 10 that you can't do the last two. If you're by yourself you have no choice but to put the bar back on the rack. But a partner standing behind you can provide just enough upward force to keep the bar moving and allow you to perform the last two reps. This is called spotting.

Besides adding to the exercise, spotters have a more basic role – ensuring safety. On the previously discussed exercises, failing to put the bar back on the rack means getting stuck under it. If it lands on your chest you'll probably be none the worse for the wear – despite how uncomfortable it feels! But numerous people have died in their homes after getting the bar stuck across their neck. Never perform bench presses alone. You can probably get away with it in a gym because someone will likely come to your aid, but the risk is not worth it.

BREATHING

It may seem strange that we're discussing one of the most fundamental of human activities, but we assure you there is a right and wrong way to breath when you exercise. Try to breathe once for every rep performed. Breath out on the lifting part of the movement and in during the lowering. For example, on the bench press, breath in as you lower the bar to the chest and out as you push it to arms' length.

The previous can be followed on all your exercises but there's a few that may require modification. The squat is a good example. If you are lifting heavy, it is impossible to give everything to the tough part of an exercise without holding your breath. This is itself not dangerous provided you don't hold your breath for more than a couple of reps. But if you find yourself holding for three reps or more, make a determined effort to breath more frequently. The body needs enormous amounts of oxygen during intense exercise. Depriving it of this life-sustaining gas will eventually lead to an oxygen debt. The first symptoms are dizziness and light-headedness followed by fainting. At the first sign of the former, stop exercising.

Our advice on breathing is to let the body take care of it for you. You won't faint because you "forgot" to breathe.

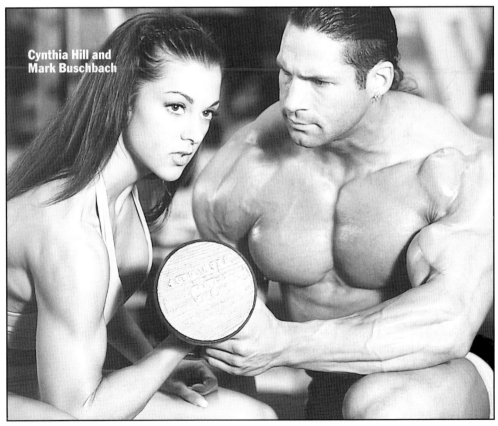

Cynthia Hill and Mark Buschbach

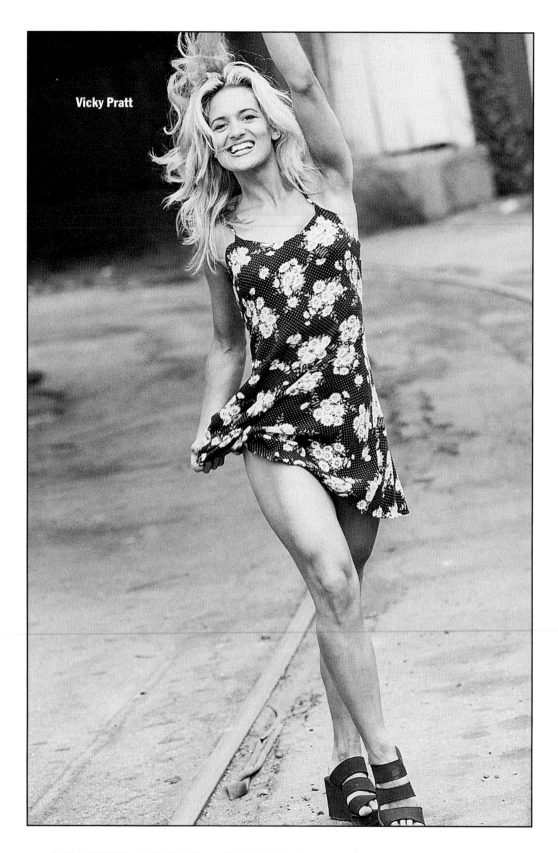

Vicky Pratt

Chapter 3

Physiology and Anatomy

I knew weight training was something special because my body responded so quickly to it. I got started in a tiny weight room at my college. It was next to the boilers and just had the basics, but it worked for me.

Ericca Kern, North American bodybuilding champion

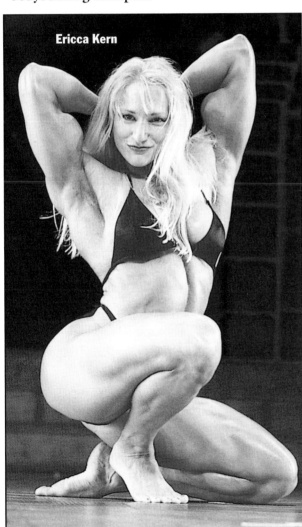

Ericca Kern

In the following chapter we'll give you a brief introduction to muscle anatomy and physiology and where possible, relate it to exercise.

MUSCLES

Muscle is the functional moving tissue of the human body. Muscle tissue can be subdivided into three categories – smooth, cardiac, and skeletal. Smooth muscle is the name given to muscle tissue found in the body's internal organs. Smooth muscle is involuntary in nature. This means you have little or no control over its functioning. For example, the movement of food through the digestive tract is under smooth-muscle control, and to all intents and purposes independent of your conscious thought. Cardiac muscle is only found in the heart and, while some people may be able to consciously slow down their heart rate, it too is primarily involuntary in nature.

When I couldn't run, I applied what I had learned from my kinesiology classes to my weight training. It was like a science experiment with my body. I learned I could change my training and my diet, and my body would change.

Vicky Pratt,
Oxygen **columnist**

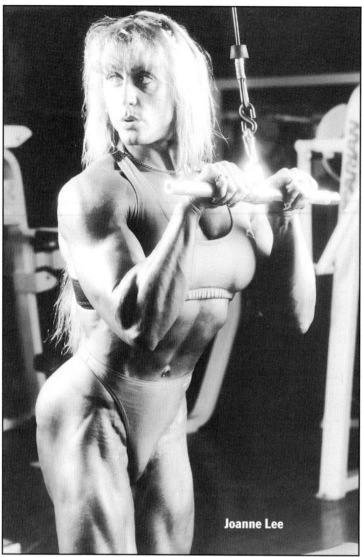

Joanne Lee

Muscle tissue has four basic properties. The first and most well-known is contractility. This involves a lengthening and shortening of the muscle belly, with the end result being movement. The second characteristic is stretchability. Muscles are not rigid structures but pliable tissues that can distend or lengthen without tearing. The third property is elasticity. This means muscles will return to their original size and shape after being stretched. The final characteristic is excitability, or the ability to be stimulated by nervous or chemical means.

While the above properties apply to all skeletal muscles, the degree of each depends on the individual muscle in question, and there is much variation with regards to contraction, duration, and function.

MUSCLE CONTRACTION

The basic subunit of muscle contraction is the motor unit. It consists of a nerve cell, called a motor neuron, and the muscle fibers connecting to it. The larger the muscle the more nerve fibers stimulated by the motor neuron.

Muscle contraction starts with a command from the brain sent to the muscle(s) in question by way of the central nervous system. Once stimulated, a network of tubes surrounding each muscle fiber (called the sarcoplasmic reticulum) cause the release of calcium. Increased levels of calcium in turn cause a cascade of reactions resulting in the two main muscle filaments, actin and myosin, sliding past one another. Movement is caused by connections (called cross bridges) on myosin tugging or pulling on the adjacent actin filament. The end result is a shortening of each individual fiber unit called the

The third category of muscle is skeletal muscle. Often called striated muscle, skeletal muscle is what we think of when we say, "Flex your muscles." With the exception of reflex arcs (the unconscious movement of a limb by a type of short-circuiting of the normal neuromuscular pathway) skeletal muscle is voluntary in nature and it allows you to stand, run, swim, and lift weights.

Skeletal muscle represents by far the largest single tissue group in the body. In an average adult about 50 percent of the body's weight is made up of skeletal muscle. There are over 600 muscles in the body, each of which move the body, or part of the body, in a certain direction.

sarcomere. A coordinated lengthening and shortening produces movement.

TYPES OF MUSCLE CONTRACTION

Although there are at least five types of muscle contraction, for the purposes of this book we'll only discuss two – isotonic and isometric.

The most familiar type of muscle contraction is isotonic. The name comes from the Greek *iso* meaning equal, and *tonic* meaning tension. The characteristics of isotonic contractions are that the muscle shortens and gets thicker. For example, as you raise and lower a barbell, the biceps lengthens and shortens but the tension remains the same.

The second type of contraction, known as isometric, comes from the Greek *iso* meaning equal and *metric* meaning length. In this case the muscle remains the same length during the contraction. For example, pushing on a brick wall causes the muscles to contract, but their length does not change.

From an exercise point of view isotonic contractions are considered far superior to isometrics. In fact, the increased blood pressure produced by isometric contractions can be dangerous.

TYPES OF MUSCLE FIBERS

Muscle fibers can be classified into two categories based on duration of muscle contraction. For example, the small muscles that control the eyes have contractions lasting only 30 milliseconds, whereas the calves – particularly the lower soleus region – have contractions lasting upwards of 3000 milliseconds. The difference has led physiologists to use the term fast twitch and slow twitch to describe both fiber types.

Fast-twitch muscle fibers are found in muscles requiring fast contractions over

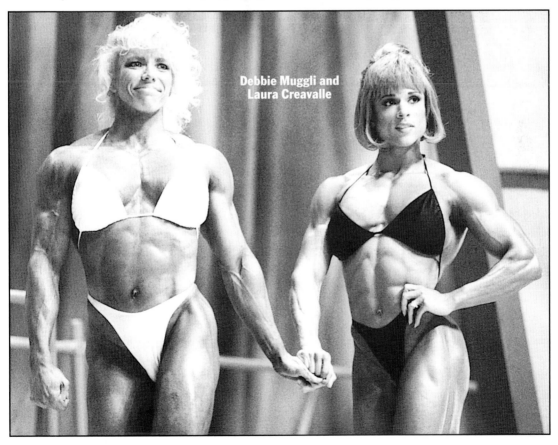

Debbie Muggli and Laura Creavalle

short periods of time. Their limited duration is due to low levels of the oxygen-binding protein myoglobin. Slow-twitch muscle fibers are found in muscles requiring slow continuous contractions over long periods of time. The lower calves, forearms, and spinal erectors are examples.

Besides contraction duration, there are differences in color. Slow-twitch muscle is red in appearance because of the high levels of myoglobin. Conversely, fast-twitch fibers with low-myoglobin levels are almost white.

NAMING MUSCLES

Muscles evolved to be functional, not categorized, and as such, the naming systems used by anatomists have their flaws. At the top of the debate is whether a structure should be named as one muscle or as many smaller muscles. For practical purposes, the body's muscles can be named based on shape, size, location, function, and number of parts. In many cases, more than one characteristic is included in the name.

NUMBER OF PARTS

Perhaps the simplest way to name a muscle is by the number of muscle bellies. A well-known example is the upper arm biceps, which consists of two "heads." The name biceps comes from the prefix *bi* meaning two, and *cep* meaning head. The opposite muscle to the biceps, the triceps, has three heads hence the prefix "tri." In a similar manner the huge upper leg muscle, the quadriceps, has four distinct muscle heads or bellies.

SHAPE

Another way to name a muscle is by its shape. Early Greeks and Romans recognized that some muscles had distinct geometric shapes. The best examples of this naming system are the upper back and shoulder muscles – the deltoids, rhomboids, and trapezius. All three names indicate the geometric shape of the particular muscle.

SIZE

Muscles can also be named according to their size in relation to other muscles. For example, the chest muscles are composed of the pectoral major and pectoral minor. Likewise, the butt muscles can be subdivided into gluteus maximus and gluteus minimus.

Deltoids
Triceps
Biceps
Chest
Obliques
Abs
Quadriceps
Gastrocnemius

Vicki Anderson

POSITION

A fourth category of naming consists of classifying a muscle according to its position on the body. The large back muscles are called latissimus dorsi because they are located on the dorsal region of the body (just think of a shark's dorsal fin).

FUNCTION

A final category of naming involves classifying according to a muscle's function. The spinal erector muscles help keep the spine erect; the levator scapula elevate the scapula (shoulder blade); and the leg adductors adduct, drawing the legs together or closer to the body.

THE MAJOR MUSCLES AND THEIR FUNCTION

As there are over 600 muscles in the human body, for practical purposes we'll only concern ourselves with the larger muscle groups. The following chart lists the major muscles and their common gym names:

Anatomical Name	Common Gym Name(s)
Pectorals	Pecs or Chest
Latissimus Dorsi	Lats or Back
Deltoids	Delts or Shoulders
Quadriceps	Quads or Thighs
Hamstrings	Hams
Biceps	Bis
Triceps	Tris
Abdominals	Abs
Gastrocnemius	Calves
Soleus	Calves

GENERAL CATEGORIES OF MUSCLE ACTION

Flexors – Muscles that bend a limb and draw the limb closer to the body's mid-line.

Extensors – Muscles that push the limb further from th body's mid-line. For example, the biceps are called flexors as they draw the forearms toward the torso, while the triceps push or extend the forearms away from the body, and hence are called extensors. The

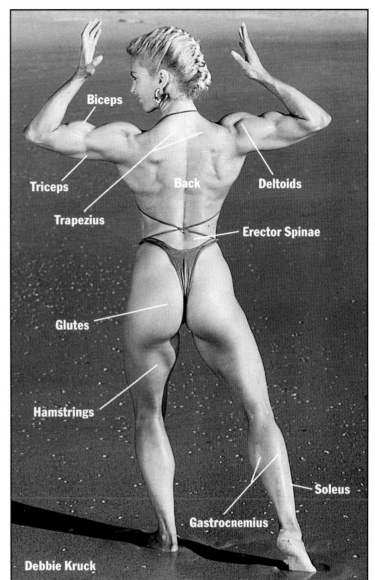

Debbie Kruck

muscles in the legs work in a similar manner. The thighs or quads are extensors and the hamstrings act as flexors.

Agonist – The muscle that contracts to produce a desired movement.

Antagonist – The muscle that relaxes, and produces the opposite movement.

These terms are relative. An agonist in one situation is an antagonist in another. Many muscles work in pairs and as one contracts the other relaxes (we say relax but there is always some tension on the muscle). The following are the most common agonist/antagonist pairs: biceps/triceps, quadriceps/hamstrings, chest/back, abdominals/spinal erectors.

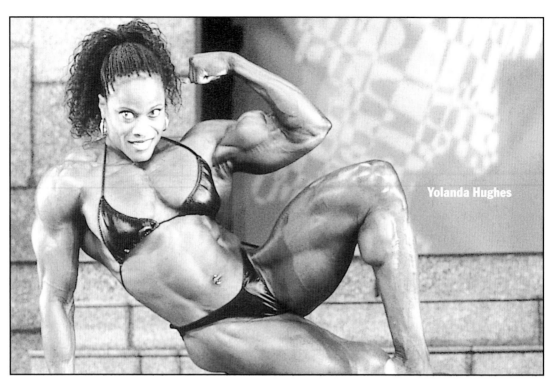

Yolanda Hughes

MUSCLE ENERGY SYSTEMS

One of the primary responses of exercise is an increase in heart rate to carry more blood to the fatiguing muscles. It's not the blood that is so important but what it carries – oxygen. The body needs oxygen to assist in the breakdown of glucose into adenosine triphosphate (ATP). This is the primary energy source in the human body. Without going into too much biochemistry, one molecule of glucose is broken down to yield two molecules of an intermediate called pyruvic acid. This in turn is broken into carbon dioxide and water.

Carbohydrate is the body's preferred fuel source during exercise. It is stored in the liver and muscles as glycogen. More than 99 percent of the carbohydrates you eat are used by the body to make ATP.

**John Parrillo,
exercise and nutrition expert**

form of respiration is called anaerobic respiration and supplies the body with energy when cellular oxygen levels are low. Eventually lactic acid builds up and begins to interfere with muscle contraction. The intense burning sensation you feel during strenuous weight-lifting is the result of lactic-acid build-up in the muscles.

Pyruvic Acid + Oxygen ⟶ Carbon Dioxide + Water + Energy

Oxygen is required to drive the above reaction, leading biochemists to use the term aerobic or "with oxygen." Aerobic respiration allows the body to exercise at a moderate level for extended periods of time.

In cases were oxygen levels are not sufficient to completely reduce pyruvic acid to carbon dioxide and water, a metabolic intermediate called lactic acid is produced. This

PHYSIOLOGICAL CHANGES DUE TO EXERCISE

A well-rounded exercise program can have numerous effects on the body. Some changes will be noticeable after the first few weeks, while others take months. It's quite possible others will first pick up the external changes. Don't despair. It won't be long before you see what they're talking about. We are going to categorize the changes to emphasize just how effective exercise is in promoting physical health.

MUSCLE CHANGES

Perhaps the most noticeable change will be seen in your muscles. Previously soft muscle tissue will become firm and toned. Muscle tone is actually the first step in growth and normally takes three to four weeks to become noticeable. Numerous factors contribute to improved muscle tone. First, the number of actin and myosin filaments increase. Second, the number of sarcomeres within each muscle fiber increase. Finally, the number of capillaries surrounding the muscle fibers increase.

Besides the muscle fibers, there are changes to the surrounding connective tissue – primarily tendons and ligaments. Both tissues thicken and enlarge like the muscle fibers they serve and protect.

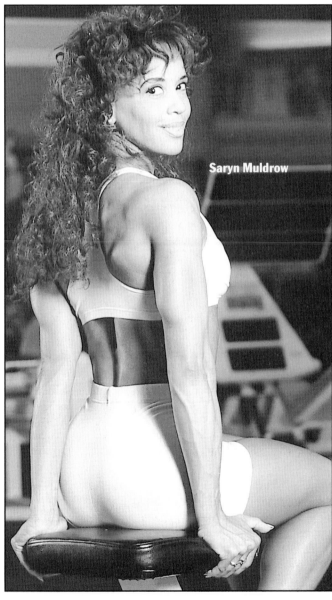

Saryn Muldrow

One of the most interesting areas of strength-training research concerns the effects of exercise on muscle-fiber types. It was originally believed that weight training had little or no effect on changing fiber types in muscle tissue. But recent research suggests muscle-fiber type can be converted in response to exercise.[1] For example, there is evidence to suggest fast-twitch muscle fiber can be converted to slow twitch. This is what makes weight training beneficial to endurance athletes; and allows power athletes to switch to endurance sports.

We should add that there is individual variation when it comes to the previous changes. Some people strengthen and grow by merely looking at a barbell. Others need months if not years for the same degree of change to occur. Because of higher testosterone levels, men gain muscle mass much easier. But don't despair. A woman can proportionally develop as much strength and muscle tone as a man. In fact, because women tend to be less active than men, those who take up weight training make "greater" gains in a shorter time period because of the initial disparity.

CARDIOVASCULAR CHANGES

The heart muscle also responds to regular exercise. Just like its skeletal counterpart, heart tissue thickens and grows in response to strenuous exercise. Besides the heart, blood vessels (particularly the arteries) also thicken and strengthen. Regular exercise also plays a role in keeping the blood vessels clear of fatty-acid build-up. So while weight training is not as effective as aerobics for stimulating the cardio-vascular system, it is still far more beneficial than originally thought.

How does weight training combat osteoporosis? Skeletal muscles are appropriately named because they are attached to your skeleton. When you stress your muscles you stress your skeleton. It becomes stronger, as do your muscles.

Will Brink,
Regular *MuscleMag* **columnist**

BONE DENSITY

One of the biggest changes seen in recent years is the number of post-menopausal women actively engaged in weight training. They are to be commended for their wisdom. Weight training does more than build muscle, it also keeps the body's bones firm and strong. The reduction in estrogen levels associated with menopause often leaves women's bones brittle and subject to easy breakage. We may laugh at a comedian's quip of "I've fallen and I can't get up," but the condition can be life threatening in elderly women. Although the process is not fully understood, declining estrogen levels cause the body's bones to lose calcium. The body doesn't seem to deposit as much calcium either. Both contribute to the cause of osteoporosis, the condition described above. While weight training doesn't cure osteoporosis, it goes a long way in treating and preventing it. Older women who regularly weight train are less susceptible to bone break-age and young women who regularly strength train are less likely to develop the condition in the first place.

Reference
1. R. Billeter and H. Hoppeler, *Muscular Basis of Strength*, (Oxford: Blackwell Scientific Publications, 1992), 52-53.

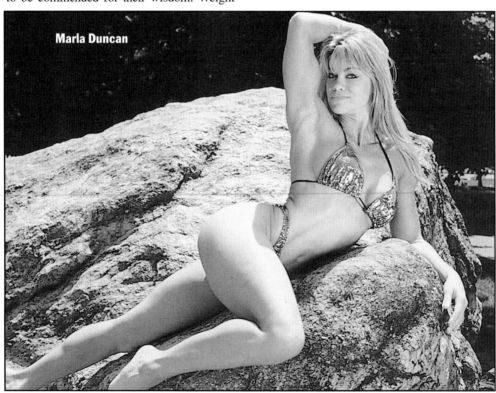

Marla Duncan

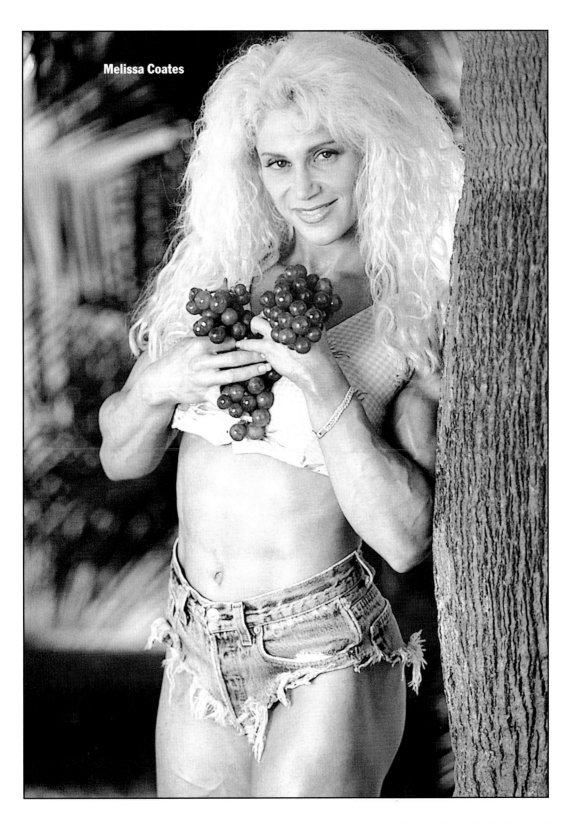

Melissa Coates

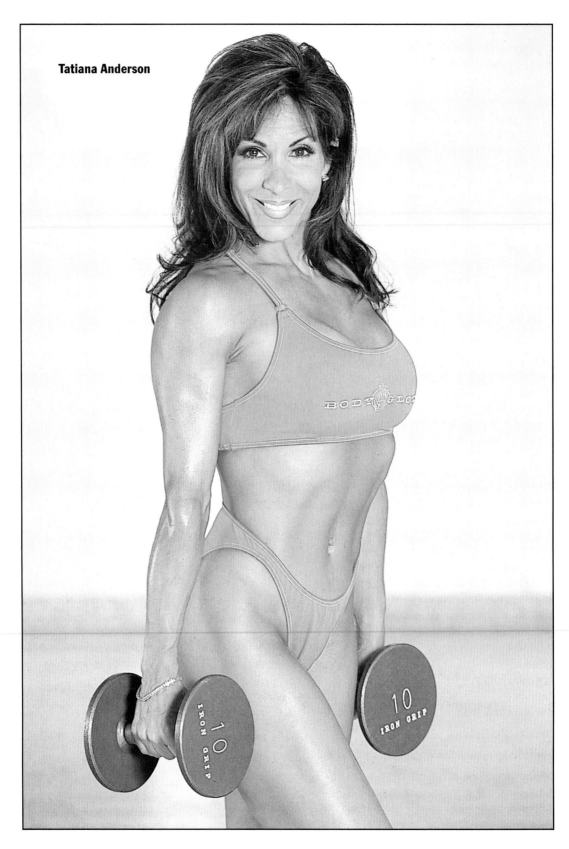

Tatiana Anderson

Chapter 4
Equipment

The fitness industry has evolved tremendously. A typical gym in the 1950s contained a few barbells, dumbells, and if you were lucky, a couple of stationary bikes or rowers. Nowadays the better gyms have million-dollar inventories containing numerous lines of strength-training equipment. They also boast dozens of computerized cardio machines. To borrow a line from the movie *Forrest Gump*, today's gym . . . is like a box of chocolates, you never know what you're going to get.

The following section is not meant to be an all-encompassing guide to gym equipment. Such an undertaking could fill an entire book. Instead, the most common pieces of equipment are highlighted – especially the ones we feel are most appropriate for your training. Like gym types, equipment can be broken down into three broad categories: free weights, machines, and cardio equipment.

FREE WEIGHTS

The simplest types of weight-training equipment are barbells and dumbells – collectively called free weights. By free we mean there's no associated pulleys, cables or handles.

The standard barbell in most gyms is a seven-foot-long spring-steel bar that is called an Olympic barbell. It consists of three main sections: the long narrow center section, and the two wider diameter end pieces called sleeves. The bar itself weighs 45 pounds (most gyms also have 20 kilogram/44-pound bars) and increasing the weight is a simple matter of placing an identical weight plate on each end. To keep the plates from sliding off you secure them with collars. The plates are designed to fit snug over the bar's sleeves with their large diameter center hole; and, therefore, will not work

with any other type of barbell. The plates come in six sizes: 2.5, 5, 10, 25, 35, and 45 pounds. By using various combinations of plates you can put any multiple of five on the bar.

Most weight trainers use barbells to work the larger muscles of the body like the legs, chest, back, and shoulders. And while some individuals also use the bars to work arms, the bar's length makes it difficult to balance.

Most gyms also have two short versions of the standard Olympic bar. Both are identical with the exception of length. One is four to five feet long and weighs 30 pounds. The reduced length makes it ideal for exercises where the longer bar is too awkward. The second version is more popular, and gets nearly as much use as its big brother. Called an EZ-curl bar, it is about three and one-half-feet long and weighs 20 to 25 pounds. Its trademark is the double S curve in the center of the bar. The size and shape of the bar

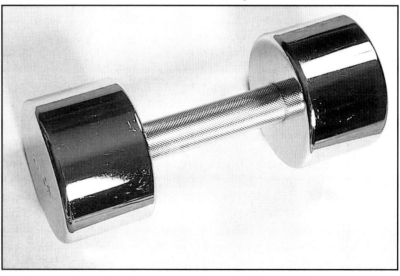

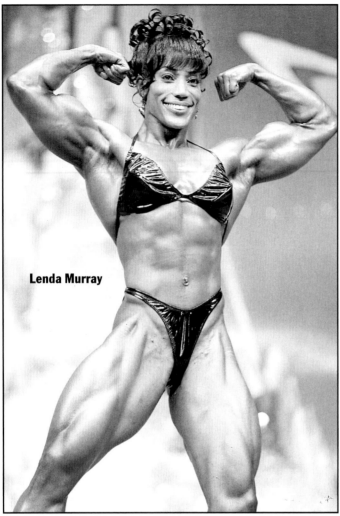

Lenda Murray

The second major type of free-weight equipment is called the dumbell. Dumbells are short (one to one and a half feet long) barbells that you hold in each hand. Although a few gyms have adjustable dumbells, most have the plates welded into place. The standard dumbell set ranges from five to 100 pounds, but some of the larger gyms have dumbells up to 150 or 200 pounds. The primary advantage of dumbells over barbells is they allow a greater range of movement. They also make it easier to isolate smaller muscle groups.

While some of the older gyms have the barbells and dumbells laying about the floor, most have them stored in specially designed holders or racks. In most gyms the dumbells are arranged in rows by the mirrors, and the Olympic bars are stored vertically in floor stands. As many of the exercises require positioning yourself under the bar, most gyms have an assortment of racks. As we'll be going into the exercises in detail later, suffice to say racks allow you to perform the desired exercise in a safe and effective manner.

Closely associated with racks are various styles of benches. Benches allow you to sit or lie down while exercising the body's torso and arm muscles. A bench may be attached to a rack or free standing, requiring you to position it yourself. Benches fall into four categories: decline, flat, incline, and vertical. As the name implies, flat benches are flat or parallel with the floor. Although there are exceptions, flat benches are primarily used for chest and triceps training. To hit the upper chest the angle must be raised or "inclined" to between 30 and 45 degrees. Most gyms have benches with fixed angles and hence the name incline bench. To really hit the lower chest the angle can be "declined" or lowered below parallel. Although it varies, most decline benches are set at around 30 degrees.

enables you to hit the biceps and triceps from just about every conceivable angle.

Besides Olympic bars, most gyms have an assortment of smaller diameter bars. Averaging four to five feet in length and weighing 10 to 20 pounds, these bars also require the use of collars to secure the weight in place. Any exercise you do with an Olympic bar you can do with one of these bars. But keep in mind most racks are designed to accommodate the longer Olympic bar. It's possible your gym has a set of such bars with the weights welded in place. This makes things very convenient, as you don't have to change plates. Just grab the barbell with the desired weight and away you go.

We should add that incline and decline are relative terms and refer to the position of your head and feet. If your head is up and your feet are down, you're inclined. Opposite this, you're in a decline position. You can make a flat bench inclined or declined by placing a wooden block under one end. The advantage of a properly designed decline bench is that it has foot holders to keep you from sliding off the bench. In fact, the popular Roman chair situp bench has two leg rollers for this purpose.

The fourth type of bench is called a vertical bench. As the name implies, it is at a 90-degree angle with the floor. The bench offers back support as you perform dumbell or barbell presses for your shoulders. Your gym may have fixed vertical benches or adjustable benches that allow any angle from 0 to 90 degrees.

Other racks and benches you'll incorporate into your workouts include squat racks, chinup bars, preacher benches, and shoulder-press racks.

MACHINES

Perhaps the biggest revolution in the strength-training industry concerns the introduction of state-of-the-art machines. Barbells and dumbells haven't changed much since the 1950s and 1960s but the quality and number of exercise machines has taken a quantum leap forward.

It started with Universal in the 1960s, progressed to Nautilus in the 1970s, and evolved to Apex, Polaris, and Hammer Strength in the 1980s and 1990s. While purists argue that no machine takes the place of free weights, the consensus among trainers and athletes alike is that a well-rounded routine

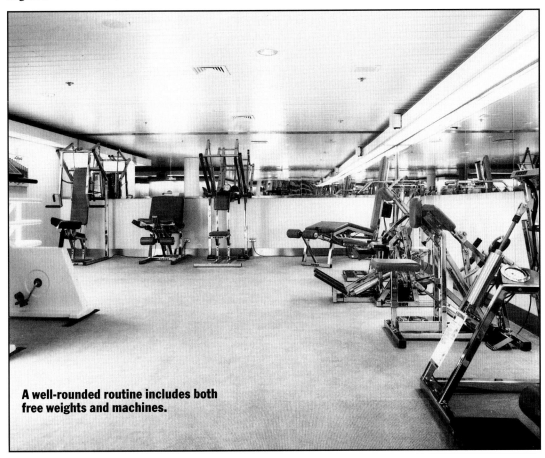

A well-rounded routine includes both free weights and machines.

should include a combination of free-weight and machine exercises. In a few cases machines are necessary, as there's no direct free-weight equivalent.

Machines can be subdivided into two broad categories – single exercise and multistation units. Most readers are probably familiar with Universal's multistation gym. Few high schools and colleges are without one of these large silver and black pieces of machinery. And while Universal machines have been replaced by more modern equipment, we have to give Universal credit for bringing strength training to the mass market.

The basic truth is that both free weights and machines are very useful strength-building tools. But they do work the body in different ways. So it's not a matter of choosing one over the other, but understanding how each works and then applying that information to help formulate a useful weight program.

**Bill Starr,
strength coach and
Oxygen contributor**

Most multistations consist of eight to 10 stations arranged around a central frame. Each station targets one or two muscle groups and it's simply a matter of moving around the unit in a circular manner to hit the entire body. The primary advantage of multistations is the small area they take up. Even the large Universal multistation could fit into a large household bedroom (with the possible exception of ceiling height).

The other category of machines is single-exercise units. Each machine targets only one or two muscle groups and you must move from machine to machine to work the whole body. While multistations are still popular, single units have seen the biggest leap forward in the weight-training field. The obvious disadvantage to single units is the space needed to accommodate a full line. You need a large room to hold eight to 10 units.

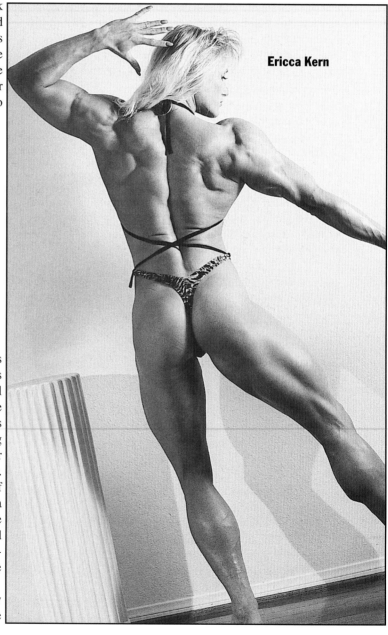

Ericca Kern

FREE WEIGHTS VERSUS MACHINES

Few topics generate as much debate in weight-training circles as comparisons between free weights and machines. Both sides have their advocates. We are not going to take sides. Instead we'll try to give an unbiased evaluation of the strengths and weaknesses of both.

I recommend you include both free weights and machines in your training program. The best-looking muscles are those exercised from all angles.

Robert Kennedy, *MuscleMag International* founder and best-selling author

The primary advantages of free weights is that they force you to both lift and balance the weight. Machines, on the other hand, are balanced and only require you to lift the weight. Having to balance the weight not only works the primary muscles but the smaller secondary muscles. Balancing also forces the weaker muscles to carry their share of the load, so they'll eventually catch up in strength with the stronger muscles. With most machine exercises the stronger side of the body will always be doing most of the work. The weaker side may never catch up. We should add that some of the newer manufacturers (Hammer Strength to name one) have attempted to get around this by designing machines that force both sides of the body to work evenly. And while they don't perfectly simulate free weights, they're the next best thing.

Another advantage to free weights is cost. For a couple of hundred dollars you could outfit your basement with enough weight to work your whole body – no matter how strong you are. To set up an equivalent machine-based gym in your basement with each unit averaging $2000, you would have to spend as much as $15,000 to $20,000.

Closely related to the previous is the amount of space taken up by free weights. Any small room or even part of a room will suffice for a barbell set, while machines require the space only gyms can provide.

Finally, free weights have it over machines when it comes to versatility. One barbell set is sufficient to work the whole body, where as you'd need eight to 10 machines to accomplish the same thing. Now having trashed machines let's see if we can rehabilitate them!

Perhaps the biggest drawing card for machines – at least for beginners – is their ease of operation. Most of the new machines can be used by sitting or lying down and pushing a leg or arm handle. Even a novice can figure out how a machine works by simply looking at it. They are self-explanatory. Not so with a barbell or set of dumbells. The average person probably knows how to do a set of curls, but for most that's it. This is one of the main

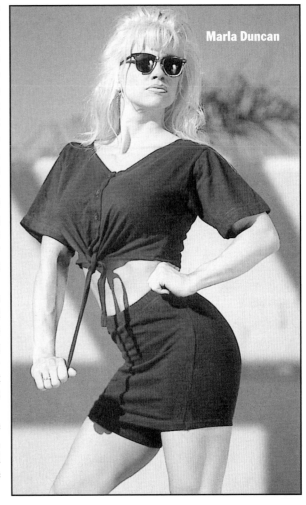

Marla Duncan

reasons why gyms have a couple of lines of machines. They allow anyone to walk in off the street and with a minimal amount of instruction do a full-body workout.

Another advantage of machines is the ease of changing the weight. While a few lines like Hammer Strength require you to put the plates on yourself, moving a small selector pin changes the weight on the majority of machines. It's only a matter of inserting the pin into the desired hole. To change the

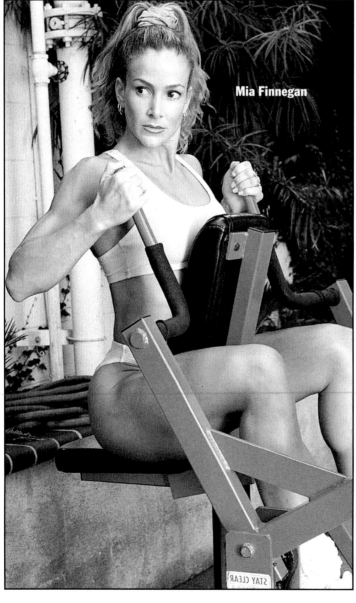

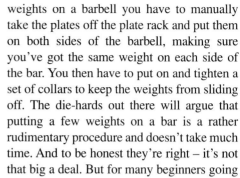

Mia Finnegan

weights on a barbell you have to manually take the plates off the plate rack and put them on both sides of the barbell, making sure you've got the same weight on each side of the bar. You then have to put on and tighten a set of collars to keep the weights from sliding off. The die-hards out there will argue that putting a few weights on a bar is a rather rudimentary procedure and doesn't take much time. And to be honest they're right – it's not that big a deal. But for many beginners going to the free-weight area of the gym, it can be a little intimidating. Throw in the obligatory groaner on the bench press and the situation becomes similar to an African safari! Despite the best efforts of gym instructors to encourage members to perform more free-weight exercises, many beginners – especially women – just don't want to have anything to do with changing weights on a barbell. If for no other reason, machines allow beginners to become more comfortable with the gym environment.

A third advantage to machines is safety. A couple of the barbell exercises can be unforgiving at times. Movements like squats place incredible stress on the knees and lower back. And while squats are probably the best lower-body exercise there is, many individuals have thrown out their knees or lower backs from such exercises. The same holds true for flat barbell bench presses – considered by many to be the best movement for strengthening the chest muscles. As mentioned earlier, a few unwise individuals have died in their basements after getting caught under the barbell while attempting a heavy single rep. If something goes wrong during a machine exercise you simply lower the weight back to the starting position and walk away. Even the worse case scenario sees you letting go of the handles or leg rollers in the middle

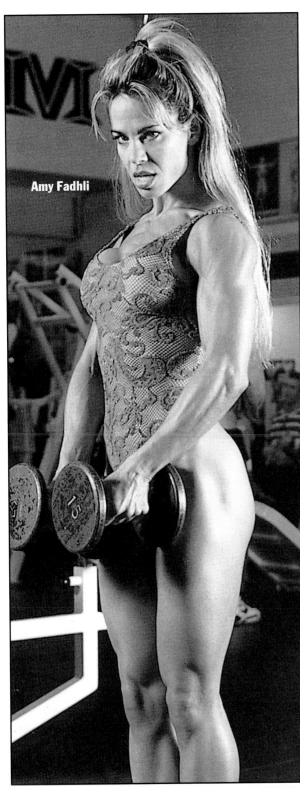

Amy Fadhli

of the movement. Granted you may make some noise, perhaps break a weight plate or two, but the odds are good to excellent that no harm will come to you. If you try the same thing with a barbell you'll probably end up in traction for three months.

A final reason for using machines is you may have to! Despite the versatility of barbells and dumbells, there are a couple of movements that can only be performed on machines. Hamstring training is one such example. While you can grab a bar or set of dumbells and perform stiff-leg deadlifts, the stress on the lower back may force you to skip the movement. On the other hand, lying leg curls can be performed by just about anyone. Even those with pre-existing back problems can usually train hamstrings in this manner. Another muscle where machines are more suited is the calves. With the primary function of the calves being to raise and lower the body on the toes, training requires you place the weight on the spine. The problem with a barbell is balance. Trying to pivot up and down on the toes with a barbell on your shoulders is both awkward and dangerous. One solution is to hold a dumbell in each hand, but eventually your calf strength will outgrow your forearm strength. In other words, you can lift more weight with the calves than you can hold in your hands. The way around this is the standing calf-raise machine. The shoulder pads allow you to easily lift the weight. At the same time the machine prevents any sideways motion.

There are also other exercises that can only be performed on machines. This is why, despite the objections of the free-weight-only advocates, the routines in this book incorporate both free weights and machines.

MISCELLANEOUS EQUIPMENT

While the previous equipment is found at most gyms, the following are items you may want to pick up yourself. Considered personal accessories, they may help your workouts go a little smoother. None are essential, and many weight trainers train for years without using any of them. Still, given their popularity, a brief description of each is provided so you can make up your own mind.

GLOVES

Like manual labor, weightlifting can play havoc with the skin on the hands – particularly the palms. The first few weeks are the worst as the skin may blister and break. In severe cases the individual has difficulty holding onto anything. Eventually the body's coping mechanisms take over and the skin thickens and deadens, producing calluses. Many weight lifters consider calluses a right of passage and prevention is out of the question. Others hate the sight and feel of the brutes and do everything possible to avoid them. Gloves are one such option and like most weight-training paraphernalia, come in many different styles.

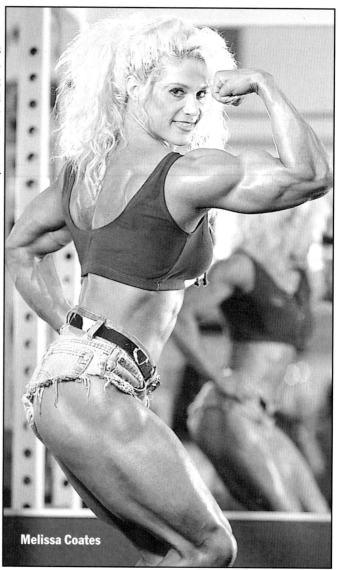

Melissa Coates

Weight-training gloves are similar in appearance to golf gloves and serve much the same purpose – to protect the soft skin from the friction produced by holding barbells and dumbells. For most individuals this occurs at the point where the fingers intersect the palms of the hands. Although there's many styles, the most popular gloves have the tips of the fingers removed and use a Velcro strip to tighten at the wrist. Most weightlifting gloves cost between $15 to $20.

Gloves have two disadvantages. For starters, they don't allow the same feel when gripping the bar. In order to be effective the glove must be a certain thickness. Unfortunately, the minimum needed for protection is too thick to get a proper feel for the bar. For many the feel of cold metal in their palms is good for a couple of additional reps.

A second disadvantage is that you may become dependant on them. If you never allow the skin to toughen up, you'll always have to wear gloves. The first time you forget them your hands will blister. Unless you have extremely sensitive skin, or need soft delicate hands in your line of work, our advice is to skip gloves and let the hands become accustomed to the weights. But the choice is yours. It all depends on your priorities.

Before leaving this topic we should touch on a variation of weightlifting gloves. Numerous ingenious individuals have saved on the expense of gloves by using pieces of soft rubber, usually tire inner tube. Simply cut a four- or five-inch diameter circle from such material and wrap it around the bar or machine handle. Not only does it provide a great grip but the soft rubber helps protect the hands.

WRAPS

Wraps are nothing more than bandages wrapped around a joint to give it a little extra security. No matter how strict your training style sooner or later one or more of your joints will start acting up. If it feels serious, stop training and see your physician. In many cases you can wrap the offending area with a first-aid bandage. The joints most prone to injury are the wrists, elbows, and knees. For the wrists and elbows use a small, two-inch-wide bandage. For the knees use a four- to five-inch bandage. Contrary to popular belief, bandages don't allow you to lift more. They keep the area warm and secure allowing you to train around a minor irritation.

Using wraps every workout is not bad for the knees. I use wraps all the time and have done so for over a decade.

Dr. Mauro DiPasquale,
MuscleMag **columnist**

STRAPS

In many exercises, the forearm muscles form the weak link in the chain. Straps are pieces of leather or woven cloth that wrap around the bar and your wrist to assist the forearms. Straps play an invaluable role when doing shrugs, deadlifts, chins, and pulldowns. Like gloves, however, straps can be abused. You can become dependant on them. Much of your forearm strength is obtained indi-

rectly from training other muscles. If you use straps for all your exercises, your forearm strength will never improve. Our advice is to limit their use to exercises where there is a big strength difference between the forearms and target muscles being worked.

If you are like most people, the limiting factor in your workout is your grip strength and forearm strength. Your poor hands and forearms get maxed-out long before your back has reached its max. That's where straps come in. They improve your grip strength, letting you hold onto, and ultimately lift, heavier weight.

Vicky Pratt, *Oxygen* **columnist**

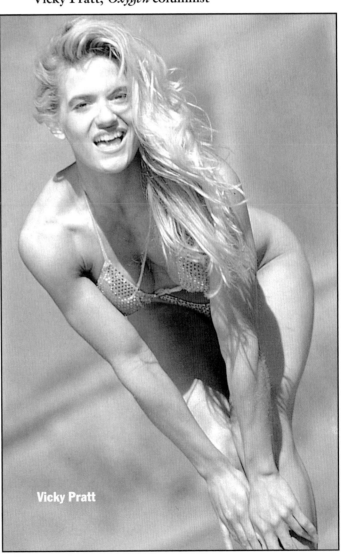

Vicky Pratt

BELTS

Next to barbells and dumbells, the most well-known piece of strength-training equipment is the weightlifting belt. Belts come in various shapes and sizes and serve to give the lower back support on such exercises as squats, deadlifts, and bent-over rows. Think of your abdominal cavity as a large balloon. For example, as you perform squats your spinal erectors and abdominals contract and increase the pressure inside the cavity. Physiologists call the pressure intra abdominal pressure (IAP). From an exercise point of view such pressure is beneficial as it helps stabilize the torso. The purpose of the belt is to give the abdominals something to press against.

When used correctly a weight belt can greatly improve performance and help keep your trunk and specifically your lower back in line.

David Sandler,
Oxygen **contributor**

ing more popular, fastened with Velcro. A word of caution about Velcro – many athletes have been right in the middle of a heavy set of squats or deadlifts when the Velcro let go. This is dangerous, as the support the belt was providing is suddenly lost. The loss of security plus the shock often disorients the lifter, and unfortunately it's the lower back that takes the brunt of the stress.

A second disadvantage to Velcro belts is their thickness. Most are no more than 1/8 of an inch thick – the absolute minimum that provides support. While Velcro belts may look more fashionable and come in a bigger variety of colors, they offer nowhere near the support of the old-fashioned four-inch thick leather belt. Our advice is to play it safe and buy something based on function not attractiveness.

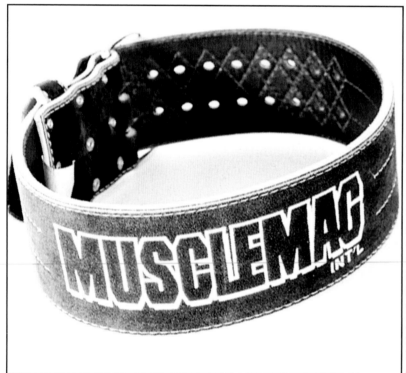

A typical belt is four- to six-inches wide and 1/8- to 1/4-inch thick. Belts don't allow you to lift more weight, they only keep the lower back secure. Belts can be buckled like a regular dress-pant belt or, as is becoming

CHALK

No doubt many readers have seen gymnasts on TV applying chalk to their hands before their routines. Weight lifters encounter the same problem when they work out – a loss of grip on the bar. This is because the increased body temperature produced by exercise causes the palms to sweat and become moist. Chalk dries the moisture allowing a better grip. Chalk is one of the cheapest weightlifting aids, costing a few dollars for a large brick-size block. If chalk has a disadvantage it's that many gyms don't allow its use. It doesn't take many chalk users to dirty the floor. Before buying chalk we suggest checking your gym's policy.

WATER BOTTLES

Although most gyms have water fountains you may want to consider bringing your own water. Let's face it, a typical gym water foun-

Chalk was always my one sure bet no matter how sweaty my hands were. I just dried my hands and then put on tons of chalk. I'd go through a few ounces of chalk every workout.

Dr. Mauro DiPasquale,
***MuscleMag* columnist and former powerlifting champion**

tain will have hundreds if not thousands of users during a typical day. A combination of volume and poor hygienic practices (spitting in the fountain) sets up a very unhealthy environment. For the sake of a few dollars you can greatly reduce the chances of catching germs by bringing your own water – either purchased daily or in a reusable container.

TOWELS

This last accessory has its advantages. Many exercises require you to sit or lie down on a piece of equipment. A couple of users and there's pools of sweat everywhere. And while most gyms encourage members to wipe up afterward, a few people never get the message. Rather than lie in someone else's sweat, bring an old towel to wipe the equipment down beforehand, as well as afterward. When you go home throw the towel in the laundry.

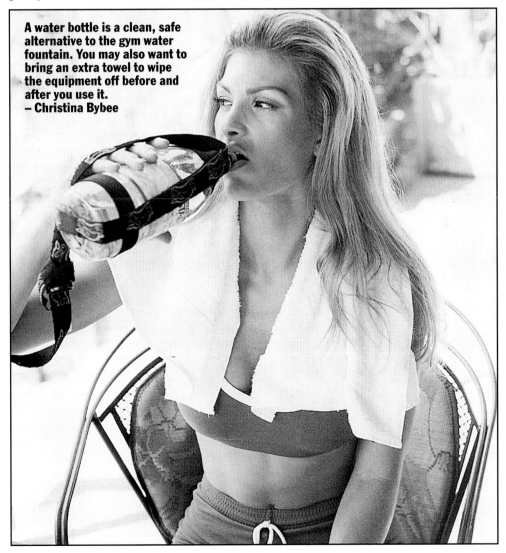

A water bottle is a clean, safe alternative to the gym water fountain. You may also want to bring an extra towel to wipe the equipment off before and after you use it.
– Christina Bybee

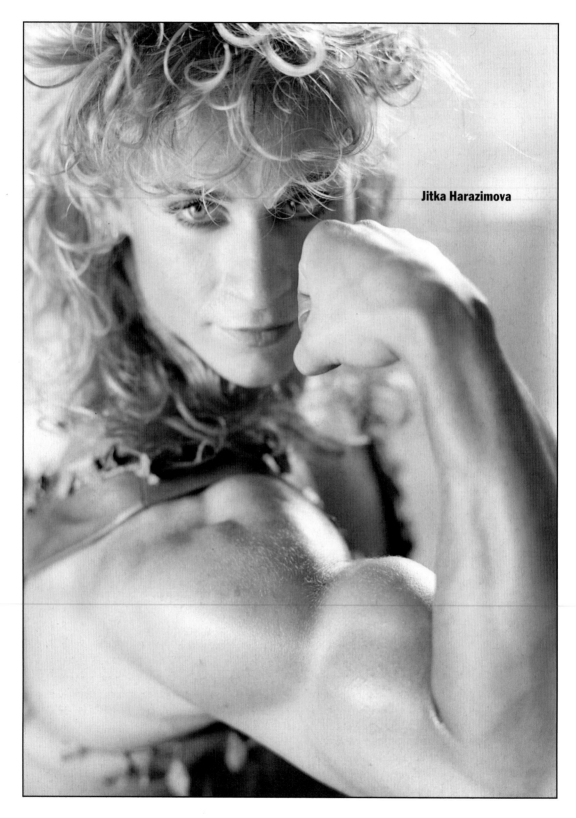

Jitka Harazimova

Chapter 5

The Exercises

The following chapter describes the core strength-training exercises that have withstood the test of time. While many exercise variations exist, your routine should always include some core movements to ensure you are hitting all the major muscle groups.

LEG TRAINING

SQUATS – You'll need a proper rack to perform this exercise. Place a bar about shoulder height on the rack and step under it so the bar rests at the base of your neck. Step back and slowly descend by bending the knees until your thighs are parallel with the floor. Return to the starting position by straightening the legs.

COMMENTS – Two of the biggest mistakes people make when performing squats are to bounce at the top and bottom of the movement. We shouldn't need to tell you the knees and lower back weren't designed to be subjected to this kind of stress. Always perform squats in a slow and controlled manner. If possible, have someone spot you in case you get in trouble.

I believe in basic exercises starting with the biggest muscle groups (legs, back, chest) and working toward the smaller groups like calves, biceps, and triceps. The purpose behind this approach is to work the larger muscles without fatiguing the secondary support muscles.

Robert Kennedy, *MuscleMag* **and** *Oxygen* **publisher**

MUSCLES WORKED – Squats are considered the king of lower-body exercises. They work the thighs, hamstrings, and glutes. Even the calves come into play as stabilizers. As a word of caution, those with severe lower-back or knee problems might want to give this exercise a pass.

My best advice for leg development is to slow down as you exercise through the full range of motion. Focus on the area being worked so you can feel a good contraction. Also, make sure you stretch after your cardio work and during training to keep your muscles lengthened.

Dale Tomita, fitness contestant

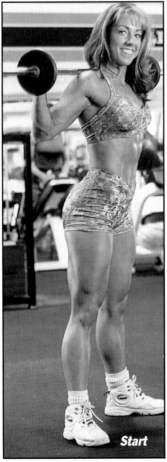

Start

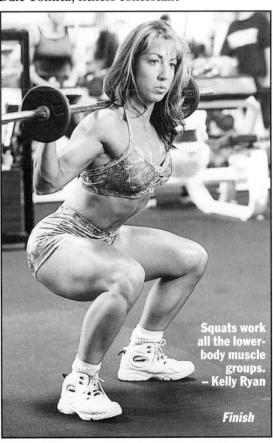

Squats work all the lower-body muscle groups.
– Kelly Ryan

Finish

SISSY SQUATS – Hold a dumbell or weight plate against your chest with one hand and grab a stationary upright for support with the other. Lean back and squat down until your thighs are parallel with the floor. Return to the starting position and repeat.

COMMENTS – Don't let the name "sissy" mislead you. The exercise is definitely not for sissies. Done properly, sissy squats are one of the best exercises for toning and separating the four heads of the quadriceps muscle. If they have one disadvantage it's that you'll eventually reach a point where your legs are capable of lifting much more weight than can be held against your chest. You can prolong the effectiveness, however, by either doing the reps in an ultra slow manner or performing them as the second exercise in a superset.

MUSCLES WORKED – Sissy squats primarily work the thighs and glutes. By changing your foot position you can target the inner and outer thighs.

LEG PRESSES – As with squats, you'll need a special piece of apparatus to do this exercise. Sit down in the machine's chair with your feet about shoulder width apart, toes pointing slightly outward. Bend the knees and lower the platform until your upper legs form an 80- to 90-degree angle with your lower legs. Press the platform back, stopping just short of locking the legs out.

COMMENTS – Like squats, bouncing at the bottom is a great way to damage the knees. The advantage of leg presses over squats is you can load the machine with additional weight without putting extra stress on the lower back. Of course many people abuse this and put so much weight on the machine they can only do partial reps.

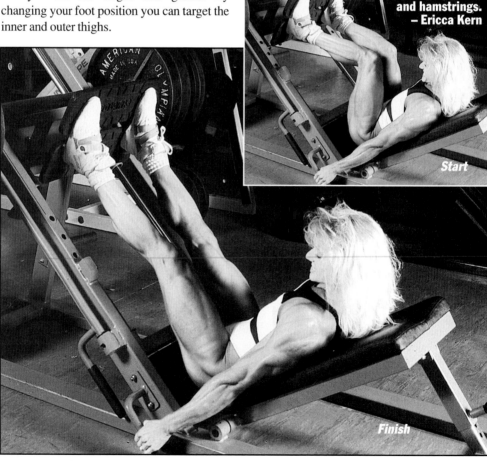

Leg press your way to shapely thighs, glutes and hamstrings.
– Ericca Kern

Start

Finish

MUSCLES WORKED – Done with the legs high and wide, leg presses primarily work the inner thighs, glutes, and hamstrings. Done with the feet low and narrow, most of the stress is placed on the outer thigh. Those with knee problems should avoid the latter as this stance increases pressure on the knees.

LEG EXTENSIONS – Sit in the machine so that your knees rest slightly forward of the chair's edge. If the machine has an adjustable leg roller set it so it rests at the tip of the tongue on your sneaker. Grasp the handles or sides of the chair for support and extend your legs until they're straight. Lower your legs until the weight plates are about an inch apart.

COMMENTS – Leg extensions are considered an isolation movement as they virtually eliminate the glutes and hamstrings from the exercise. Leg extensions are a great way to firm and separate the individual muscles of the thighs. You'll find different opinions regarding locking out at the top of the movement. Some individuals find they have to lock out to fully flex the thighs, others find locking out too painful on the knees. Our advice is to try a full extension and see how it feels. If it's too stressful, stop the movement a few degrees from lockout.

MUSCLES WORKED – Leg extensions primarily work the thighs. The hips and glutes only come into play as stabilizers – unlike squats and presses where the muscles play an active role.

HACK SQUATS – Lie back on the incline board with the pads resting on your shoulders. With your back kept straight, descend until the thighs are parallel or slightly lower than parallel with the floor. Return to the starting position.

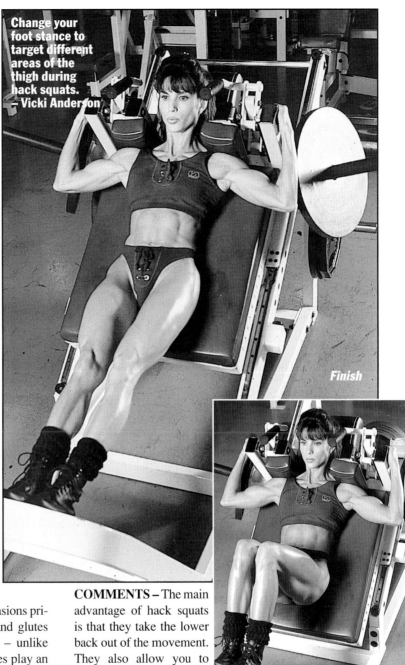

Change your foot stance to target different areas of the thigh during hack squats.
– Vicki Anderson

Finish

Start

COMMENTS – The main advantage of hack squats is that they take the lower back out of the movement. They also allow you to target different parts of the thigh by changing your foot stance.

MUSCLES WORKED – Hack squats primarily work the thighs, but the hamstrings and glutes come into play as you descend close to parallel.

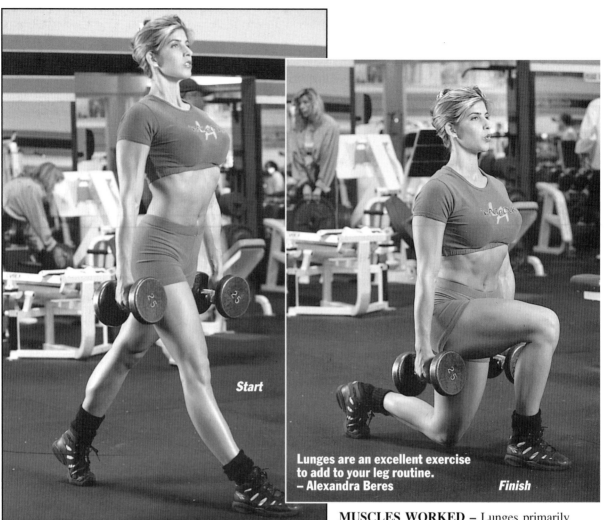

Lunges are an excellent exercise to add to your leg routine.
– Alexandra Beres

Start

Finish

LUNGES – Hold a dumbell in each hand and adopt a runner's stance with one leg forward and one back. Descend slowly by bending the knee of the forward leg. Pause at the bottom and then return to the starting position.

COMMENTS – As with squats, be careful not to bounce at the bottom of the exercise. Also, your knee on the bending leg should not go past your toes. This puts awkward pressure on the knee ligaments. For variety you can perform lunges with a barbell resting on your shoulders. We recommend learning the movement with dumbells, because losing your balance with dumbells doesn't leave you in the same precarious situation as a barbell would. Eventually your legs will be capable of lifting much more weight than your forearms can hold on to. At this point the barbell will be your only option.

MUSCLES WORKED – Lunges primarily target the thighs and glutes, but the hamstrings are brought into play as well.

LOW KICKBACKS – Stand against the kickback machine with one ankle hooked in the adjustable attachment. With both hands holding on for support, kick the leg back and upward as far as possible. Slowly return to the starting position.

COMMENTS – If your gym doesn't have a kickback machine, the low pulley on the cable crossover unit makes a good substitute. As a word of caution, try to keep the torso as upright as possible. The nature of the movement may put pressure on the lower back so stay slow and controlled. No bouncing at the top or bottom.

MUSCLES WORKED – Although primarily a glute exercise, the hamstrings also receive some benefit.

LEG CURLS – Lie face down on the machine with the leg roller resting above your ankles. Hold the handles or end of the bench for support and curl your lower legs upward until they're perpendicular with your upper legs. Lower to the starting position and repeat.

COMMENTS – Depending on the gym, you may have a choice of machines. Some lying-leg-curl machines force you to keep the knees on the bench; others allow you to keep them a couple of inches off the bench. If you have a choice, use the latter. Your knees will thank you for it down the road!

Besides the lying leg curl, many gyms have standing leg curls that allow you to work the legs one at a time. Many individuals find the standing version provides a better contraction in the hamstrings.

MUSCLES WORKED – Leg curls are probably the best exercise for working the leg biceps, more commonly called the hamstrings. The calves and glutes also play a role as stabilizers.

STIFF-LEG DEADLIFTS – You can do this exercise holding either a barbell or two dumbells. With the knees slightly bent, bend at the hips, lowering your torso until it's parallel with the floor. Return to the starting position with the torso held erect.

COMMENTS – The name stiff-leg is misleading, as you should never do the movement with the legs completely stiff. Always keep them slightly bent. This helps alleviate much of the stress on the lower back.

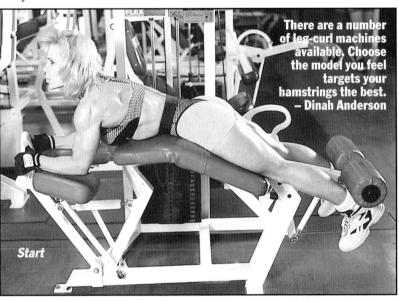

There are a number of leg-curl machines available. Choose the model you feel targets your hamstrings the best.
– Dinah Anderson

Start

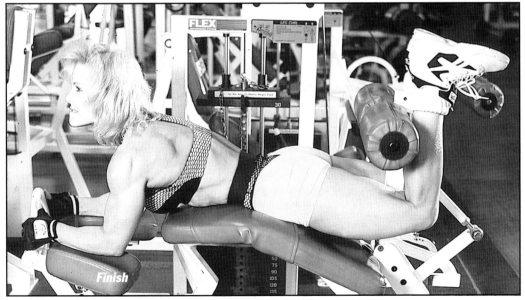

Finish

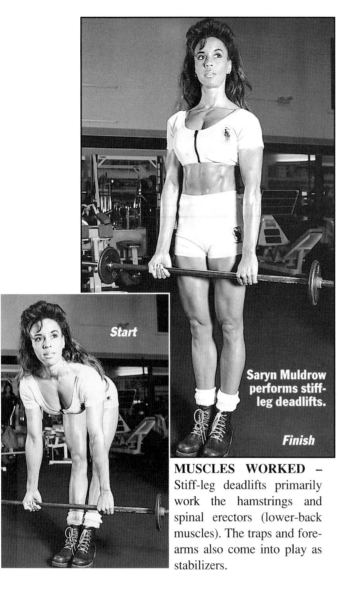

Start

Saryn Muldrow performs stiff-leg deadlifts.

Finish

Also, some individuals make the mistake of bouncing at the bottom of the movement. True, this will allow you to lift more weight but it places tremendous stress on the Achilles tendon. If the exercise has a disadvantage it's that all the weight is resting on the spine. Those with weak or injured lower backs should skip the machine version of this exercise.

MUSCLES WORKED – Standing calf raises primarily work the beautiful heart-shaped calf muscles known as the gastrocnemius. Secondary stress is placed on the lower soleus region.

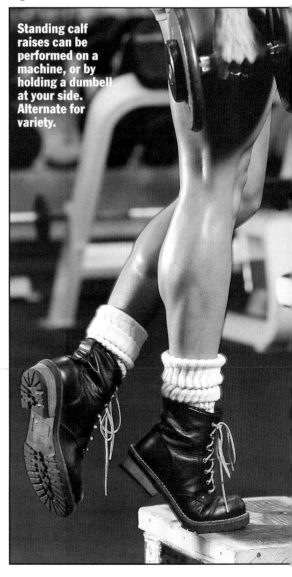

Standing calf raises can be performed on a machine, or by holding a dumbell at your side. Alternate for variety.

MUSCLES WORKED – Stiff-leg deadlifts primarily work the hamstrings and spinal erectors (lower-back muscles). The traps and forearms also come into play as stabilizers.

STANDING CALF RAISES – If you have access to a machine, position yourself under the shoulder supports, placing the balls of your feet on the narrow platform. With your feet six to eight inches apart and legs straight, lower your heels as far as you can. Return to the starting position by raising up on your toes as far as possible, flexing your calves at the top of the movement.

COMMENTS – Standing raises are as much of a stretching exercise as a strength-training exercise. It's much safer to use medium poundages, and a full range of motion, than heavy weight and a partial range of motion.

SEATED CALF RAISES – Although you can do this exercise with a barbell or dumbell placed on the knees, the machine specially designed for the job is much more convenient. Sit down on the seat with your knees under the pads, and the balls of your feet on the rest. Release the weight support (on most machines it's a simple matter of pushing a lever) and lower the heels and then raise up on the toes as far as possible.

COMMENTS – As with standing calf raises, go for maximum stretch. If you don't have access to a machine you can lay a barbell or large dumbell on the knees. Unfortunately your calves will eventually reach the point where it's extremely awkward lifting the weight into position. Not to mention the pressure of the bar resting on the thighs. One solution is to get a partner to lay a couple of barbell plates on the knees. They are a bit more comfortable than a bar, but once again it won't be long before you'll need to use three, four, or more, 45-pound plates.

MUSCLES WORKED – By bending the knees the large upper gastrocnemius part of the calves is taken out of the exercise, forcing the lower soleus to do most of the work.

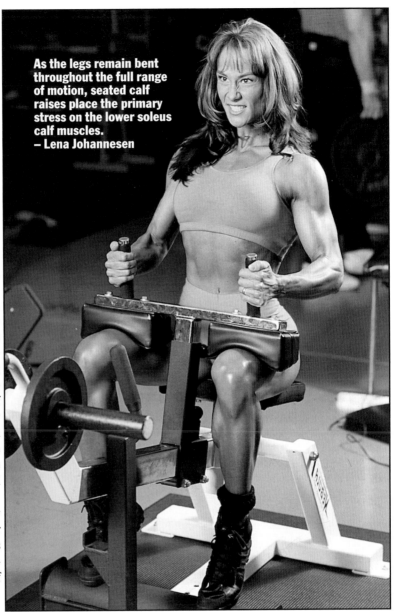

As the legs remain bent throughout the full range of motion, seated calf raises place the primary stress on the lower soleus calf muscles.
– Lena Johannesen

TOE PRESSES – Using the leg-press machine, place your toes on the lower edge of the platform and straighten your legs. Instead of bending the knees, flex the platform up and down using only the ankle joint and hence the calf muscles.

COMMENTS – If this exercise has a disadvantage it's that some individuals find it hard on the knees. On the other hand, its primary advantage is that you don't have any weight pressing down on the spine. Some leg presses have platforms that don't allow you to place your toes on the lower edge.

MUSCLES WORKED – Despite the seated position, the exercise primarily works the upper gastrocnemius muscle, as the legs are straight throughout the movement. Remember, it's not the position of the body that determines which part of the calf is worked but whether the legs are bent or straight.

DONKEY CALF RAISES – If your gym doesn't have a machine for this exercise, you'll need a willing partner to help with this one. Bend over so your elbows are resting on a waist-high support with the balls of your feet on a two- to three-inch block of wood. Have your partner straddle your back close to your hips. From here the movement is identical to standing calf raises. Stretch up and down as far as possible.

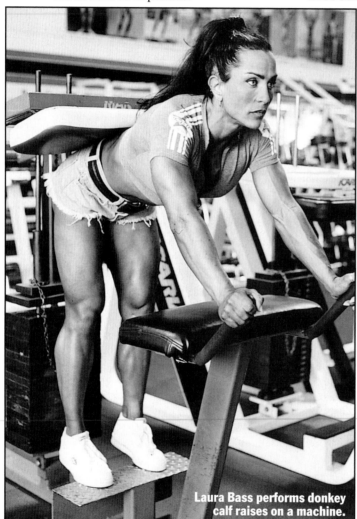

Laura Bass performs donkey calf raises on a machine.

COMMENTS – For safety and effectiveness your partner should not sit in the center of your back. Not only does this take some of the weight off the calves but it could overstress the spine. Perhaps the biggest disadvantage to donkeys is the position involved. The odds of doing the exercise without a few snickers and comments is slim. Most of these comments come from the less informed (something you probably wouldn't run into in a hardcore bodybuilding gym); therefore, the exercise can be intimidating. While many gyms now have donkey calf machines to get around this problem, they're still not standard issue.

MUSCLES WORKED – Donkeys primarily work the large gastrocnemius muscle of the calf. Bending the knees slightly bring in the lower soleus.

CHEST TRAINING
FLAT-BENCH
BARBELL PRESSES – Lie under the bar with your head between the barbell supports. Hold the bar six to eight inches wider than shoulder width and lift it off the rack. Lower the bar to the center of the chest, and then push it to arms' length.

COMMENTS – Although once considered the king of chest exercises, its value has been debated in recent years. We are not going to say it's the best exercise, but "one of the best." As with leg extensions you may want to experiment with locking out at the top. Also, don't bounce the bar off your chest. You may be able to lift more weight, bit it's a great way to damage the rib cage.

MUSCLES WORKED – Primarily a lower/mid chest exercise, flat-bench presses also hit the front shoulders and triceps.

INCLINE BARBELL
PRESSES – With the exception of the angle, this movement is performed identical to the flat version.

COMMENTS – Angles between 30 and 45 degrees work the best. As soon as the angle goes above 45 degrees the front shoulders do most of the work.

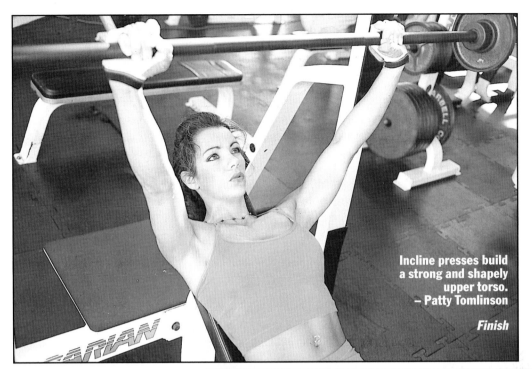

Incline presses build
a strong and shapely
upper torso.
– Patty Tomlinson

Finish

MUSCLES WORKED – Incline presses primarily work the upper chest, but the front shoulders and triceps are also brought into play.

FLAT AND INCLINE DUMBELL PRESSES – For variety, use two dumbells instead of the barbell when you perform presses.

COMMENTS – The advantage of dumbells over barbells is that you can lower the dumbells further at the bottom of the exercise. Many individuals also find dumbells easier on the wrists. A barbell locks you in one position, while dumbells allow for greater flexibility. For inclines, set the angle between 30 and 45 degrees.

FLAT FLYES – Grab a pair of dumbells and lie back on a flat bench. With the arms held to the sides at 90 degrees to the torso, elbows slightly bent and palms facing inward, lower the dumbells until the upper arms are about 20 degrees below parallel. From this position squeeze the dumbells up and inward in a hugging fashion, touching them at the top.

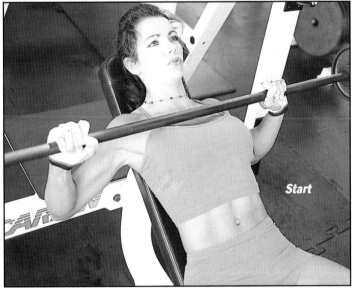

Start

COMMENTS – When lowering, don't bounce at the bottom of the movement as it places tremendous stress on the chest-shoulder tie in. Always execute this movement in a slow and controlled manner.

MUSCLES WORKED – Flyes are a great way to work the chest muscles without putting too much stress on the triceps and front shoulders. Presses are considered a compound movement, while flyes are considered an isolation movement.

CHAPTER FIVE – THE EXERCISES   71

INCLINE FLYES – With the exception of the angled bench, incline flyes are identical to the flat version.

COMMENTS – As with presses, incline flyes should be performed on a bench kept below 45 degrees. For a few individuals even 30 degrees is too steep, and they may have to set the angle at 20 to 25 degrees.

MUSCLES WORKED – Incline flyes primarily work the upper chest. The front shoulders and triceps act as stabilizers.

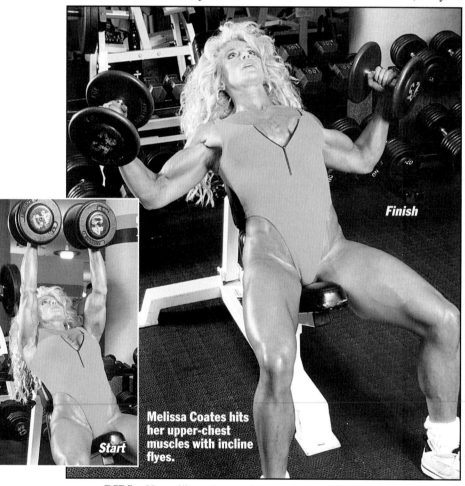

Finish

Start

Melissa Coates hits her upper-chest muscles with incline flyes.

DIPS – You will need a special set of bars to perform this exercise. If the bars in your gym are V-shaped grab the handles so your hands are about shoulder width apart. Lower yourself between the bars until the upper arms are about parallel with the floor. Return to the starting position.

COMMENTS – The disadvantage of dips is that you have to use your entire bodyweight from day one – an impossibility for many people. Your gym may have addressed the problem by purchasing a special machine that assists as you do the exercise.

MUSCLES WORKED – Dips are one of those exercises that depend on body position. Lean forward, elbows out, chin on the chest, and the chest muscles do most of the work. Lean back, body straight, elbows in, and the triceps do most of the work. In both versions the front shoulders are also involved.

PEC-DEKS – Depending on the machine you may have to sit up straight (Apex) or lie back at a 45-degree angle (Nautilus). For the Apex version grab the vertical handles and with the hands, shoulders, and elbows in a straight line, squeeze them forward in a hugging motion. The Nautilus machine requires you to place your elbows on two pads and push forward.

COMMENTS – Pec-deks are basically the machine version of flat dumbell flyes. Don't let the angle on the Nautilus fool you either. Even though you are leaning back on an incline bench, the design of the machine puts most of the stress on the lower and inner chest. Like the dumbell version, be careful not to bounce at the bottom of the exercise.

MUSCLES WORKED – The pec-dek primarily works the chest, but the triceps and front shoulders also come into play.

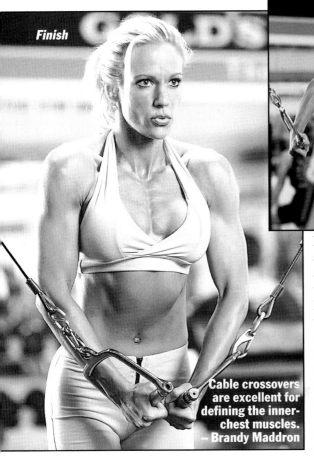

Finish

Start

Cable crossovers are excellent for defining the inner-chest muscles. – Brandy Maddron

CABLE CROSSOVERS – Grab a handle in each hand and stand in the middle of the cable crossover machine with a slight bend in the knees and the feet positioned towards the front of the unit. Bend slightly at the waist and draw the hands forward and downward at about a 45-degree angle with the body.

COMMENTS – One of the biggest mistakes you can make on this exercise is using so much weight you have to swing your upper body to get the weight moving. If you can't lift the weight by using the arms and hence the chest muscles, drop the weight a few plates.

MUSCLES WORKED – Cable crossovers primarily work the center chest but the front shoulders are also worked.

DUMBELL PULLOVERS – Grab a dumbell and lie face up across a flat bench. With the arms slightly bent, stretch the dumbell back until it's fully extended behind the head. Bring the arms forward until they're above the chest.

COMMENTS – To get the maximum benefit try not to bend the arms excessively. If you have shoulder problems you may want to avoid this exercise. For variety you can sub-stitute an EZ-curl bar in place of the dumbell, and instead of lying across the bench lie lengthwise.

MUSCLES WORKED – Pullovers are one of those exercises that are hard to classify as working one muscle group. For some the exercise primarily hits the lats, while for others it's a great chest exercise.

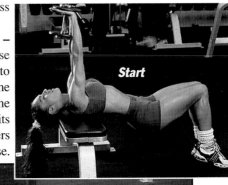

Start

Correct form is essential for maximum muscle stimulation. – Tsianina Joelson performs dumbell pullovers.

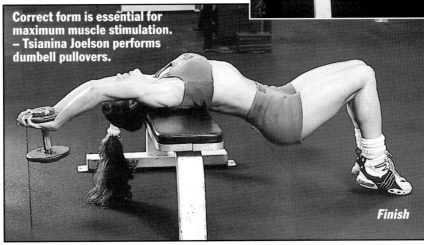

Finish

For those working both muscles on the same day, use pullovers to finish one muscle and warm up the other.

MACHINE PULLOVERS – We'll describe this exercise as your gym may have one. Sit down in the machine and depending on the arrangement, either place your upper arms on the pads, or grab the overhead crossbar. Pull the pads or bar down until your elbows are by your sides. Return to the starting position.

COMMENTS – Machine pullovers are great for those who find it awkward lying across a bench. They also offer an advantage in that they keep the tension on the chest and back muscles throughout a greater range of motion.

MUSCLES WORKED – Like the dumbell or barbell version, machine pullovers primarily work the chest and back, with the rear delts and triceps playing a minor role.

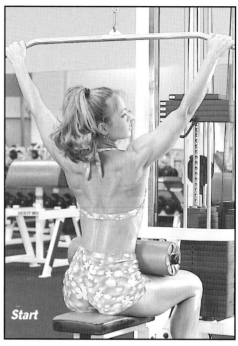

Start

BACK TRAINING

WIDE-GRIP PULLDOWNS – Take a slightly wider than shoulder-width grip on the machine's bar and sit down with your knees under the pads. Lean back slightly and pull the bar down so that it touches the upper chest. Return the bar to the starting position, and repeat.

COMMENTS – Make sure you don't sway and throw the upper body into the movement to move the weight. You should be able to pull the bar down with just your arm and lat muscles. For variety, you can pull the bar down behind your head, but we caution against this. Numerous individuals have torn rotator-cuff muscles in this manner.

MUSCLES WORKED – Front pull-downs primarily work the lats (large back muscles). They also strongly affect the biceps and forearms. Secondary stress is placed on the rear delts, teres (major and minor), and rhomboids. Behind-the-head pulldowns primarily work the teres, rhomboids, biceps, and upper lats.

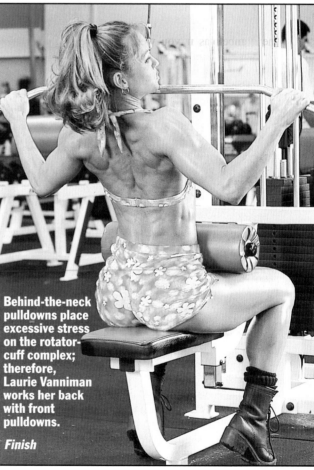

Behind-the-neck pulldowns place excessive stress on the rotator-cuff complex; therefore, Laurie Vanniman works her back with front pulldowns.

Finish

NARROW-GRIP PULLDOWNS – Either grab the long lat bar with a narrow (eight- to ten-inch) grip or use one of the short attachments that most gyms have. Lean back slightly and pull the bar to the chest.

COMMENTS – If using the long bar you can vary the grip by facing the palms up or down.

MUSCLES WORKED – Narrow-grip pulldowns primarily work the lower lats where the muscles attach to the lower torso. Gripping the bar with an underhand grip brings the biceps into play.

ONE-ARM ROWS – Grab a dumbell in one hand and place one knee on a flat bench for support. Bend at the hips so that the torso is almost parallel with the floor. Lower and raise the dumbell as if you were sawing wood with a handsaw.

COMMENTS – To really stretch the lats, raise and lower the dumbell on an angle. In other words, stretch the

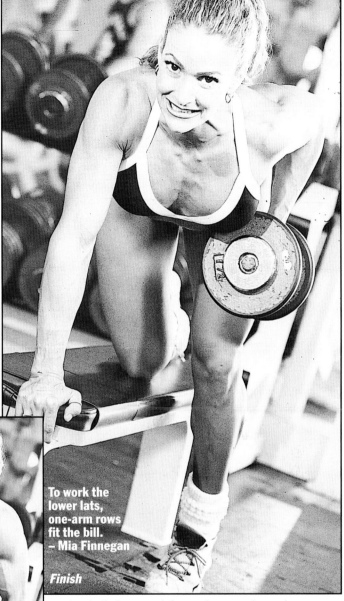

To work the lower lats, one-arm rows fit the bill.
– Mia Finnegan

Start

Finish

dumbell down and forward as you lower it. For those with weak or injured lower backs, a variation called two-arm rows can be performed. Lie face down on a bench set at 25 to 30 degrees. Hold a dumbell in each hand and raise and lower them in the same manner as the one-arm version.

MUSCLES WORKED – One- and two-arm rows work the lower lats, but the rear delts and biceps also come into play.

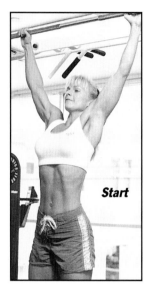

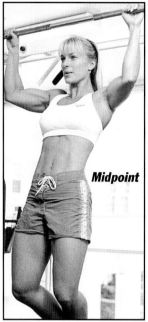

Start

Midpoint

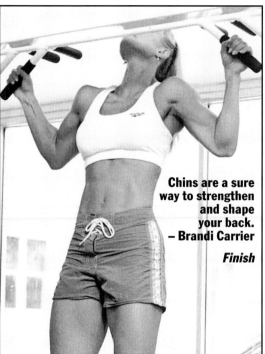

Chins are a sure way to strengthen and shape your back.
– Brandi Carrier

Finish

SEATED ROWS – Sit on the platform with your feet resting on the foot support. With your knees slightly bent, grab the V-bar attachment and pull it into the lower rib cage. Return to the starting position by stretching the torso forward. Try to time it so that the bar reaches the rib cage as soon as the torso is vertical.

COMMENTS – As you pull the bar towards the chest squeeze the shoulder blades and arch the chest slightly. Make sure you don't bounce at the bottom as you stretch forward. Those with lower-back problems may want to skip this exercise.

MUSCLES WORKED – Seated rows work most of the muscles of the back, particularly those of the center back. The forearms and biceps are also involved.

CHINUPS – With a slightly wider than shoulder-width grip grab hold of a chinning bar. Pull your body up to the bar, leaning slightly backward.

COMMENTS – Chins are one of the easiest exercises to do in theory but hardest in practice. Like dips, chins require you to use your entire bodyweight – an impossibility for many individuals. If you fall into this category don't despair. Many gyms these days have special machines called assisted chin machines that help you perform the exercise.

The more weight you put on the stack the easier it gets. Unlike most machines your goal on a chin machine is to use less and less weight.

MUSCLES WORKED – Done to the front of the head, chins primarily work the lats, but the rear delts, teres, and biceps also come into play. Done to the rear of the head, chins put most of the stress on the teres, rear delts and biceps. Like behind-the-head pulldowns, chins to the rear place excessive stress on the rotator-cuff complex.

STRAIGHT-ARM PUSHDOWNS – Stand in front of the lat pulldown machine with your hands placed about shoulder width on the bar. With your arms straight, elbows locked, push the bar down to the thighs. Let the bar raise back up until the plates on the machine are about an inch apart, or when your arms are one to two feet above the forehead.

COMMENTS – This exercise is a good substitute for those who don't have access to a pullover machine. Try to keep the elbows locked throughout the movement. As soon as the elbows bend, the triceps come into play. In fact this is a good way to determine if you've put too much weight on the bar.

MUSCLES WORKED – Straight-arm push-downs primarily work the lower lats. There is some rear-delt and serratus involvement.

SHOULDER TRAINING

FRONT BARBELL PRESSES – Position the bar on the specially designed rack and sit down with your back against the back support. Grab the bar with a slightly wider than shoulder-width grip and lift the bar off the rack so it's positioned above the bridge of your nose. Lower the bar to the top of the chest. Push the bar straight back up to arm's length.

COMMENTS – As you lower the bar be careful not to strike your collarbone, or excessively arch your lower back. As with most barbell exercises you may want to experiment with locking or not locking the arms at the top of the movement.

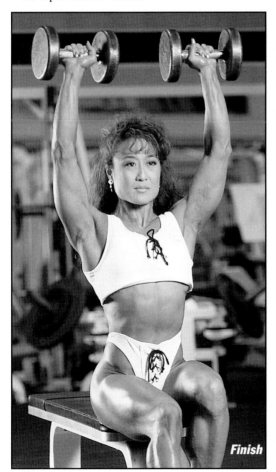

Finish

Some individuals lower the bar behind the head thinking it switches the stress to the side delts, but this is not the case. The front delts are still the primary muscles being exercised. As well, behind-the-head presses place tremendous stress on the rotator-cuff complex. Front presses will give you all the benefits of the behind-the-head version without the negative aspects.

MUSCLES WORKED – Front barbell presses primarily work the front deltoids. There is also some side-shoulder involvement. At the top of the exercise the triceps come into play, especially if you lock out.

DUMBELL PRESSES – As with chest training you can substitute dumbells in place of barbells to work your shoulders. Either use a bench with a vertical back or set an adjustable bench at 80 to 90 degrees. Lift the dumbells to shoulder height with your palms facing forward. Press the dumbells up and slightly forward and then lower them to the starting position with the upper arms about 20 degrees below parallel.

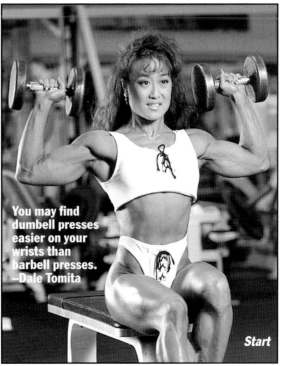

You may find dumbell presses easier on your wrists than barbell presses. —Dale Tomita

Start

COMMENTS – Dumbells allow for a greater range of motion at the bottom of the exercise than a barbell. For many people dumbell presses are much easier on the wrists.

MUSCLES WORKED – Dumbell presses primarily work the front delts with the triceps and side delts playing a secondary role.

LATERAL RAISES – Sit on the end of a flat bench holding a dumbell in each hand. With the palms facing inward and a slight bend in the elbows, raise the arms to the side until they're parallel with the floor. Lower the dumbells to the starting position and repeat.

COMMENTS – You can add to the exercise by bringing the dumbells together in front of the body. The knees will be in the way while sitting, so you'll have to stand for this. If doing the standing version, don't make the mistake of swinging the dumbells up by using the lower back. Only the arms should be moving.

MUSCLES WORKED – Side laterals primarily work the side deltoids but the rear deltoids and trapezius also come into play.

BENT-OVER LATERALS – Sit on the end of a bench with the torso bent forward at a 30- to 45-degree angle. With a slight bend in the elbows raise the dumbells to the side, stopping at shoulder height.

COMMENTS – Some individuals do this exercise standing, with the knees slightly bent, but standing increases the stress on the lower back. For extra back security try resting your head on a waist-high support. The padded cushion on many hyperextension machines can be used in this manner. For those with weak or injured lower backs we suggest reverse pec-deks as an alternative.

MUSCLES WORKED – Bent-over laterals primarily work the rear deltoids, but the traps and rhomboids also come into play.

REVERSE PEC-DEKS – You'll need a version of the pec-dek that has vertical handles rather than flat pads. Sit down facing the machine's back support, and grab the handles

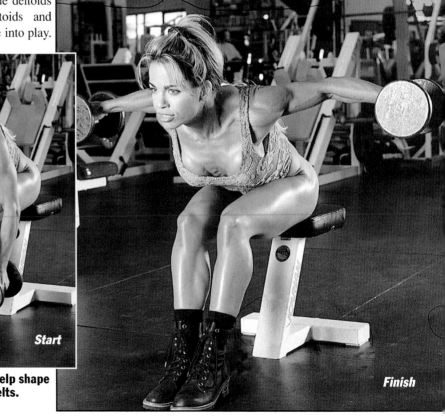

Start

Bent-over laterals help shape and tone the rear delts.
– Amy Fadhli

Finish

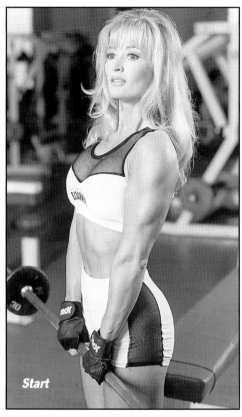

Start

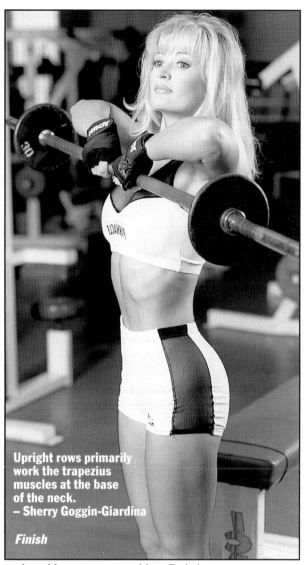

Upright rows primarily work the trapezius muscles at the base of the neck.
– Sherry Goggin-Giardina

Finish

so the hands, elbows, and shoulders are in a straight line. Pull the handles back until they're slightly behind your torso. Return to the starting position.

COMMENTS – As this machine is also used for chest training, you may have to adjust the handles so that they are all the way back. Having them forward in the chest-training position won't allow the full range of motion. Reverse pec-deks have two main advantages over bent-over laterals; they put little or no stress on the lower back, and sitting upright makes it easier to breath.

MUSCLES WORKED – Reverse pec-deks primarily work the rear deltoids but the traps and rhomboids also come into play.

UPRIGHT ROWS – Grab a short barbell or EZ-bar with a shoulder-width grip. Lift the bar straight up, following the midline of your body. Keep your elbows bent out to the sides.

COMMENTS – If you find the barbell hard on the wrists try using the triceps rope attachment. Hook the rope onto the low pulley of the cable-crossover machine. Grab the rope so your hands face backward, and pull up. The rope allows the wrists to rotate slightly, thus reducing the stress on the joints.

MUSCLES WORKED – Upright rows primarily work the trapezius muscles at the base of the neck. They also bring all three heads of the deltoids into play. (A wider grip engages the shoulders to a greater degree.) The rhomboids are also stimulated.

SHRUGS – Hold a dumbell in each hand with the palms facing the thighs. With your knees slightly bent shrug your shoulders. Try to keep the arms straight. Any elbow bending brings the biceps into play.

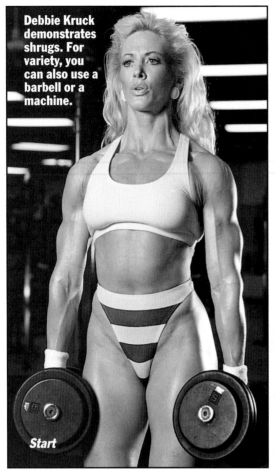

Debbie Kruck demonstrates shrugs. For variety, you can also use a barbell or a machine.

Start

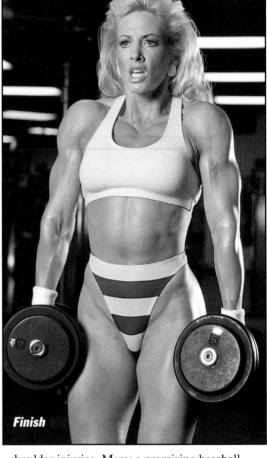

Finish

COMMENTS – For variety you can do the same exercise with a barbell or machine. For example, serious weight lifters use the Universal bench press station as much for shrugs as chest training.

MUSCLES WORKED – Shrugs primarily work the trapezius. They indirectly work the spinal erectors and forearms.

LATERAL ROTATION – Sit down on the preacher (Scott) bench with one elbow resting on the wedge-shaped pad. Hold a dumbell in your hand with the forearm at 90 degrees to your upper arm. With the arm kept rigid, lower the dumbell sideways until it's about an inch from the bench.

COMMENTS – Although the deltoids receive most of the attention, it's the smaller rotator muscles that are the cause of most shoulder injuries. Many a promising baseball career has been cut short by rotator tears. While the same exercise can be performed standing, the seated version makes it stricter. If the seated preacher curl is in use, you can substitute an incline bench and stand behind it with one arm resting on top.

MUSCLES WORKED – Lateral rotations are one of the few exercises that work the rotator complex without bringing the large deltoids into play.

BICEPS TRAINING
STANDING BARBELL CURLS – Hold a straight barbell with a shoulder-width grip, keeping the elbows close to the sides of the body. Raise the bar about three quarters of the way up and then lower to within a couple of inches of the thighs.

COMMENTS – Barbell curls are one of the most popular weight-training exercises, but they're also one of the most abused. Don't swing the bar using the lower back. This is both ineffective and dangerous. For those who find the straight bar hard on the wrists try substituting an EZ-curl bar. The bar's angles allow the hands to rotate inward slightly, reducing the stress on the wrists.

MUSCLES WORKED – Standing barbell curls primarily work the biceps, but the front delts and forearms are also brought into play.

INCLINE CURLS – Grab a pair of dumbells and sit in a 45-degree incline chair. With the palms facing up raise the dumbells until the forearms are just short of perpendicular with the floor. Lower to the starting position.

COMMENTS – You can perform the movement with both hands moving simultaneously or alternating one up, one down. Some individuals start with the palms facing inward and rotate them upward as the dumbells are raised. In theory this makes sense, as one of the functions of the biceps is to supinate the forearm. Unfortunately, you can supinate much more weight than you can curl. In other words, a 20-pound curl probably means you can supinate 40, 50, or even 60 pounds. Supinating the hands while curling doesn't really add much more to the movement. Still, given the number of people who swear by this movement, you may want to give it a try.

MUSCLES WORKED – Because of the angle, incline curls tend to shift most of the stress to the upper biceps. Like barbell curls, the forearms and front shoulders are also brought into play.

As popular as they are, barbell curls are one of the most abused exercises. Keep the movement slow and controlled throughout the full range of motion. – Melissa Coates

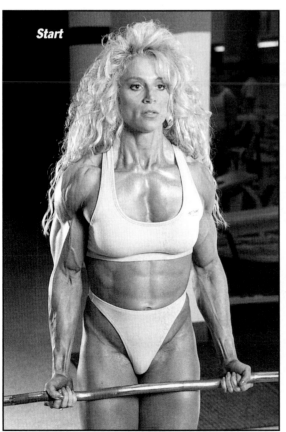

Start

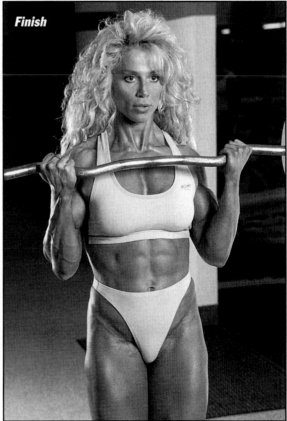

Finish

PREACHER (SCOTT) CURLS – Sit down on the bench with both elbows resting on the pad. Take a shoulder-width grip on a barbell and curl upwards until the forearm is just short of perpendicular with the floor. Lower the bar to the starting position.

COMMENTS – It's very important you don't bounce at the bottom of the movement. Numerous athletes have torn biceps tendons in this manner. Like barbell curls, substitute the EZ-curl bar if the straight bar is too stressful on your wrists.

MUSCLES WORKED – Preacher curls primarily work the lower biceps. The forearms are also brought into play.

CONCENTRATION CURLS – Sit at the end of a bench and brace one elbow on the inside of your knee. Curl a dumbell about three quarters of the way up, then lower and repeat.

COMMENTS – As with all biceps exercises, don't bounce at the bottom of the exercise.

MUSCLES WORKED – Concentration curls can be considered a good overall biceps exercise. This exercise also stresses the forearms.

CABLE CURLS – Connect a short straight bar to the low pulley of the cable-crossover machine. With a shoulder-width grip, curl the bar up three-quarters of the way. Lower the bar stopping a few inches from the thighs.

COMMENTS – While not ranked as high as barbell curls, cable curls offer the advantage of being easier on the wrists. They also provide tension throughout the full range of motion.

MUSCLES WORKED – Cable curls work the entire biceps as well as the forearms. The front delts play a secondary role for stabilization.

HAMMER CURLS – Grab a set of dumbells and with the palms facing inward curl the dumbells upward as if doing a standard dumbell curl. Lower to the starting position.

COMMENTS – If standing, try not to lift the weight by swaying the torso.

MUSCLES WORKED – Keeping the palms facing inward brings the large brachialis muscle into play. This is the forearm muscle that fills in the gap between the lower biceps and upper forearm. Hammer curls also stress the biceps and other smaller forearm muscle.

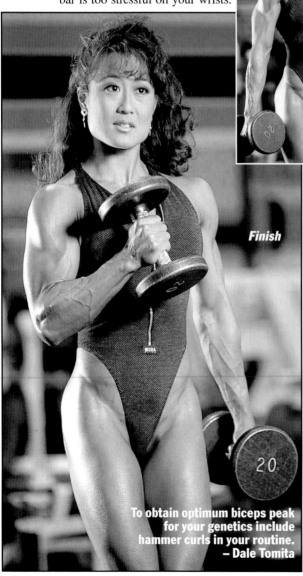

Start

Finish

To obtain optimum biceps peak for your genetics include hammer curls in your routine.
– Dale Tomita

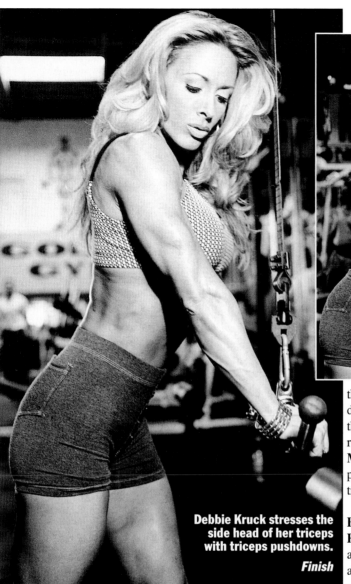

Debbie Kruck stresses the side head of her triceps with triceps pushdowns.

Finish

Start

the rest of the fingers gives a few extra degrees of tension. For variety try using the different attachments (short bar, rope, V-bar, etc.).

MUSCLE WORKED – Pushdowns primarily stress the side head of the triceps muscle.

BEHIND-THE-HEAD DUMBELL EXTENSIONS – Sit on a bench with a back support and hold a dumbell above your head with the palms facing upward. Lower the dumbell behind your head to a comfortable stretch and then push upward to a locked-out position.

COMMENTS – The grip on the dumbell should look like the standard volley position when playing volleyball (palms upward, fingers facing backward, thumbs forward). If your gym has a variety of dumbells use the ones with the smaller diameter weights on the handles. This gives more clearance when you lower the weight behind the head. A variation of this exercise is to use a lighter dumbell and lower behind the head with one hand. While the exercise is equally effective, most find the two-hand version easier to coordinate.

TRICEPS TRAINING

TRICEPS PUSHDOWNS – You can use a standard pulldown or cable-crossover machine for this exercise. Place your hands palms down, about six to eight inches apart on the bar with your elbows tucked into your sides. Push downward, locking the arms out at the bottom. Raise the forearms until they're at a right angle to your upper arms.

COMMENTS – Keep the elbows tucked close to your sides. Flaring them outwards only brings the larger torso muscles into play. Although not a necessity most individuals find placing the thumbs on top of the bar with

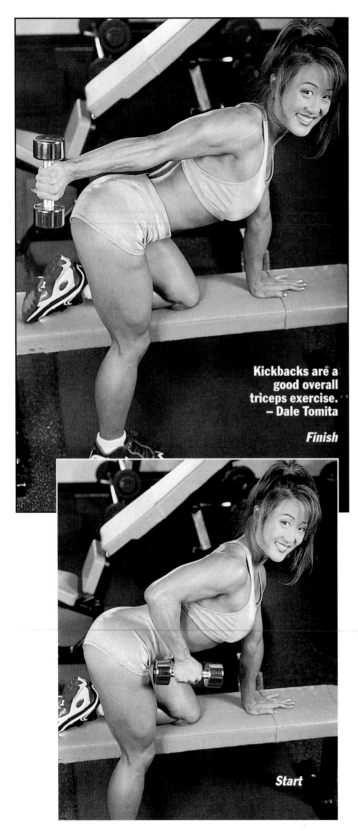

Kickbacks are a good overall triceps exercise.
– Dale Tomita

Finish

Start

MUSCLE WORKED – Dumbell extensions primarily stress the long rear head of the triceps. Kinesiologists say you can't target the heads separately but weight trainers experience otherwise.

LYING EZ-BAR EXTENSION – Place an EZ bar at one end of a flat bench and lie down so the bar is positioned above your head. Reach back and grab the bar, placing the palms an inch or two apart. Raise the bar above the forehead and with the elbows kept inward, lower the bar to the forehead. Press the bar up until the arms are straight.

COMMENTS – Try to keep the elbows as close to your sides as possible. Try not to lower the bar behind the head as this brings the chest and back into play. As reaching back and grabbing the bar is the hardest part of the movement, it is best to have someone pass the bar to you. For variety you can substitute dumbells in place of the bar. The dumbells are easier on the wrists and can be lowered to the sides of the head allowing for a greater range of motion.

MUSCLES WORKED – Lying extensions primarily work the long head of the triceps, but the nature of the exercise allows you to use more weight than most other exercises so the other two heads are stressed as well. The front shoulders come into play as stabilizers.

KICKBACKS – Place one hand on a flat bench for support, keeping the torso parallel with the floor or slightly above. Hold a dumbell in the other hand and lock the upper arm in line with the torso. Keeping the elbow close to your side, extend the lower arm back until it reaches the locked-out position. Return to the bent position, forearm pointing to the floor.

COMMENTS – The only part of the body that should move is the forearm. If you have to swing the upper arm you're using too much weight. Those with weak or lower-back injuries may want to avoid this exercise.

MUSCLES WORKED – Kickbacks are a good overall triceps exercise.

DIPS – Although the chest version also works the triceps, you can modify the movement to target the triceps more fully. Position two flat benches parallel to one another about four feet apart. Place your heels on one and your hands on the other so you're sitting between the two. With your weight supported on your hands, bend the elbows and lower between the two benches. Return to the starting position by straightening the arms.

COMMENTS – Some individuals find the exercise stressful on the shoulders or wrists so use your best judgement. Others may need to have a partner place weight on their thighs to make the exercise harder.

MUSCLES WORKED – Dips are considered one of the best exercises for overall triceps development.

NARROW PRESSES – Position yourself as if preparing for standard flat barbell bench presses. However, instead of the wide grip, place your hands about 10 to 12 inches apart. Lift the bar off the rack and lower it down to the chest. Push it back up until the arms are locked out.

COMMENTS – The narrow grip takes most of the stress off the chest and places it on the triceps. As with chest training, don't bounce the bar off the chest.

MUSCLES WORKED – Narrow presses primarily work the triceps but the chest and front shoulders also come into play.

ABDOMINAL TRAINING

CRUNCHES – Sit on the floor with the knees bent and feet flat on the floor. Place the hands behind the head and point the elbows outward. Lift the upper torso off the floor about eight to 10 inches and then lower to the floor.

COMMENTS – Contrary to popular belief the abdominal muscles only move the upper body eight to 10 inches. Lifting the torso right up to the knees primarily works the hip flexors, placing incredible stress on the lower-back ligaments. Crunches take the hip flexors out of the exercise while reducing stress on the spine.

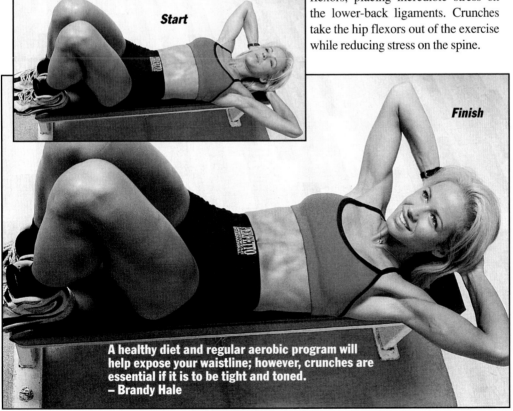

Start

Finish

A healthy diet and regular aerobic program will help expose your waistline; however, crunches are essential if it is to be tight and toned.
– Brandy Hale

MUSCLES WORKED – Crunches primarily work the upper abdominals but the lower region is stimulated as well. The obliques come into play when you twist side to side as you rise.

REVERSE CRUNCHES – Lie on the floor with your knees bent, keeping your lower legs parallel with the floor. Draw the knees toward the upper body. Now extend the legs until they are nearly straight.

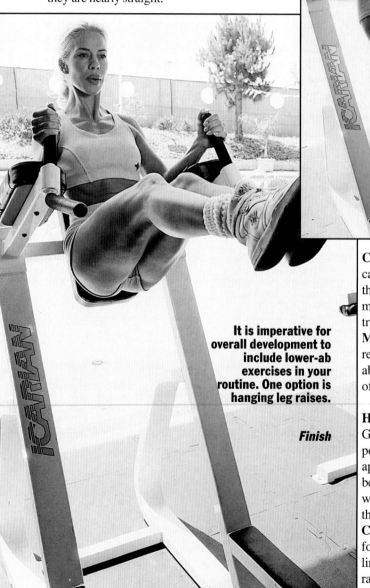

Start

It is imperative for overall development to include lower-ab exercises in your routine. One option is hanging leg raises.

Finish

COMMENTS – Although you can straighten the legs completely, this may stress the lower back. To make the exercise more difficult, try doing it on an incline board.
MUSCLES WORKED – While reverse crunches work the entire abdominal region they place most of the stress on the lower abs.

HANGING LEG RAISES – Grab an overhead chinup bar or position yourself on a leg-raise apparatus. Raise the legs, knees bent, until the thighs are parallel with the floor. Lower the legs to the start position.
COMMENTS – When performed on a chinup bar, the limiting factor with hanging leg raises is forearm grip. Your forearms may give out before your

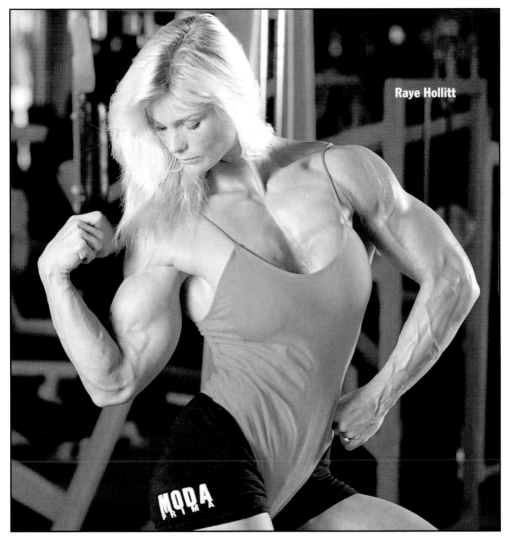

Raye Hollitt

abs. As a suggestion, leave this exercise toward the end of your ab routine. This way your already fatigued abs should give out before your forearms.

MUSCLES WORKED – Hanging leg raises work both the abdominals and hip flexors; however, kinesiologists say they're almost entirely a hip-flexor exercise. The consensus among bodybuilders is that they're a great way to hit the lower abs so we're including them in our list of exercises.

TV AB MACHINES – Given the popularity of these gizmos we thought we'd mention them. Position your head on the padded headrest and your feet flat on the floor, knees bent. Lift the torso forward as if doing a standard crunch, then lower until your shoulders just touch the floor.

COMMENTS – The main advantage of portable ab machines is that they support the head throughout the exercise. For many this alleviates neck stress. Their main disadvantage is the cross bar. It begs for you to push forward with the arms, but the arms should only go for the ride and nothing more. You are trying to work the abs, not the chest and shoulders.

MUSCLES WORKED – Like crunches, ab machines are designed to place most of the stress on the abs – particularly the upper abs. You can bring the lower abs into the movement more by elevating the legs as if getting ready to do reverse crunches.

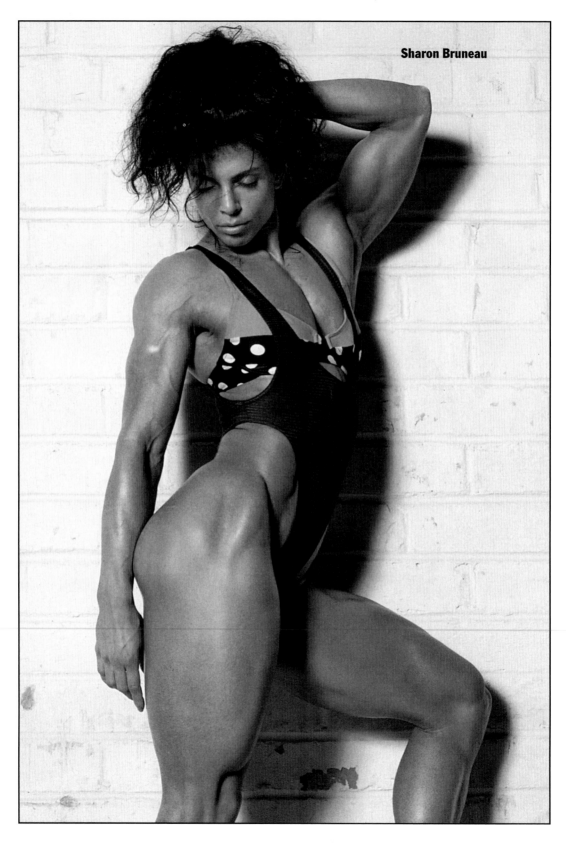

Sharon Bruneau

Book Two

Framing the Physique

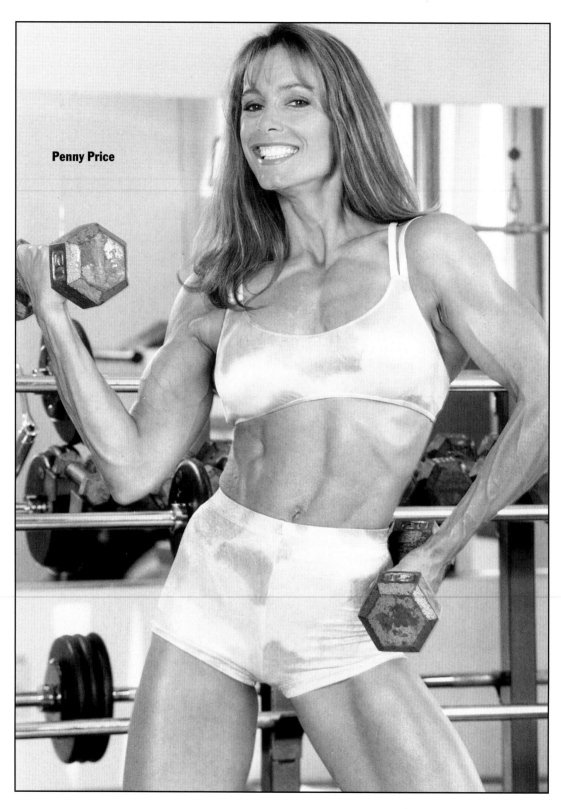

Penny Price

Chapter 6
Introductory Routines

The title of this chapter may mislead you. Don't let the word introductory deceive you. For someone unaccustomed to physical exercise the routines will be more than strenuous enough. In fact those who have never worked out before, or have been inactive for any length of time, should get clearance from their physician before starting a routine. It's not that we think you'll collapse from a heart attack, but let's face it, it makes far more sense to detect potential problems in the physician's office rather than under a barbell!

The following routines are designed to be followed two to three times per week. We strongly suggest alternating a day of exercise with a day of rest. This gives the body a minimum of 48 hours before the next workout. Don't make the mistake of training two or three days in a row. At this stage your recovery system will be taxed to the max after only a couple of weeks. There will be enough time down the road for such advanced training.

I have good size on my arms already, so I work on just refining them and making them look more detailed for competition.

Dale Tomita, fitness pro

For beginners, dumbells may be a lighter alternative, but a barbell can be more stable. Try both to see which is more comfortable.

Mia Wallace,
***Oxygen* contributor**

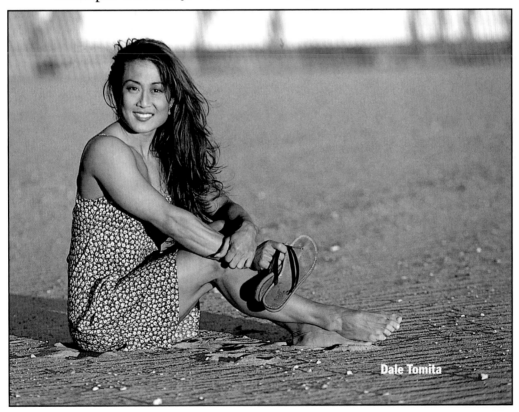

Dale Tomita

The exercises have been selected assuming you have access to a fully equipped gym. You may have to make substitutions depending on the equipment available.

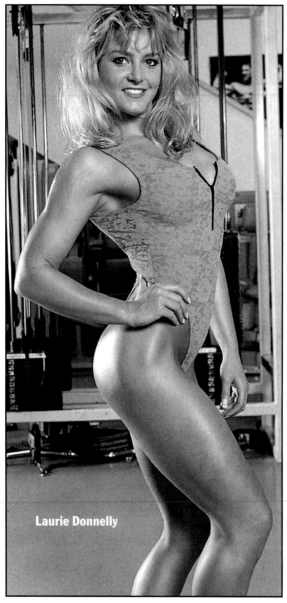

Before you can get started in a specific program, goals have to be determined. It is possible to wander forever without a destination in mind.

Laurie Donnelly, top fitness competitor and *Oxygen* contributor

ROUTINE 1

EXERCISE	SETS	REPS
Leg extensions	2-3	10-12
Leg curls	2-3	10-12
Standing calf raises	2-3	10-12
Flat-bench barbell presses	2-3	10-12
Front pulldowns	2-3	10-12
Dumbell presses	2-3	10-12
Incline curls	2-3	10-12
Triceps pushdowns	2-3	10-12
Crunches	2-3	20-25

ROUTINE 2

EXERCISE	SETS	REPS
Leg presses	2-3	10-12
Stiff-leg deadlifts	2-3	10-12
Seated calf raises	2-3	10-12
Incline dumbell flyes	2-3	10-12
One-arm rows	2-3	10-12
Lateral raises	2-3	10-12
Barbell curls	2-3	10-12
Kickbacks	2-3	10-12
Reverse crunches	2-3	20-25

ROUTINE 3

EXERCISE	SETS	REPS
Lunges	2-3	10-12
Adductions	2-3	10-12
Leg curls	2-3	10-12
One-leg calf raises	2-3	10-12
Pec-deks	2-3	10-12
Seated rows	2-3	10-12
Machine presses	2-3	10-12
Preacher curls	2-3	10-12
EZ-bar extensions	2-3	10-12
Hanging leg raises	2-3	10-12

ROUTINE 4

EXERCISE	SETS	REPS
Hack squats	2-3	10-12
Sissy squats	2-3	10-12
Standing leg curls	2-3	10-12
Toe presses	2-3	15-20
Incline barbell presses	2-3	10-12
T-bar rows	2-3	10-12
Lateral raises	2-3	10-12
Concentration curls	2-3	10-12
Dumbell extensions	2-3	10-12
Ab roller	2-3	20-25

ROUTINE 5

EXERCISE	SETS	REPS
Squats	2-3	10-12
Lunges	2-3	10-12
Dumbell deadlifts	2-3	10-12
Donkey calf raises	2-3	10-12
Incline dumbell presses	2-3	10-12
Front chins	2-3	10-12
Upright rows	2-3	10-12
Cable curls	2-3	10-12
Bench dips	2-3	10-12
Rope crunches	2-3	20-25

GENERAL COMMENTS

The above routines have been designed to allow you to train the entire body during one workout. At 10 exercises, three sets per exercise, one minute to do each set and one minute between sets, the workout is about 60 minutes. However, this doesn't allow for setting up equipment or waiting for others to finish their sets. If you're pressed for time, rather than skip some of the exercises, only perform two sets per exercise. Don't think that only performing two sets is diminishing your workout. Research suggests two sets per exercise is 90 to 92 percent as effective as three sets. For a savings of 15 to 20 minutes you can still make decent gains.[1]

With regards to the exercises, most gyms have the equipment referred to. There may, however, be a few exceptions. For example, the standing leg curl machine is not found in all gyms. You may have to use the lying version – a piece of equipment few gyms go without. Likewise, the abductor machine is not standard issue in all gyms. In this case attach an ankle strap to the low pulley on the cable crossover machine and perform cable leg raises.

Finally, the donkey calf raise may present problems. Many gyms don't have the machine version, and many readers may have reservations about having a partner jump on their back. In either case, use the standing calf machine or perform toe presses on the leg-press machine.

You are a beginner. You must train like a beginner. Follow a three-times-a-week training program – either Mon-Wed-Fri, or Tues-Thurs-Sat. This split gives you an extra day's rest between workouts, plus weekends off.

Greg Zulak, former *MuscleMag* **editor and columnist**

Reference

1. W. Wescott, "Advanced Strength Exercise: Recommendations and Results," seminar (Toronto, ON: Can Fit Pro Conference, September 1997).

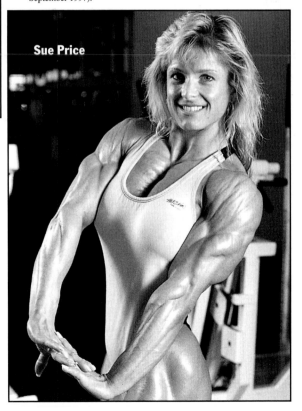

Sue Price

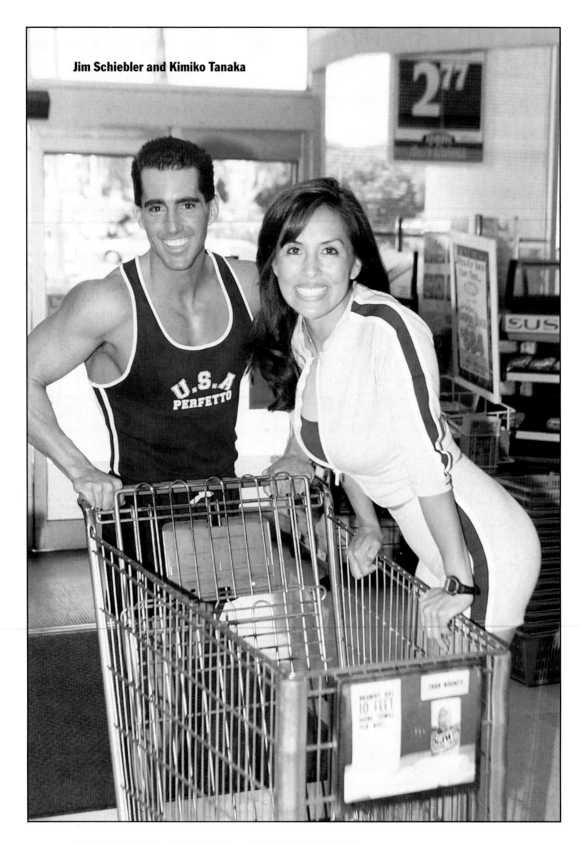

Jim Schiebler and Kimiko Tanaka

Chapter 7
Nutrition

Just as you wouldn't put cheap gasoline in an expensive sports car, consuming junk food is not going to fuel your body for peak performance. Some experts suggest that athletic success is 80 percent nutrition. This number may be debated; nevertheless, the old adage "you are what you eat" is sound advice.

Nutrition can be defined as the "art of eating correctly," or consuming adequate amounts of the right nutrients. They key words in the previous sentences are "adequate" and "right." Eat too many empty calories and you gain unwanted bodyfat. Eat too few good nutrients and the body starts suffering from malnutrition. Chocolate bars, soft drinks, and French fries should not be the cornerstone of your daily diet!

The best way to shrink and control the spread of cellulite is to adopt a healthy lifestyle. This includes a good, clean diet high in fiber and protein, and very low in fat. A regular exercise regimen is also important and should include both weight training and cardiovascular activities.

Marla Duncan,
Oxygen columnist

The following chapter is meant to be a general guide to healthy eating, not a step-by-step eating plan. Such a volume of information could fill an entire book – and there are thousands of them out there. If you are unsure of your eating habits, consult a nutritionist, especially one who is knowledgeable on athletic requirements.

FOOD NUTRIENTS

PROTEIN

Protein is essential in building and maintaining a lean, mean, fighting machine. Protein is the building tissue of the human body. Just as a bricklayer needs bricks to construct a strong foundation, your body needs protein to remain strong and healthy.

Protein is formed from amino acids. Amino acids have a central carbon atom with an amine group on one end and an acid group on the other. Two additional side groups, usually hydrogen atoms, make up the amino-acid molecule.

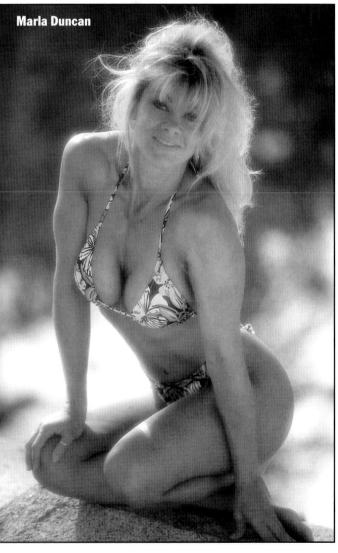

Marla Duncan

Of the twenty amino acids, we can synthesize 11 ourselves, but we must consume the other nine, so they are called "essential amino acids." Animal proteins contain all the amino acids we need. Different sources of plant proteins need to be combined to ensure all of the amino acids are present.

The best sources of animal proteins are meat, fish, and poultry. Of the three, fish and poultry are considered healthier as they have a lower fat content. Despite what some media reports say, one or two servings of red meat a week is healthy.

If there is a debatable issue related to protein, it's how much we need. Depending on the source consulted, it may range from .75 gram per pound of bodyweight to over two grams per pound of bodyweight. Some experts argue that athletes receive all the protein they need from everyday eating. Others contend that hard-training athletes need more. Our opinion lies somewhere in between. It is possible to receive adequate protein in the diet, but how many people eat properly? Unfortunately, not many. We are not going to suggest that females need anywhere near two grams per pound of bodyweight, but on the other hand the RDA values which are down in the .70 to .75 gram range are probably only suited to sedentary (non-exercising) individuals. Although it varies, most athletes need one to one and a half grams of protein per pound of bodyweight. For a 120-pound female this works out to:

$$120 \times 1 = 120 \text{ grams}$$
$$120 \times 1.5 = 180 \text{ grams}$$

The range for this individual would be from 120 to 180 grams of protein per day.

If your eating schedule allows you to eat this amount of protein, you don't need protein supplements, despite what the manufacturers say. On the other hand, it's much easier to drink extra protein than to eat it, and you don't have to worry about extra calories either. To get a rough idea of your protein intake, record your food intake for a week and then consult a good calorie/nutrient food guide.

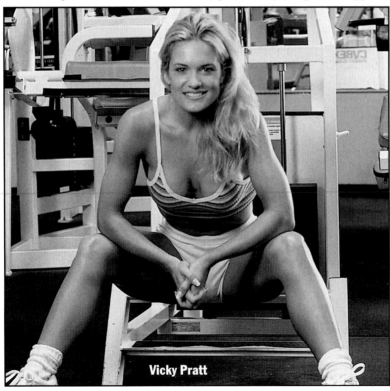

Vicky Pratt

If you are below the recommended level, add a good protein supplement to your diet. (see the section on supplements in Chapter Seven)

FATS

Just the mention of the word fat sends shivers up the spines of most individuals. But should it? No nutrient has received as much bad press as fats. And while certain fats deserve such trashing, others are just as vital to life as protein, vitamins and minerals.

This study only reaffirms what I have been saying in the pages of MuscleMag *for years – a) high-carb diets suck, especially for bodybuilders, and b) fat is not the enemy of bodybuilders. Certain fats can be used to lose weight, increase muscle and improve health, while other fats do the opposite.*

Will Brink, *MuscleMag* **columnist**

Fats are highly concentrated forms of energy. They are also essential in transporting vitamins A, D, E and K. Fats add taste to food, and because they take longer to digest, they decrease feelings of hunger. But our bodies have been designed to cherish and store fat because of its metabolic value. After millions of years of evolution, the human body cannot be convinced that famine is not around the corner.

Biochemically, fats can be divided into two categories, saturated and unsaturated fats. Saturated fats are solid at room temperature and are found in dairy products, meat, and such oils as coconut and palm oil. These fats are the ones linked to heart disease, stroke, and obesity. Your goal in life should be to keep the intake of such fats to a minimum.

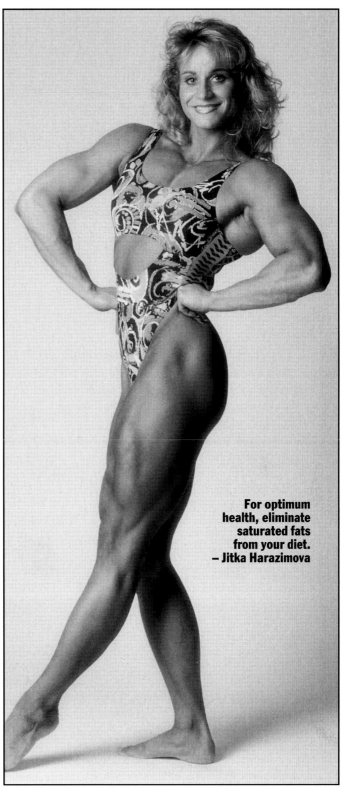

For optimum health, eliminate saturated fats from your diet. – Jitka Harazimova

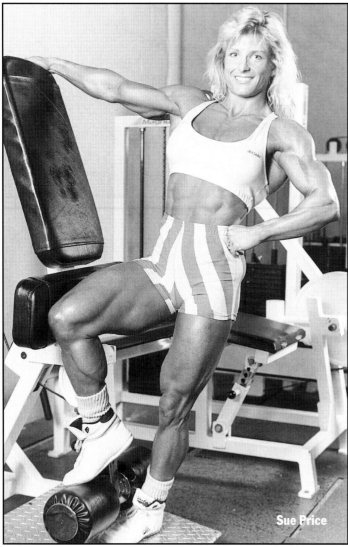
Sue Price

Some writers object to the term fatty acid as EFAs are very similar to vitamins and protein in that they are essential to life. For example, EFAs are needed by the body for the repair and growth of nerve tissue. A lack of EFAs will interfere with proper nerve conduction. Also, over 90 percent of the brain is composed of fats, of which EFAs are a main component. EFAs also play a role in the composition of cell membranes, and in the proper functioning of white blood cells.

From a health perspective, another type of fatty acid, omega-3 fatty acid, is very important. Found in such deepwater fish as tuna, salmon, and herring, omega-3s have been shown to reduce the risk of heart attacks by reducing the body's blood-clotting action. They also play a role in the formation of prostaglandins, hormone-like substances that modulate many of the body's major systems.

HOW MUCH FAT?

Depending on the source consulted, fat intake should be kept between 10 and 30 percent of daily dietary intake. Of this the vast majority should come from unsaturated sources. Recent research suggests the risk of heart disease and stroke can be greatly reduced if saturated fat is kept below 10 percent of fat intake.

In recent years there has been much debate in athletic circles regarding decreasing carbohydrate intake in favor of more fat (the popular Zone Diet makes heavy use of this concept). The theory is that increasing fat intake causes the body to decrease fat storage and also give up fat stores for energy sources; restricting fat causes the body to go into a survival mode, storing everything as fat for future use.

Our advice is to keep fat intake in the 20 to 25 percent range. And those with a history of heart disease should make a special effort to eliminate saturated fats from their diet.

Unsaturated fats are liquid at room temperature and are mainly found in plant oils. Unsaturated fats can themselves be broken down into two main categories, monounsaturates (monos) and polyunsaturates (polys). Monos are found in olive oil, canola oil, almond oil and avocados. Polys are found in safflower oil, sunflower oil, corn oil and soybean oil.

ESSENTIAL FATTY ACIDS

A category of fat that has become the subject of much attention in recent years is essential fatty acids (EFAs). Like essential amino acids, they cannot be made by the body and must be consumed in the diet.

CARBOHYDRATES

Carbohydrates (carbs) can be friend or foe depending on who you talk to. A few of the latest theories suggest that 60 to 70 percent of a diet coming from carbs is too high, and should be cut back in favor of more fat. The contrary opinion suggests carbs are the body's preferred fuel source and should constitute the largest part of the diet.

Many people eat too many carbohydrates in a day. Unless you are very active most of the excess carbohydrate will end up deposited on your physique. When this occurs on a regular basis, the combination adds up to a fatter figure.

Dwayne Hines II, *Oxygen* **contributor**

As the name implies, carbohydrates are composed of carbon and "hydrate" or water. The primary role of carbs is to provide short-term energy (less than an hour) for the body. Carbs can be classified as simple or complex, both of which are converted by the liver into glycogen for storage. Most people know carbs by another name – sugar!

Simple sugars, such as fructose, sucrose, and glucose enter the bloodstream very quickly and serve as an immediate fuel source. Foods high in simple sugars include candy, chocolate bars, jams, and soft drinks. Although a small amount of simple sugar is fine, most of your carb intake should come from complex sources. The reason is that simple sugars cause a rapid increase in insulin, the body's primary storage hormone. The more insulin floating around, the more calories that get stored as fat.

Complex carbs are digested and absorbed slower than simple carbs. Rather than produce a short burst of energy, complex carbs produce energy for longer periods of time. They're also kinder on insulin levels. The best food sources for complex carbs are rice, pastas, beans, and breads.

HOW THEY'RE USED

After being consumed in the diet, complex carbs are broken down into simple sugars and transported to the liver where they are converted into the stored form of sugar called glycogen. Some of the glycogen remains in the liver, while the bulk of it goes to the body's muscles. We should add that excess amounts of carbs will be stored as fat. This is why we feel the old range of 60 to 70 percent is too high for most individuals. A better range would be 45 to 50 percent with the remaining 50 to 55 percent being split between fat and protein.

VITAMINS

Vitamins can be defined as chemical compounds that are necessary for growth, health and normal metabolism. They may be essential parts of enzymes (organic compounds that control the rate of chemical reactions), or they may be essential parts of hormones (chemical messengers of the body).

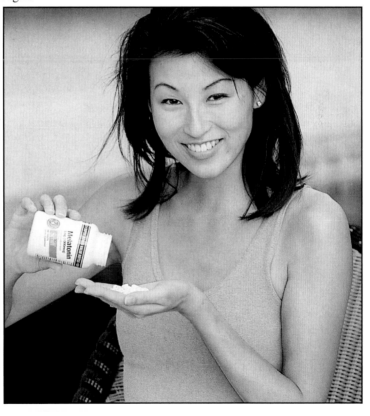

At one time the medical establishment believed that a well-balanced diet eliminated the need for vitamin supplementation. But soil exhaustion, pesticide use, and an extended shelf life have decreased the amount of vitamins found naturally in food. And a better understanding of the role of vitamins in preventing disease has led many researchers to reconsider their traditional position.

FAT-SOLUBLE VITAMINS

These vitamins are stored in bodyfat, hence the name. Excessive concentrations of these vitamins can be toxic. The following are the principal fat-soluble vitamins:

VITAMIN	NATURAL SOURCES
Vitamin A (retinol)	Carrots, green and yellow vegetables, fish, liver, milk and eggs
Vitamin D (cholecalciferol)*	Cod-liver oil, egg yolks, fortified milk
Vitamin E (alpha-tocopherol)	Vegetable oil, green leafy vegetables, fresh nuts, whole-grain cereals and wheat germ
Vitamin K (menadiol)	Green leafy vegetables and root vegetables, cheddar cheese, fruits seeds, yogurt, cow milk and liver

*Vitamin D is also formed when ultraviolet rays from sunlight act on chemicals naturally present in the skin.

WATER-SOLUBLE VITAMINS

Water-soluble vitamins cannot be stored in the body. The daily amount needed must be provided in the diet. The amount of vitamins a person needs may be increased by heavy training and excessive water consumption.

VITAMIN	NATURAL SOURCES
Vitamin B1 (thiamine)	Yeast, whole-grain cereals, nuts, eggs, pork and liver
Vitamin B2 (riboflavin)	Yeast, whole-wheat products, peanuts, peas, asparagus, beets, eggs, lamb, veal, beef and liver
Vitamin B3 (niacin)	Yeast, whole-grain breads and cereals, nuts, beans, peas, fish, meats and liver
Vitamin B5 (pantothenic acid)	Whole-grain products, yeast, green vegetables, cereal, egg yolks, kidney, liver and lobster
Vitamin B6 (pyridoxine)	Yeast, whole-grain cereals, spinach, tomatoes, yellow corn, yogurt, and salmon
Vitamin B9 (folic acid)	Wheat, wheat germ, barley, fruits, rice, soybeans, green leafy vegetables and liver
Vitamin B12 (cyanocbalamin)	Clams, meat, liver, kidney, cheese, eggs chicken and milk
Vitamin H (biotin)	Chicken, yeast, liver, egg yolks, kidneys tuna and walnuts
Vitamin C (ascorbic acid)	Citrus fruits, green leafy vegetables, potatoes, and tomatoes

Below is a list of some important vitamins and their functions:

VITAMIN	FUNTIONS
Vitamin A (retinol)	Aids night vision and helps prevent eye disease, promotes bone growth in infants and children, and helps maintain the mucous membranes in the ears, nose and intestinal lining.
Vitamin B1 (thiamine)	Helps regulate appetite, maintain a responsive nervous system (necessary for the synthesis of acetylcholine, a neuro-transmitter), and releases energy from carbohydrates (acts as a coenzyme for 24 different enzymes involved in the carbohydrate metabolism of pyruvic acid to CO_2 and H_2O.
Vitamin B2 (riboflavin)	Aids food metabolism (component of certain coenzymes involved with carbohydrate and protein metabolism), promotes healthy skin, and helps the body use oxygen.
Vitamin B3 (niacin)	Involved in fat metabolism (during lipid metabolism it inhibits the production of cholesterol and aids in fat breakdown), tissue respiration, and the conversion of sugars to energy (essential coenzyme concerned with energy-releasing reactions).
Vitamin B5 (pantothenic acid)	Acid is a part of co-enzyme A, which is essential for the transfer of pyruvic acid into the Kreb's cycle during protein metabolism. It is also involved in the trans-formation of amino acids and fats into glucose and the formation of choles-terol and steroid hormones.
Vitamin B6 (pyridoxine)	An essential coenzyme for amino-acid metabolism and may function as a coenzyme in fat metabo-lism. It assists in the production of circulating antibodies.
Vitamin B9 (folic acid)	Part of the enzyme systems which synthesize the purines and pyrimidines built into RNA and DNA. This vitamin is necessary for normal production of red and white blood cells.
Vitamin B12 (cyanocbalamin)	A coenzyme necessary for red blood cell formation and to manufacture the amino acid methionine and the neurotransmitter pre-cursor choline. It is also responsible for the entrance of some amino acids into the Kreb's cycle during the metabolism of proteins. This vitamin has a positive effect on the metabolism during exer-cise, particularly when oxygen levels are low. Certain drugs interfere with B12 and may limit its effectiveness: codiene, oral contraceptives, the antibiotic neomycin, chloramphenicol, aspirin and aspirin substitutes.

Vitamin B15	Aids metabolism in the myocardium (the thick inner layer of the heart wall) by increasing creatine levels in the layer while dilating the venous vessels. This vitamin also helps prevent the deposition of fat in the liver. A recommended dosage based on European standards is 100 mg daily.
Vitamin C (ascorbic acid)	Helps form collagen, the substance that binds body cells together. This acid promotes many metabolic reactions, particularly protein metabolism, and is essential to the growth and repair of teeth, gums and blood vessels, and specialized bone cells. This vitamin works with antibodies and, as a coenzyme, may bind with poisons, rendering them harmless.
Vitamin D (cholecalciferol)	Vital for absorption and utilization of the minerals calcium and phosphorus from the GI tract. There is also evidence to suggest the vitamin may work with the parathyroid hormone which regulates calcium metabolism.
Vitamin E (alpha-tocopherol)	Involved in the manufacture of RNA, DNA and red blood cells. It behaves as a cofactor in several enzyme systems. Vitamin E works as an antioxidant and prevents the enzyme action of peroxidase on the unsaturated bonds of cell membranes, and protects red blood cells from dissolving.
Vitamin H (biotin)	A vital coenzyme for the conversion of pyruvic acid to oxalocetic acid and in manufacturing purines and fatty acids.

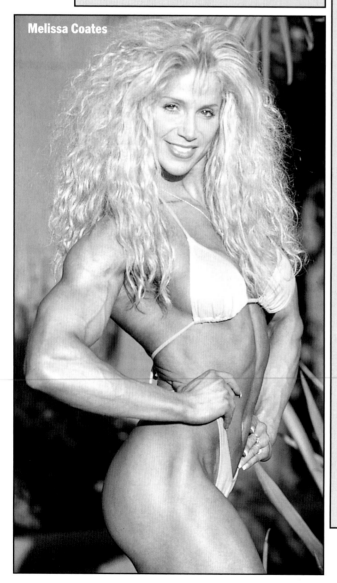

Melissa Coates

MEGADOSING

Megadosing is the practice of consuming supplements in dosages far beyond what is recommended. DNA-helix co-discoverer and Nobel prize winner, Dr. Linus Pauling, advocates megadosing of vitamin C. He consumes 18,000 milligrams daily, or 300 times the RDA. While most excess water-solubles are simply excreted, research indicates that excessive vitamin C can result in diarrhea, cramps, nausea, kidney stones, gout, and headache. If vitamin B6, another water-soluble vitamin, is taken in amounts of 100 times the RDA (two milligrams), or more, there is a risk of nerve damage.

Fat solubles are an even more controversial subject, because megadosing with fat-soluble vitamins such as A and D can cause bone deformities and damage the liver.

Another important point to consider is that a large dose results in decreased absorption and increased excretion. For example, it is better to take vitamin C in dosages of 50 milligrams compared to 100 milligrams because less will be absorbed with the higher dosage. Therefore, vitamin supplements should be taken at low dosages throughout the day.

MINERALS AND TRACE ELEMENTS

Minerals play a crucial role in the body even though they are only used in minute amounts. If the body requires more than 100 milligrams of an element each day then the substance is called a mineral. If the daily requirement is less, than it is called a trace element. Minerals and trace elements can be defined as inorganic substances. They may appear in combination with each other, or in combination with organic (carbon-based) compounds. Minerals constitute about four percent of the body's total weight, and they are concentrated most heavily in the skeleton.

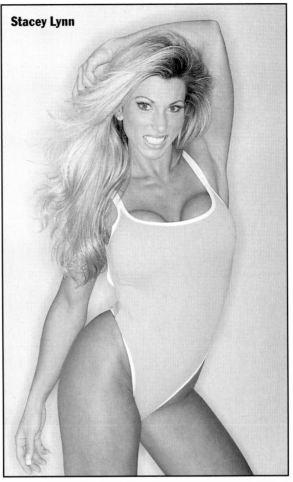

Stacey Lynn

MINERAL	NATURAL SOURCES
Calcium	Green leafy vegetables, shellfish, egg yolks, sardines with bones, and milk
Chlorine	Meat, fish and table salt
Magnesium	Wheat germ, soybeans, green leafy vegetables, nuts, sunflower seeds and fish
Phosphorus	Nuts, dairy products, fish, poultry and meat
Sodium	Meat, fish and table salt
Sulphur	Beans, egg yolks, cheese, fish, poultry, lamb, beef and liver

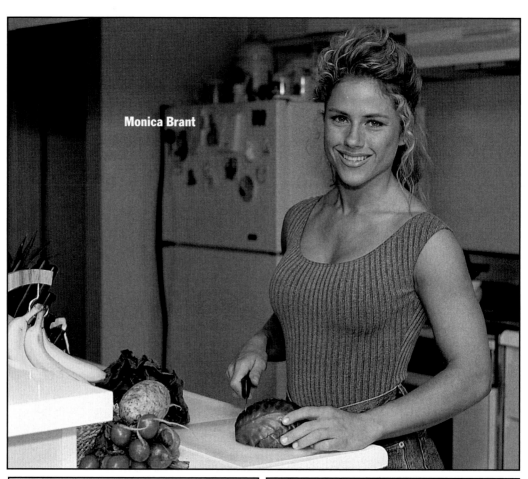

Monica Brant

TRACE ELEMENT	NATURAL SOURCES
Cobalt	Clams, meat, liver, kidney, cheese, eggs and milk
Copper	Barley, mushrooms, oats, whole-wheat flour, beans, asparagus, spinach, beets, eggs, fish, and liver
Iodine	Cod-liver oil, iodized table salt, seafood, sunflower seeds
Iron	Whole-grain products, cashews, beans, dried fruits, cheddar cheese, egg yolks, shellfish, meat and liver
Zinc	Yeast, whole-grain products, soybeans, sunflower seeds, fish, poultry and meat
Chromium	Whole-grain products, fresh fruit, potato skins, seafood, poultry and meat
Manganese	Barley, bran, buckwheat, ginger, coffee, spinach, peas and peanuts
Molybdenum	Whole grains, peas and liver
Selenium	Whole grains, seafood and liver

METABOLIC ROLE

Minerals and trace elements are required for growth, maintenance and repair of the body. In addition, minerals participate in the proper functioning of the nervous and muscular systems. A diet that does not contain any minerals is fatal. This is because when the body excretes wastes, it must also excrete a certain amount of salt. It is important to eat a well-balanced diet, so that the mineral salts (approximately 30 grams) lost daily through excretion are replaced. Because most minerals are widely distributed in foods, severe mineral deficiencies in the general population are unusual in developed countries, although they are seen in specific groups. The following are examples of minerals and trace elements and their functions:

MINERAL	FUNCTIONS
Calcium	Essential for blood clotting, muscle and nerve activity, bone and teeth formation.
Chlorine	Maintains water balance, pH balance of the blood, and forms HCL in the stomach and is involved in maintaining cellular osmotic pressure.
Magnesium	Part of many coenzymes, essential for muscle and nerve activity, involved in bone formation, and required for protein and carbohydrate metabolism.
Phosphorus	Involved in the transfer and storage of ATP, buffer system for the blood, essential for muscle contraction and nerve activity, component of DNA and RNA, involved in bone and teeth formation.
Sodium	Part of the bicarbonate buffer system, strongly affects distribution of water in the extracellular fluid.
Sulphur	Part of many proteins, hormones (including insulin) and some vitamins (including biotin and thiamine); thus, it helps regulate bodily activities.

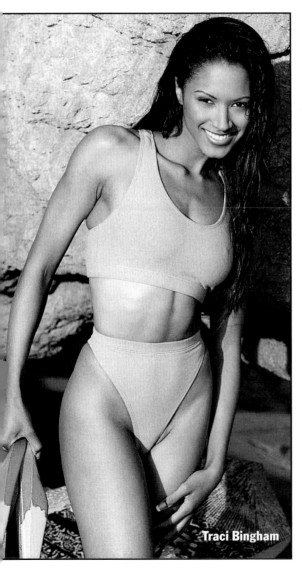

Traci Bingham

TRACE ELEMENTS	FUNCTIONS
Cobalt	Component of B12, needed for the production of red blood cells.
Copper	Part of an enzyme required for melanin-pigment formation, essential for the synthesis of haemoglobin.
Iodine	Needed by the thyroid gland to form two hormones that regulate metabolic rate: triiodothyronine and thyroxin.
Iron	Part of the coenzymes that form ATP from catabolism, and part of the haemoglobin that carries oxygen to cells.
Zinc	Part of enzymes involved in growth.
Chromium	Enhances the effect of insulin in glucose utilization, and helps the transport of amino acids to heart and liver cells.
Manganese	Necessary for growth, reproduction, lactation, haemoglobin synthesis, and is essential for the activation of several enzymes.
Molybdenum	Forms part of the enzyme xanthine oxidase, which oxidises hypoxanthine to xanthine and then to urate. Urate is the final product of purine degradation and is excreted in the urine.
Selenium	Involved in a number of enzyme systems and the metabolism of vitamin E.

SUPPLEMENTS

Should you take supplements? At one time, the answer would have been no, provided you consumed a balanced diet of the essential food groups. But with changes in farming practices (soil depletion and heavy chemical use), international sources (which means produce must have an extended shelf life, causing a loss of nutrients) and a greater knowledge of the role of diet in the disease process, we now understand that some form of supplementation is necessary. A daily intake of low-dosage multivitamins will help ensure your metabolic needs for vitamins are being met. Evening primrose oil, which has wonderful rejuvenating effects on the skin, is another essential for fitness contestants. We recommend Efamol Calcium – evening primrose oil with calcium and fish oil. The Efamol Company is based in the Canadian province of Nova Scotia, and their products are standardized. A problem with many supplements is that there is very little regulation, hence poor quality control. As always, consult your doctor and your pharmacist before taking supplements.

FIBER

Make sure you incorporate fiber into your diet. You should be consuming generous portions of fruit and vegetables every day. Fiber can reduce both your risk for heart disease and stroke, as well as haemorrhoids and colon cancer. On the other hand, a high-fiber diet can cause problems of a social nature in the form of unwanted gas. You may want to take an anti-gas medication like Beano if you suffer from this condition.

ENERGY BARS, WHY NOT MAKE YOUR OWN?

Flip through any fitness magazine, and you'll see plenty of advertisements for energy bars. These are convenient energy-rich snacks that can give you a much-needed "boost" during a workout. They sound great (because they are great), but they cost an arm and a leg! If you're buying these expensive supplements because of their low-fat levels, you should realize that

10 grams of fat either way is not going to make or break your physique. If you're a professional and getting ready for a competition, spend the extra cash. But if you're a normal athlete who just wants to look and feel good, put your money back in your wallet and pay attention. For a fraction of the cost, you can make your own energy bars. Here are two recipes:

THE CARB INJECTOR

1 cup dried fruit pieces
1 cup quick-cooking oats or rice
1/2 cup crushed nuts (almonds, or your preference)
1/4 cup low-fat butter
1/3 cup honey
1/2 tsp ground cinnamon
Optional – Add 2 cups whey protein.

Combine honey, cinnamon and butter in a pan. Bring to a boil and boil for one minute, stirring constantly. Turn off the heat, and add remaining ingredients while stirring. Pour the mixture into an eight-inch pan. Let cool, and refrigerate. Makes 24 energy bars. This costs about five to eight dollars. The same number of name brand, low-fat energy bars would have cost you more than 72 dollars! With the money you saved, you can buy yourself some good quality creatine.

ARABIAN DELIGHT

6 oz of dried apricots, finely chopped
6 oz dried figs, finely chopped
6 oz dried dates, finely chopped
5 tbsp fruit juice
1 orange rind, grated
2 oz ground nuts
320 g of creatine

Combine the ingredients in an eight-inch square pan and refrigerate. Makes 16 bars.

STAY HEALTHY WITH CRANBERRY JUICE

When training, and during the rest of the day, you should make sure that you are drinking plenty of fluids. One glass of water an hour is a minimum. When working out, you should have a water bottle handy, and drink between sets. Besides filtered water, one of the best drinks going is cranberry juice. Long a hospital favorite, cranberry juice is effective at treating and preventing urinary tract infections (UTIs). Women are 25 times more likely to develop UTIs than men. One of the causes is believed to be dehydration. So simply increasing your fluid intake can help prevent a UTI. Cranberry juice is believed to work by preventing bacteria from adhering to the walls of the bladder. So if you're training heavy, make sure to include cranberry juice in your diet.

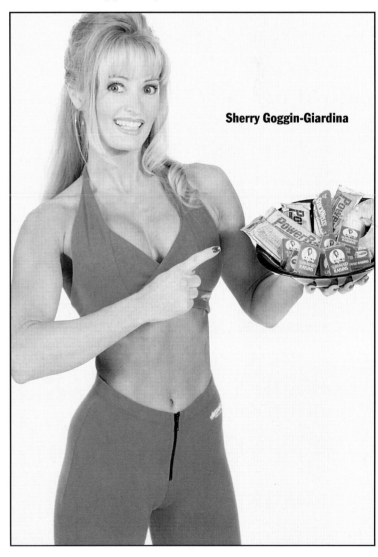

Sherry Goggin-Giardina

TIPS FOR THOSE FOOD CRAVING DAYS

Oxygen magazine contributor Kathleen Engel offers the following tips to keep you on the right path when it comes to sound nutrition on bad food days.

1) Opt for protein sources that are a tad higher in fat. For example, substitute chicken for turkey, salmon for cod, etc. And don't be afraid to toss in an extra egg yolk or two with your breakfast.

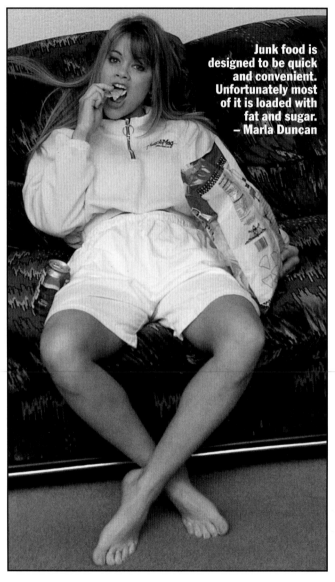

Junk food is designed to be quick and convenient. Unfortunately most of it is loaded with fat and sugar.
– Marla Duncan

2) On those high-appetite days, increase the volume of fibrous food eaten. Such foods don't substantially increase the calorie count, but do fill you up.

3) Always start the day with a large nutritious breakfast. One of the reasons food cravings attack later in the day is because you skipped breakfast.

4) Drink lots of water. As simple as this sounds, water not only helps the body's systems operate smoother, it also depresses appetite.

5) On those days where time is a factor and junk food seems inevitable, be prepared and bring your own healthy meal or snack. Junk food is designed to be quick and convenient. Unfortunately most of it is loaded with fat and sugar. You can avoid all this by preparing small healthy meals that can be carried with you no matter where you go.

6) Plan for sweet-tooth days. We all have them and cutting loose once in a while is not a big deal. Instead of chocolate or candy try cinnamon or artificial sweeteners with your meals.

7) Although food is preferable, make use of meal-replacement powders when time is limited. They're quick, easy to mix, and the better ones are low in fat.

8) Try not to eat high levels of carbs by themselves. This causes the release of insulin, which is the primary fat-storage hormone in the body. Try to balance your food intake evenly between carbs, protein, and to a lesser extent, fat.

9) Determine if you are eating out of habit or actual hunger. Many people eat by the clock whether hungry or not. Unless absolutely necessary, try to eat when the body says so, not by some mechanical device on the wall.

10) Keep nighttime snacking under control. Some experts say no eating after supper but this often leaves the body famished by three or four in the morning. A small, high-fiber snack will help cut down on the those early morning refrigerator raids.

When used as part of a balanced diet, beer is beneficial for human health.

Dr. David Williams, professor of chemistry at the University of Wales

11) Try to only eat fresh food. Studies have shown that the low-nutrient content of old food causes individuals to compensate by eating more.

12) Don't despair if you abandon good eating for that occasional chocolate bar. Unless you make a habit of it, one or two candy bars a week is not going to make much difference to your overall health and fat stores.

RECIPES THAT ARE HEART-SMART AND TASTY

Eating healthy also means eating delicious foods. Long gone are the days when women were condemned to bowls of plain cottage cheese and tap water. You can still lose weight, or maintain what you have, and still enjoy exotic flavors. But before we get cooking, let's examine why we eat the way we do.

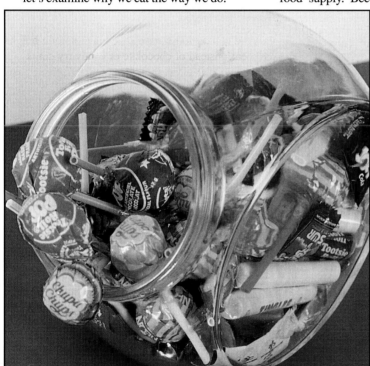

Obviously, the most important factor is cultural. Our early eating habits are a major influence on the way we deal with food as adults. Fortunately, cultural behavior is learned, which means it can be unlearned, or changed. Those of us who grew up on meat and potatoes can soon learn to enjoy liver soup and chicken pilaff, if given the opportunity. Another factor that bares mentioning is a recent theory developed by anthropologists. In researching the environment and food supply of early humans, scientists discovered that our ancestors had a diet deficient in fat. Game animals were very lean, and roots and berries were not always in season. In other words, our ancestors were designed to find fat, and consume it. Bodyfat would keep people alive through periods of hunger. Thus, organ meats such as the liver and kidneys, rich sources of nutrients and fat, were held in high regard. It is only in the last 100 years in the developed world that famine has been eradicated. We are only four generations ahead of ancestors who did not have a secure food supply. Becoming educated about our bodies and the foods we consume can help us make the intelligent choices that will satisfy our craving for taste, and our goal of long-term health.

BEFORE YOU EAT

There are a few tricks to ensure that you don't lose control at the dinner table. You can begin by having desert, or something sweet. Sound like heresy? Yes, but when the stomach detects the presence of fat and sugar, it stops screaming for more. You'll feel less hungry and eat less in the long run.

Try bread dipped in olive oil. The oil is heavy (and healthy), and your pangs of hunger will quickly subside. Drink water with every meal. Last but not least, always leave something on your plate. But with the recipes we've got for you here, that last one is not going to happen!

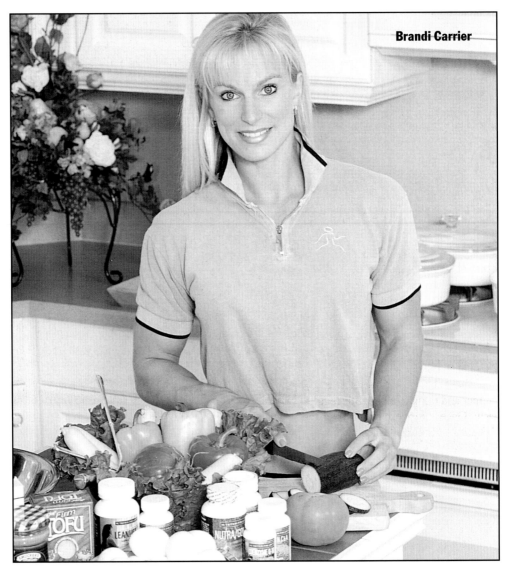

Brandi Carrier

LIVER DISHES

Our recipes reduce the amount of meat so that it is merely a flavoring component, but liver is so rich in minerals and vitamins, go ahead and indulge yourself.

CHICKEN LIVERS IN RED WINE

1/2 kilo chicken livers
1/2 cup red wine
1 cup low-salt chicken broth
1 onion
1 clove garlic
1 tsp black pepper
4 tbsp low-fat butter
2 tbsp whole-wheat flour
1 tbsp fresh dill

First, add the butter and livers to a frying pan, and pan-fry until the livers are cooked (about 5 minutes at high heat). Place the livers in a casserole dish and cover to keep warm, leaving the melted butter and juices in the pan. Add the flour to the pan, stirring gently. While stirring with a wire whisk, add the chicken broth. Once a thick sauce has been formed, you are ready to combine the rest of the ingredients. The onion and dill should be finely chopped, and the garlic crushed, then add the three to the pan. Add pepper and the red wine, and stir constantly for about five minutes. Add the chicken livers to the pan, and stir for another five minutes. Liver will no longer be a dirty word in your home.

LIVER AND RICE

1/2 kilo chicken livers
4 tbsp of low-fat butter
4 large tomatoes
2 large onions
2 cups rice
2 cups filtered water
2 tbsp dill
2 tbsp cranberries
2 tbsp almonds
1 tsp black pepper

Place the butter in a pan and pan-fry the chicken livers. Remove the livers and cover. Finely chop the onions and pan-fry one of them. Remove the onion and combine it with the livers. Finely chop the tomatoes and almonds, and together with the remaining onion, add to the pan. Add the cranberries, rice, water and pepper and bring to a boil. Stir regularly. Once the rice has absorbed the water, reduce the heat and lay the liver and chopped onion on top of the rice, cover and heat gently. Finely chop the fresh dill and sprinkle over the meal just before serving.

FRIED LIVER

400 g beef or lamb's liver
100 g Turkey-Bacon slices
1/2 tsp black pepper
4 tbsp extra-virgin olive oil
3 tbsp fresh parsley
2 tbsp whole-wheat flour
1 tsp of paprika
2 cups rice
1 orange

Cut the liver into 1/4-inch slices. Dust the liver with paprika. Finely chop two tablespoons of parsley, and add it to the flour and salt. Roll the liver slices in the flour mixture until the slices are coated well. Finely chop the Turkey-Bacon slices, and pan-fry with the coated liver slices. Boil the rice, lay it on a plate and lay the pan-fried meat on it. Garnish with parsley and orange slices.

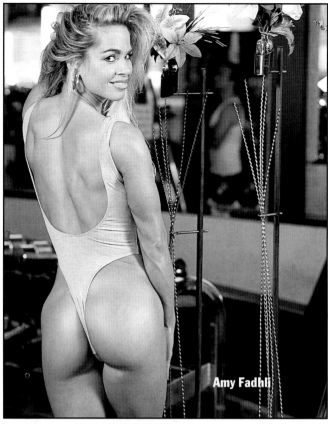

Amy Fadhli

GRILLED LIVER

1/2 kilo beef liver
2 large onions
2 cloves garlic
1 tsp black pepper
2 tsp mint leaves
1 lemon
4 tbsp extra-virgin olive oil
2 cups white vinegar
2 green peppers
2 cups rice
1 can tomato juice

Crush the garlic and dried mint leaves. Mix both with the pepper and two tablespoons of olive oil in a bowl. Cut the liver into thin slices, and add the liver and vinegar to the bowl. Stir, and place in the fridge overnight. When ready to grill, remove the liver and skewer the slices. Slice the onions and peppers, and place slices between each piece of liver. Grill over a barbecue, turning regularly until nicely browned. Boil the rice in tomato juice. Lay the rice on a plate, and place the grilled liver and vegetables on the bed of rice. Sprinkle lemon juice on the liver, and serve.

TURKEY LIVER IN SOYA SAUCE
1/2 kilo turkey livers
2 large tomatoes
2 tbsp low-salt soya sauce
2 tbsp low-fat butter
2 cups brown rice
1 large green pepper

Slice the livers and pan-fry in butter and soya sauce. Remove the livers and pan-fry the previously boiled rice. Remove the rice and pan-fry the finely chopped tomatoes and green pepper. Combine the ingredients on a bed of fried rice.

LIVER SOUP
1/2 kilo lamb's liver
4 large Spanish onions
4 large tomatoes
2 cloves garlic
6 cups low-salt beef broth
1 tsp black pepper
1/4 tsp dried, crushed marjoram
5 tbsp low-fat butter
1 cup rice

Slice the liver and lightly pan-fry in butter. Remove the slices and finely chop them. Now finely chop the onions and pan-fry. Add the liver and the rest of the ingredients, and while stirring, bring to a boil. Reduce the heat and let simmer for 45 minutes. Serve and enjoy.

EGGS
Despite all the bad press, eggs are a complete source of protein, and wonderfully nutritious. For those who remain unconvinced, genetic engineering has helped create a new product for the market, BORN 3, a politically-correct egg. A regular egg has 216 milligrams of cholesterol, while a BORN 3 egg has 100 milligrams. BORN 3 eggs also contain vitamin E and beneficial omega-3 oils (the good oils found in fish). BORN 3 eggs are two to three times more expensive than regular eggs, but as the market expands and competition increases, expect the price to come down. Whether eggs are regular or engineered, they are a versatile ingredient, as you will discover from the following recipes:

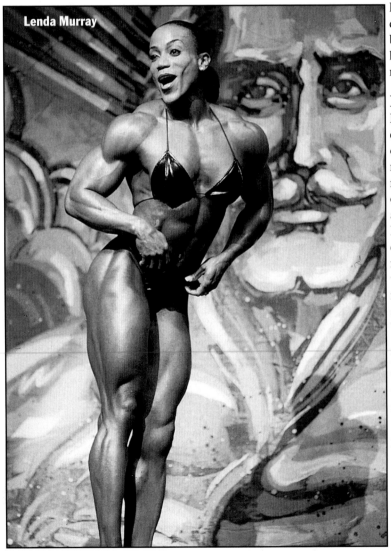

Lenda Murray

RICE OMELET

2 eggs
1/2 tbsp whole-wheat flour
1 large tomato
1 small onion, finely chopped
1/2 cup rice
2 tbsp low-fat butter
1/2 tsp black pepper
1 tsp fresh dill

Slice the tomato and coat in a flour-pepper (1/4 teaspoon of pepper) mixture. Pan-fry the slices in butter, then set aside. Lightly pan-fry the onion, then remove from pan. Boil the rice and drain. Beat the eggs. Add the eggs, the onions and 1/4 teaspoon of pepper to the rice. Pan-fry the mixture. Serve with tomato slices surrounding the omelet.

EGGPLANT OMELET

2 eggs
100 g of eggplant
2 large tomatoes
1 small onion
2 tbsp low-fat butter
1 tsp fresh dill
1/8 tsp saffron
1/4 tsp black pepper

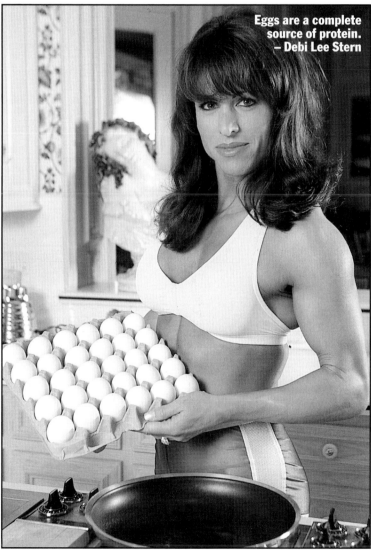

Eggs are a complete source of protein.
– Debi Lee Stern

Peel, remove the seeds, and finely chop the eggplant. Pan-fry with finely chopped tomatoes and onion. Once the eggplant is tender, remove the mixture and mash. Beat the eggs and add the saffron and pepper. Pan-fry the omelet. Remove the omelet, spoon the eggplant mixture onto the eggs, and serve.

GREEN GARDEN OMELET

8 eggs
4 large Spanish onions
500 g spinach leaves
3 tbsp chives
1 tbsp fresh dill
1/2 tsp black pepper
4 tbsp low-fat butter
2 tbsp fresh parsley
1 head of Boston lettuce
1/8 tsp saffron

Finely chop the onions, spinach leaves, chives, lettuce, parsley, fresh dill, and combine with the eggs, flour and pepper in a bowl. Mix thoroughly and pan-fry in the butter. Flip once. When browned on both sides and cooked through, serve.

YOGURT

Yogurt is a marvelous food with a long history in many cultures. Yogurt is made from milk that has had specific bacterial cultures added to it. It is a good source of calcium, potassium, B vitamins and protein. In the past it has been used as a traditional remedy for treating diarrhea and yeast infections. Yogurt is also lactose-free. But you don't have to just eat it cold. Why not try it in soup?

YOGURT SOUP

2 cups plain yogurt
200 g ground lamb
4 large Spanish onions
500 g spinach
1/2 cup yellow split peas
1 cup rice
2 tbsp fresh dill
1 tbsp olive oil
6 cups filtered water
1 tsp black pepper

Finely chop the onions, spinach, and combine with lamb, pepper, peas and water. Boil, then let simmer for 45 minutes. Add the rice. Continue simmering for 30 minutes, stirring occasionally. Add the yogurt and stir for one minute. Remove the pan from the stove. Pan-fry the dill for one minute in olive oil. Add to the soup. Stir and serve.

CUISINE FROM AROUND THE WORLD

ZUCCHINI DUMPLINGS

1 large zucchini
1 large Spanish onion
2 eggs
1 tsp Cayenne pepper
1 tbsp olive oil
1 tbsp fresh dill
200 g ground lamb
1 cup flour
oil for deep frying

Peel, remove the seeds, and finely chop the zucchini. Finely chop the onion and dill and

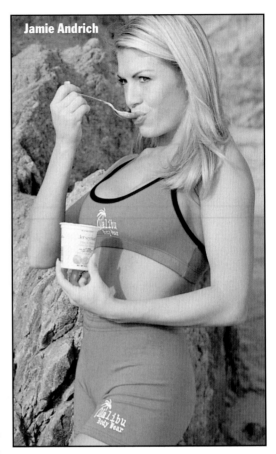
Jamie Andrich

combine with the zucchini in a bowl. Add the eggs, olive oil, pepper, cream cheese, 3/4 cup of flour and lamb. Mix thoroughly. Shape the mixture into balls, and coat with flour. Place in your deep fryer (the only safe way to deep fry food), and cook for five minutes at 190° C (375° F). Drain and serve.

PORK IN MANDARIN RICE

200 g ground pork
1 cup rice
3 Mandarin oranges
1/2 cup low-salt vegetable stock
1-1/2 cups filtered water
1 cup mushrooms
1/4 cup fresh parsley
1 large Spanish onion
1/2 tsp paprika
1/4 tsp cumin
1 cup celery
1/2 tsp black pepper
1 green pepper
1 tbsp fresh dill

Finely chop the green pepper, mushrooms, parsley, and onion. Peel and blend the oranges. Place all the ingredients in a pot (except for the dill), and bring to a boil. Reduce heat and let simmer while stirring regularly until the rice has absorbed most of the water. Serve garnished with chopped dill and a side order of chilled carrot and celery sticks.

CHICKEN PILAF

200 g chicken
2 cups low-salt chicken broth
1 large Spanish onion
1 large tomato
3/4 cup frozen peas
1 cup rice
dash saffron
1 tbsp parsley
1/2 tsp black pepper
3 tbsp chopped walnuts
2 tbsp low-fat butter
1 head lettuce

Remove the skin and finely chop the chicken. Pan-fry until lightly browned, and remove. Finely chop the onion, pan-fry until browned, then add the peas, chicken, walnuts, saffron and finely chopped parsley and tomato. Now add the rice and broth, and bring to a boil. Reduce the heat and let simmer until the rice absorbs all the water. Serve on a bed of fresh lettuce leaves.

WRAPPED PORK SLICES ON FRIED RICE

200 g pork
2 large Spanish onions
2 tbsp low-salt butter
3 large tomatoes
3 tbsp fresh parsley
1/2 tsp black pepper
2 cups low-fat beef broth
1 lemon
1 cup rice

Finely chop the onions and pan-fry in butter until brown. Finely chop the tomatoes and parsley, and add to the onions. Add the pepper. Once cooked remove and let cool. Slice the pork into 10 thin slices. Spoon the cooled mixture onto each slice, and roll the slice, securing it with a toothpick. Place the slices in a pot, and pour in the beef broth. Bake in a covered pot at 190° C (375° F) for 35 minutes. Be sure to occasionally baste the slices. Remove the slices and pour the broth into a pot. Boil the rice in this pot (if need be, add water). Once boiled remove the rice and fry it in the original frying pan. Serve the rolled slices on a bed of fried rice.

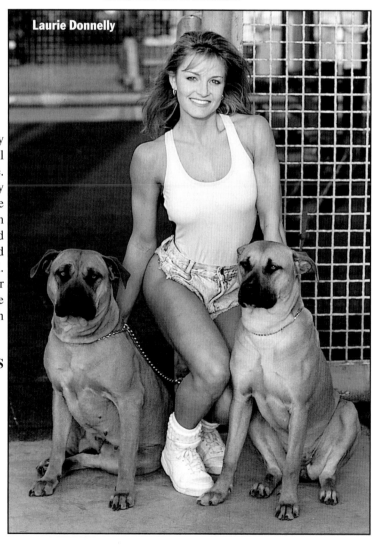
Laurie Donnelly

STUFFED PITA

1 bag whole-wheat pita bread
1 L can tomato sauce
1 cup fresh mushrooms
1 large onion
1 large green pepper
1 tsp oregano
1/4 tsp garlic
100 g low-fat cheddar cheese

De-seed the pepper, and finely chop the onion, pepper and fresh mushrooms. Finely grate the cheddar cheese, and mix all the ingredients in a bowl. Spoon the mixture into each pita bread, and lay on a pan. Place in the oven at 100° C (200° F) for three minutes. Enjoy.

TEQUILA CHICKEN SURPRISE

Tex-Mex cuisine has made real inroads into the American mainstream. Here's our interpretation of one such delight.

200 g chicken
1/2 cup tequila
worm from the bottle
(SURPRISE!) – optional
2 cups rice
2 tbsp lemon juice
1/2 tsp pepper
1 tbsp fresh parsley
1/2 cup olive oil
1 large onion
1 hot chili pepper
2 tbsp low-fat butter

Remove the skin and fat from the chicken and chop into tiny cubes. Finely chop the parsley. Combine the chicken, tequila, lemon juice, pepper, parsley and olive oil. Refrigerate and let marinate overnight. Boil the rice until cooked. Finely chop

the onion and chili pepper. Pan-fry the chicken in butter until golden brown, add the onion, chili pepper and rice. Pan-fry and stir until done. If your bottle has a worm, and you're so inclined (or drunk, let's be honest), add the worm and let your guests figure out who got it.

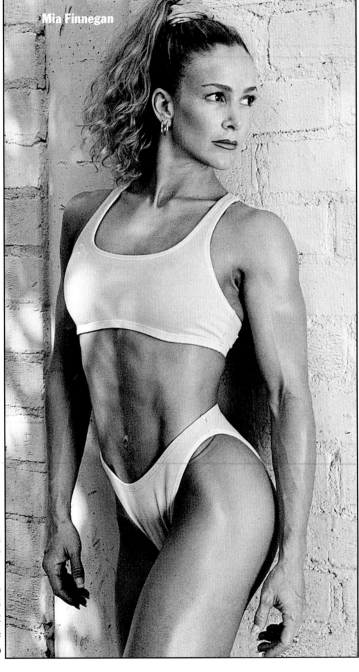

Mia Finnegan

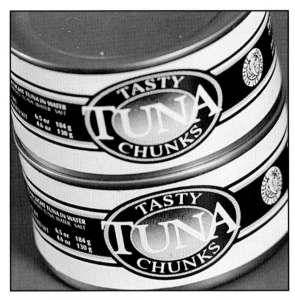

COLD FAJITAS

4 whole-wheat soft tortillas
1 carrot, shredded
4 finely chopped scallions
1 zucchini, thinly sliced
4 tbsp nonfat Philadelphia cream cheese
2 tbsp low-fat Parmesan cheese, shredded
2 tbsp low-fat cheddar cheese, shredded
4 tbsp fresh cilantro, finely chopped
1 red pepper, finely chopped

Combine the ingredients in a bowl, mix and spread onto the tortillas. Roll up the tortillas. Refrigerate and serve cold.

TUNA AND RICE SALAD

Estonia is a tiny country that rests on the eastern edge of the Baltic Sea. This maritime nation has long enjoyed the bounties of the sea. This salad is one of their wonderful creations.

1 can water-packed tuna
2 cups rice
1 cup green peas
1 green pepper, finely chopped
4 scallions, finely chopped
1/2 cup low-fat mayonnaise
2 hard-boiled eggs, finely chopped
1 tsp pepper

Combine the cooked rice and cooked green peas with the rest of the ingredients in a salad bowl and mix thoroughly. Refrigerate before serving.

EAT YOUR GREENS

Popeye had the right idea after all. Spinach can make you strong. Our hero liked to eat it straight from the can, but we suggest a more subtle approach:

SPINACH SOUFFLÉ

1 cup spinach
1 large onion
1 tbsp low-fat, Parmesan cheese
1 tbsp light Philadelphia cream cheese
2 eggs
1 tsp lemon juice
1/4 tsp pepper

Boil the spinach until it reaches the texture you enjoy. Finely chop the spinach and onion, and combine all the ingredients in a blender. Once blended to a creamy consistency, pour into a large bowl, cover, and microwave on high for three minutes. Let sit for three minutes, then uncover and serve.

LAZY SALAD

Some of our readers may find that because of their former eating habits, they find themselves getting ravenous. What do you do when craving a midnight snack? Try this recipe.

1 cabbage, finely chopped
2 cups vinegar
1 cup extra-virgin olive oil

Combine the ingredients in a salad bowl and mix thoroughly, then refrigerate. Anytime you need to snack between meals, help yourself. This is the ONLY food you're allowed to eat in front of the TV. Don't worry – it tastes good. Okay, not that good, but it's not bad.

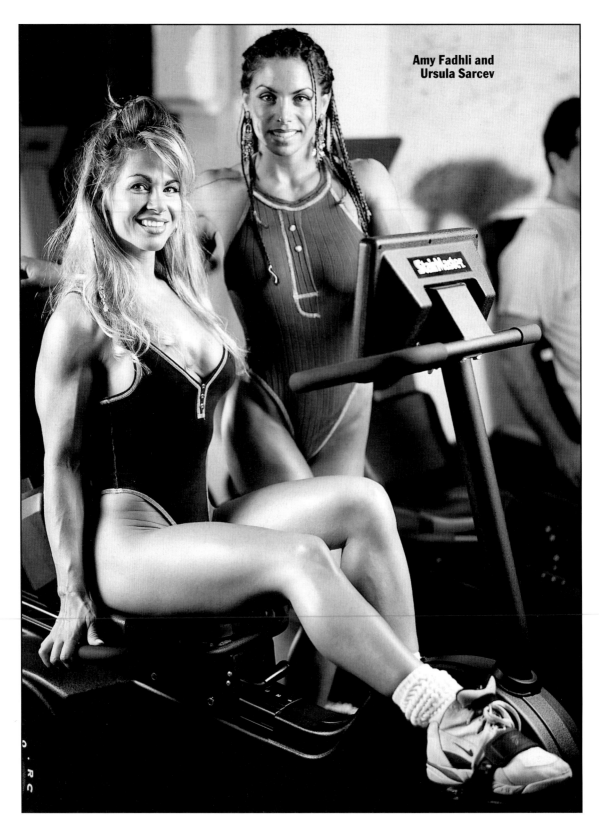

Amy Fadhli and
Ursula Sarcev

Chapter 8

Cardio Training

While the authors are biased towards strength training, we'll be the first to admit it's only half the battle. No matter how intense your strength-training routine, it is of limited value for cardiovascular stimulation. To get the most from your conditioning program you need to perform a minimum of two to three, 30-minute cardio sessions per week. In the following chapter we'll give an overview of the cardiovascular system and how it relates to exercise. To conclude we'll briefly discuss the various categories of cardio equipment found in better gyms.

For starters, all the cardio in the world won't undo the damage of sloppy eating habits. Do you want definition or donuts? You can't have both, at least not on a regular basis.

Kathleen Engel,
Oxygen
contributor

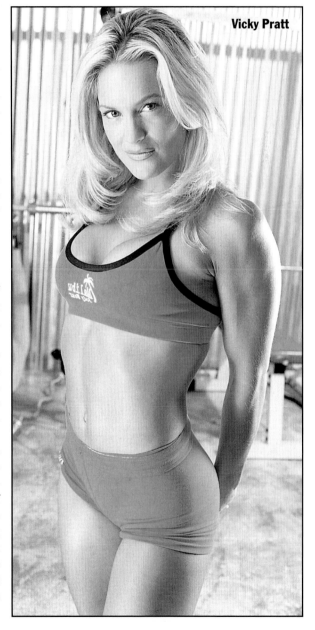

Vicky Pratt

THE CARDIOVASCULAR SYSTEM

The cardiovascular system can be thought of as the transport system of the human body. It is composed of the heart and associated blood vessels called arteries, veins, and capillaries. The heart is a pumping organ divided into four chambers, two chambers per side. The heart is really a double pump with one side (right) pumping deoxygenated blood to the lungs, and the other (left) pumping oxygenated blood to the rest of the body.

The main function of the heart is to pump blood around the body. The average number of beats per minute is 70 to 72 – pushing or expelling about 70 milliliters of blood per beat. Over the average life span the heart will beat 2.5 million times circulating 225 to 230 million liters of blood throughout the human body. Maximum heart rate is the maximum number of beats per minute. It depends on such variables as age and fitness level.

CARDIOVASCULAR ENDURANCE AND FITNESS

The two most important factors governing cardiovascular fitness are intensity and duration. The two are interrelated. High-intensity exercise is usually performed in shorter durations, while low-intensity exercise is usually performed in longer durations. Generally speaking, cardiovascular conditioning requires a minimum of 20 minutes duration, three times per week.

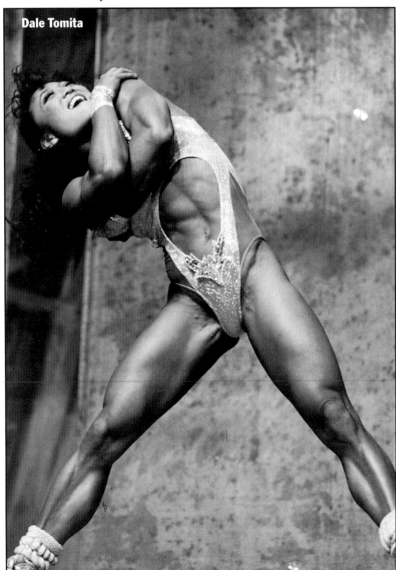

Dale Tomita

Aerobic exercise provides the finishing touch to a beautiful physique. Engaging in some form of aerobic work is almost an unwritten guarantee for a leaner body. It is the third ingredient in a good fitness regime which also includes resistance training and a sound diet.

Nina Simone, *Oxygen* contributor

While there's no fool-proof way to determine the most efficient exercise level, the most popular and easiest to use is heart rate. As mentioned earlier maximum heart rate is the maximum number of beats per minute that an individual's heart can beat. Exercise physiologists use a simple formula to predict maximum heart rate. It involves subtracting the person's age from the theoretical maximum of 220 beats per minute. For example, a 25-year-old female would have a maximum heart rate of 195 beats per minute (220 - 25 = 195).

Research has shown that if people exercise at 60 to 90 percent of this value they can adequately stimulate their cardio systems without overstressing the body.[1] The two values obtained give what is called the target heart-rate zone. The previous 25-year-old's target heart rate zone (THRZ) would be between 117 and 175 beats per minute (60% x 195 = 117 and 90% x 195 = 175).

If the individual exercises below 117 beats per minute she is not adequately stimulating her cardio system. Above 175 beats per minute, and the workout is probably too strenuous. Most gyms have target heart-rate zone charts to save you the trouble of calculating the values.

I found that I needed a variety of ways to get cardiovascular conditioning. When you have to prepare for three or four contests a year, you have to find ways to keep your interest up. Doing one type of cardiovascular training would drive me crazy.

Dale Tomita, top fitness competitor

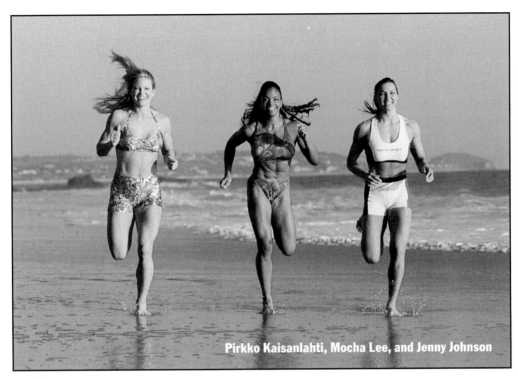

Pirkko Kaisanlahti, Mocha Lee, and Jenny Johnson

TWO TARGET HEART-RATE ZONES

In recent years exercise physiologists have broken the target heart-rate zone into two zones – one for fat loss and the other for cardio. While the evidence is preliminary, keeping your heart rate between 65 and 75 percent of your theoretical max is better for burning fat calories, while 75 to 90 percent is better for stimulating the cardiovascular system. Keep in mind there is much overlap between the two. The lower level will stimulate the cardio system, and the upper level will burn fat. Therefore alternate periods of high-intensity training (upper zone) with periods of moderate-intensity training (lower zone).

> *You can run, rollerblade, play sports, or work the stairmaster. Just do it three to five times a week.*
>
> **Aliś Willoughby, fitness competitor**

TAKING YOUR PULSE

If the cardio machines you have access to don't have built-in heart monitors, you'll have to do things the old-fashioned way. The best places to take your pulse are the neck (carotid) and wrist (radial). It may take a bit of practice to find your pulse. Rather than counting the number of beats for a full minute, take it for 10 or 15 seconds and multiply by six or four respectively. This will give you a value accurate to one or two beats per minute. As a word of caution, feel for your pulse using one or two fingers. Don't use the thumb as it has its own pulse and you may confuse the two.

WHEN TO DO CARDIO

It doesn't matter as long as you do it! You can do your cardio on the same day as your strength training (a must if you're training five to six days per week) or on alternate days. The advantage to alternate days is you'll only be doing one form of exercise each day. The drawback is you'll be exercising six to seven days per week. Doing it on the same day as strength training gives you two to three days off from exercise entirely.

If you do cardio on the same day that you weight train you can get up early and do it before breakfast, or you can combine it with your strength training later in the day (not counting those who weight train early in the

The fact is, walking offers the same benefits as running, but without the wear and tear on your joints and muscles, because it is a low-impact aerobic exercise. When you walk the impact of each step is one to one and a half times your weight. Compare these numbers to running which yields an impact of three to four times your bodyweight.

Suzanne Levine, podiatrist and author of *Walking It Off*

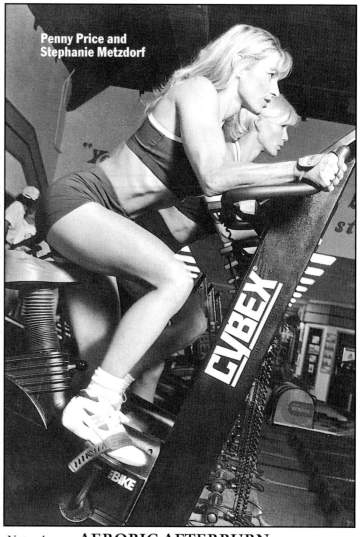

Penny Price and
Stephanie Metzdorf

morning). If you plan to do both at the same time of day, you have two options. Most find it easier to do cardio first and then finish with the weight training. But you might want to experiment and try it after. From a biological point of view there's little difference. If doing cardio first has a slight advantage, it serves as a good warmup for weight training.

TYPES OF CARDIO

Cardiovascular stimulation can take many forms. You can exercise outdoors, (jogging, skiing, swimming), or you can take part in an indoor activity (aerobics, handball, or floor hockey). Another option is to use one of the many cardio machines found in the gym. The choice is yours. For variety most people participate in more than one activity. Not only is this more productive but it's also more fun. The following is a comparison of common cardio exercises (performed at high intensity) and the calories burned per hour.

ACTIVITY	CALORIES PER HOUR
Walking	400-500
Running	750-800
Swimming	550-600
Skipping rope	750-800
Skiing	550-600
Aerobics	550-600
Stationary bike	650-700
Racquetball	450-500

AEROBIC AFTERBURN

Afterburn can be defined as the elevation in metabolic rate after exercise. When you stop exercising your metabolic rate does not suddenly drop to base level. Instead, it stays elevated for a period of hours, with some studies suggesting up to 15 to 20 hours. This means that even though you finished exercising for the day your body is still burning calories at a higher rate.

Although duration seems to play a role, intensity contributes the most to afterburn. If you want to maximize calorie burning after you leave the gym, try alternating periods of moderate cardio training with short periods of high-intensity training.

CARDIO EQUIPMENT

Unless you're working out at an old, hardcore bodybuilding gym, chances are your gym has a good selection of cardio equipment. The more popular pieces of equipment are described here. For updates on new equipment pick up a recent copy of *Oxygen* magazine.

TREADMILLS

Treadmills are one of the most popular pieces of cardio equipment. Nowhere is this more apparent than in the home-fitness business. Each year millions of treadmills are placed under Christmas trees in the hopes that the winter months will be spent running off those extra pounds. While the intentions are usually sincere, mid-January finds most of the machines in the attic or garage.

Treadmills can be subdivided into two categories, motorized and unmotorized. As the name implies, motorized treadmills are self-moving and require you to keep pace with the belt. Most brands go from one to 15 miles per hour. The better brands also have incline features which allow you to simulate an uphill trek. In most cases the angle will increase to 15 degrees. Motorized treadmills are the most expensive and a top of the line model by Quintin will set you back $8000 to $10,000. Such units are generally designed for the high volume use of commercial gyms. You can pick up a decent house model for $800 to $1000. Just remember, you get what you pay for. Top of the line models have great warranty packages, are programmable, and in many cases, are cushioned (so they are easier on the joints).

The other category of treadmills are unmotorized. The belt is dependant on you for movement. You push the belt with your feet as you run. Most of these versions are designed with home use in mind and wouldn't last long in a gym given the high-volume usage. If they have a redeeming feature it's their cost – as little as $200 when on sale.

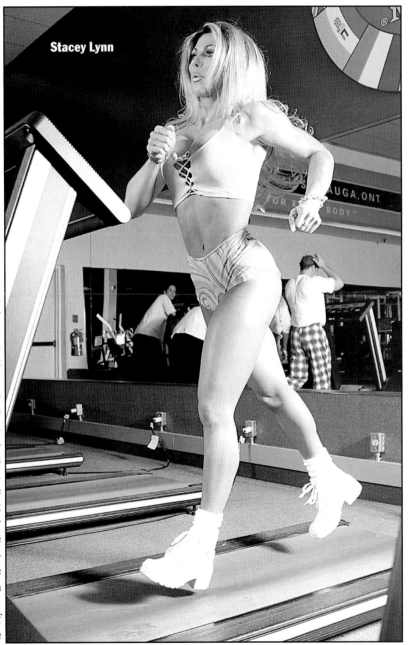

Stacey Lynn

STEPPERS

Steppers are very popular with women because the exercise primarily involves the hip and thigh muscles. But remember you cannot spot reduce these areas. When you perform an intense cardio routine, the body takes the stored calories from everywhere – hips, thighs, arms, shoulders, etc. So while the stepper is a great way to burn extra calories, it doesn't slim the hips and thighs anymore than say, a rowing exercise.

Stair climbing is great because the effect put forth is just enough to cause the body to burn fat, but it doesn't really throw the body into the same exhausted state that running does.
Dwayne Hines II, *MuscleMag* contributor and co-author of *Hot Legs!*

If steppers have a disadvantage it's that they place a lot of stress on the knees. Let's face it, most of your bodyweight is bouncing up and down on the knee joints in this exercise. As many people have weak knees to begin with, this movement can aggravate the condition. Our advice is to use a rower or cycle for a few weeks before trying the stepper. Not only will this still give the cardiovascular system a good workout, but it will give the muscles around the knees a chance to strengthen if you have just started a weight-training program.

ROWERS

The third category of cardio machines are rowers, or ergometers. These machines require you to sit in a sliding chair and grab a set of handles similar in appearance to the upper section of boat oars. Although steppers and treadmills seem to be more popular, the rower might well be the best of the bunch. This is because the exercise brings both the lower and upper body into play, whereas the other two only involve the lower body. The more muscles in motion the more calories burned; therefore, it stands to reason that you'll burn more calories per unit of time with the rower.

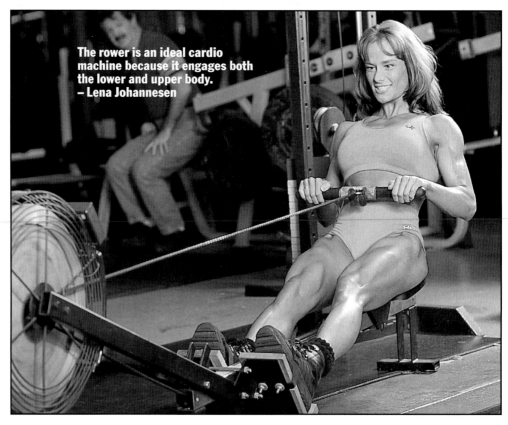

The rower is an ideal cardio machine because it engages both the lower and upper body.
– Lena Johannesen

CARDIO CYCLES

Cardio cycles have come a long way since the stationary bikes of the 1950s and 1960s. Cardio cycles are stationary bikes that mimic the ride on a real bike. The cheaper versions have one tension setting, while top of the line models can be programmed to vary the tension as you peddle. The latest bikes by LifeCycle will even take your pulse and vary the tension to keep your heart rate in the most efficient training zone. The nice thing about cycles is that you can give the cardiovascular system a great workout without putting excessive stress on the knees.

For those who find the standard bike uncomfortable on the lower back, manufacturers have come out with recumbent bikes that allow you to sit back and peddle similar to the paddle boats at an amusement park. Virtually all the stress is taken off the lower back and kept on the hips and thighs.

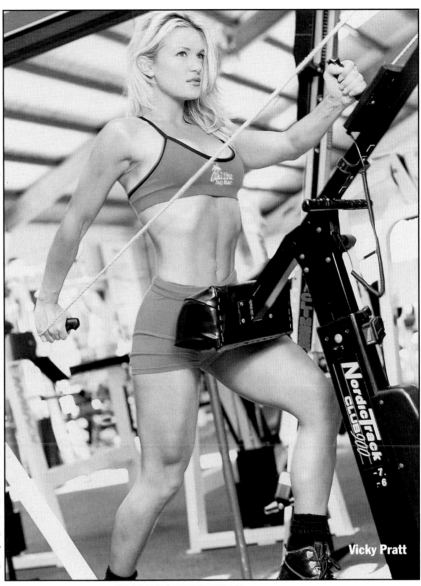

Vicky Pratt

SKATERS OR SLIDERS

One of the arguments against most cardio machines is that they only work the body in a forward/backward motion. But the legs and arms also move laterally. A few manufacturers have addressed this by designing equipment that works in both directions. Nautilus has come out with a skate machine that's ideal for those involved in such sports as hockey, soccer, and tennis. If you regularly play sports involving lateral movements we suggest giving such machines a try.

SKI MACHINES

For those who want to stay in ski shape year-round, NordicTrack and others have developed just the machines. Instead of stepping or running you place your feet on a ski-like apparatus and slide forward and backward. Those who don't ski might want to give the machines a try because cross-country skiing is one of the best forms of cardiovascular training.

Reference
1. YMCA Canada Fitness Leader: Basic Theory Manual, (Canada, 1995), 93-94.

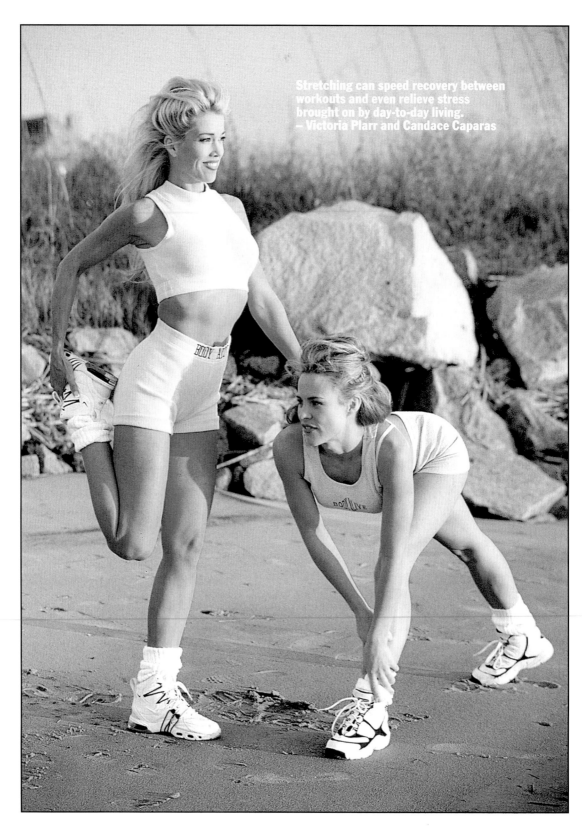

Stretching can speed recovery between workouts and even relieve stress brought on by day-to-day living.
— Victoria Plarr and Candace Caparas

Chapter 9
Stretching

*I*t's amazing the number of people who spend years contracting their muscles yet fail to stretch. Stretching is one of the most important variables in overall physical conditioning.

WHY STRETCH?

There are numerous reasons for incorporating stretching into your conditioning program. For starters, stretching is one of the best ways to prevent injuries. Think of your muscles as elastic bands. The more stretchable and pliable the rubber the less chance of a breakage or tear. Your muscles react the same way. Regular stretching gives the muscles a greater range of motion to prevent injuries.

What many people don't realize is that the flexibility that comes with stretching also helps increase their muscle power and efficiency.

Norman Zale,
MuscleMag
contributor

Another benefit to stretching is that it can speed recovery between workouts. It does this by speeding the removal of lactic acid from exercised muscles. Evidence suggests that not only does lactic acid reduce a muscle's contractibilty but also slows down its recovery ability.

A third benefit to stretching is that it may increase the growth potential of the muscle. Research is sketchy at present but evidence is mounting that regular stretching somehow encourages muscle bellies to become fuller.

A fourth benefit to stretching is psychological in nature. Virtually everyone who incorporates stretching into his or her routine reports feeling much more energized and refreshed. Some even go as far as to say it helps relieve tension and stress brought on by day-to-day living.

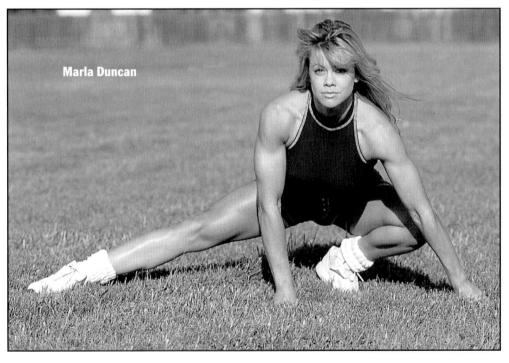

Marla Duncan

WHEN TO STRETCH

A cold muscle is not as pliable as a warm one. It makes more sense to perform some light cardio first to get the heart rate elevated and muscles warmed up. You can then do some light stretching before beginning your weight training. Save the rigorous stretching till after your workout when the muscles are fully warmed up. As a final suggestion, many of the stretches can be done during your workout. For example, thigh and hamstring stretches can be performed between squats and leg curls. Stretching doesn't take much out of you energy wise so it won't interfere with your sets. It can actually make your workout more efficient as stretching helps rid the muscles of lactic-acid build-up.

We need to be able to stretch for almost everything we do. Whether running, bending, dancing, or lifting, the human body must be limber enough to handle both mundane and intricate movements. Some people are quite flexible thanks to a daily stretching routine, while others are as stiff as boards.

Mia Wallace,
Oxygen **contributor**

HOW TO STRETCH

Although it varies, most exercise kinesiologists recommend holding the stretch position for 15 to 20 seconds and then relaxing for an equal period of time. To give the muscles a good stretch we suggest a minimum of two to three "sets" per muscle group. As with weight training, don't bounce at the bottom of a stretch. This puts tremendous stress on the muscle and surrounding tissues.

THE STRETCHES
QUAD STRETCH

This is one of the easiest stretches to perform. Start by planting one foot on a flat surface and grabbing a stationary upright for support. Curl the

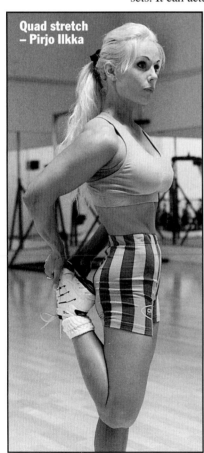

Quad stretch
– Pirjo Ilkka

other leg behind you and grab your foot with your free hand. Gently pull the foot toward the glutes, keeping the knee pointing toward the ground. This is a great stretch to perform between sets of squats, leg presses and leg extensions.

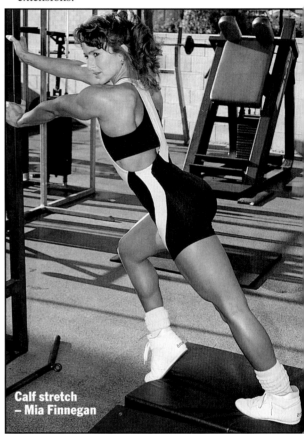

Calf stretch
– Mia Finnegan

CALF STRETCH

Adopt a runner's stance with the forward leg bent and back leg straight. With the rear foot flat on the floor, press your hands against a wall. As you push gently on the wall try to force your rear leg back while keeping the foot flat on the floor. Perform this stretch between sets of standing and seated calf raises.

HAMSTRING STRETCH

Place one foot on a waist-high chair or other flat surface. With the toes pointing upward, gently stretch forward with the upper body. Repeat for the other side. You can do this one between leg curls and stiff-leg deadlifts.

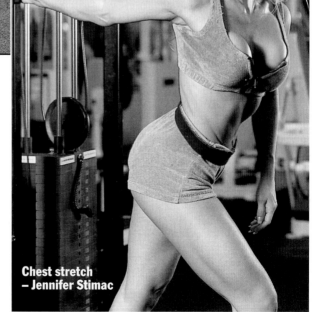

Before you stretch you should raise your core body temperature by participating in at least five minutes of low-intensity cardiovascular exercise.

Dr. Christine Lydon,
Oxygen columnist

CHEST STRETCH
Stand next to a stationary upright and hold onto it with one hand. Keeping your arm as straight as possible, gently rotate or twist the torso away from the gripping hand. This exercise primarily stretches the chest but the upper and outer lats also receive some benefit.

TRICEPS STRETCH
Place one hand behind the head so your elbow is pointing straight upward. With your free hand gently push your elbow backward until you feel a good stretch.

Hamstring stretch

V-STRETCH OR SPLITS
This is one of the better known stretches for the hamstrings and adductors. Ask someone off the street to demonstrate their flexibility and chances are they'll try and do the splits. The key to this exercise is to ease into it gently. Numerous over-enthusiastic athletes have pulled adductors doing this stretch. We should add that not everyone who practices the splits will get to the point of resting both legs fully on the floor pointing in opposite directions. To fully "split," the tendons and muscles have to be attached in just the right positions. Be patient, everyone who practices this movement will increase their flexibility by a substantial degree.

Chest stretch – Jennifer Stimac

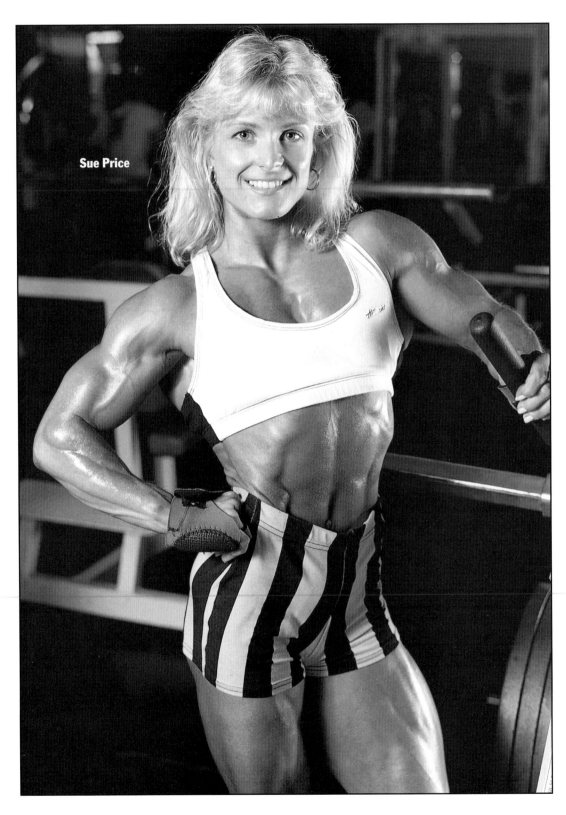

Sue Price

Chapter 10
Staying Motivated

No matter how hard the weightlifting bug bites, sooner or later you'll find yourself making excuses to miss workouts. When going to the gym becomes a chore and not a passion, it's time to employ strategies to address the problem. The following are suggestions to overcome the training blues. You may have to utilize more than one to regenerate your initial enthusiasm.

TAKE TIME OFF

This may seem contradictory but one of the main reasons for low motivation levels is overtraining. There is a limit to how much physical activity the human body can endure. Sooner or later you can overtax your recovery system. The body usually starts giving you warning signals, one of which is low-motivation levels.

Personally, I think a week's rest should be taken every four to six weeks of training, even if it's only active rest.

John Grimek, former Mr. America and Mr. Universe

Unfortunately, many ignore these signals and force themselves to work out. This may work for a short period of time but sooner or later the body becomes physically exhausted. As soon as you find yourself so exhausted and making excuses to miss workouts – take some time off. A week will do wonders to recharge the batteries. But chronic overtraining may necessitate avoiding the gym for a couple of weeks.

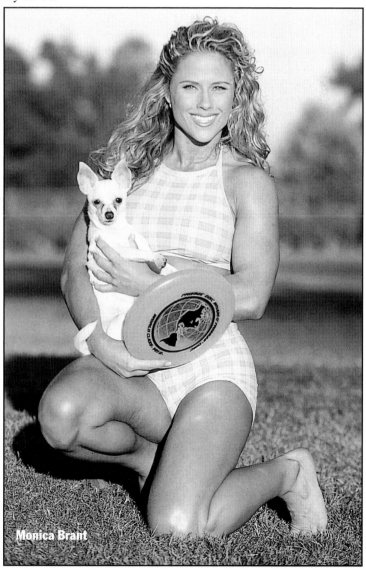
Monica Brant

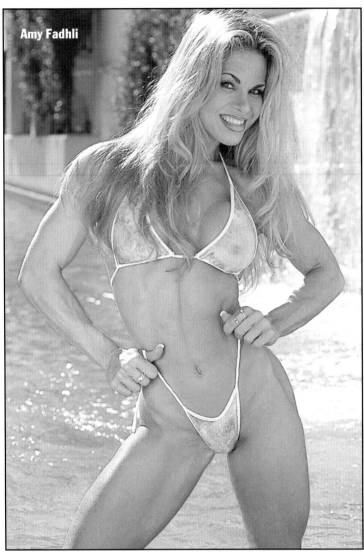

Amy Fadhli

Your body needs to rest. Rest = recuperation = growth. Overtraining is not conducive to muscular growth. It is however conducive to muscle atrophy.

Amy Fadhli, *Oxygen* **columnist and fitness champion**

even have to revamp your whole workout schedule. In a nut shell do something different to get out of the training rut. Not only will your motivation levels rise, but the change of pace will stimulate your muscles to new progress.

CHANGE GYMS

The following suggestion only applies if you live in an area that has multiple training establishments. Sometimes the easiest way to spice up your workouts lies with a change of scenery. Many of the top fitness competitors have memberships in two of the most famous gyms in the world, Gold's and World Gyms. Switching gyms has many advantages. For starters, with few exceptions, no gym has every piece of equipment. Changing gyms often gives you access to equipment that you otherwise wouldn't be able to use. Some gyms have better leg-training equipment while others may have a bigger selection in upper-body training.

Changing gyms also puts you in contact with new people. Who knows, changing gyms may put you in contact with a top athlete, enable you meet a new trainer or training partner, or lead you into a new friendship or relationship.

Changing gyms is not always as expensive as it sounds. Many gyms offer month-by-month memberships. For the sake of $30 to $50, you can experience a whole new training environment.

CHANGE YOUR ROUTINE

The main reason people stop weight training is lack of variety – in short, they get bored. While every hockey or baseball game is different, weight training can be monotonous, especially if you continue to perform the same exercises day in day out. Even the top fitness competitors and bodybuilders get tired of doing the same routine over and over. The old saying "variety is the spice of life" applies just as much to weight training as to any other daily activity. As soon as you find your workouts becoming stale change things around. At the very least change the exercises. You may

FIND A TRAINING PARTNER

Have you ever noticed how you tend to do that extra rep when someone's watching or spotting you? Now think what an improvement it would make to your workouts if this happened on each and every set. This is where training partners come in. A training partner is someone who matches you set for set during a workout. A good training partner knows when to take the bar and when to make you do that extra rep. He or she also serves to motivate you on those lazy days, and you can reciprocate on his or her down times.

Most training relationships are not planned but happen by accident. Two people training at the same time each day, doing much the same routine, start spotting one another, and before they know it they're training partners. For those who don't have a training partner but kind of like the idea here's a few suggestions:

1) Choose a partner who works out at about the same time each day. As long as you arrive at the gym within 15 to 20 minutes of one another, things should work out.
2) Pick someone who is following a similar routine. Unless one of you is willing to drastically change your workout schedule, it doesn't make much sense to train together if you perform completely different exercises – it will only waste time.
2) Hook up with someone who's close to you in strength levels – say within five to ten pounds on most exercises. A few extra pounds on leg exercises is no big deal but it doesn't make sense to be continuously loading and unloading the barbell.

Closely related to the previous is the issue of intensity level. A beginner teaming up with an advanced trainer will eventually encounter problems. Tagging along for a few workouts is fine (you'll learn a lot), but jumping into a six-day-a-week routine with only a

I like training both ways, but a training partner gives you motivation not to skip workouts, and you probably will train harder because of friendly competition.

**Marjo Selin,
former *MuscleMag* columnist**

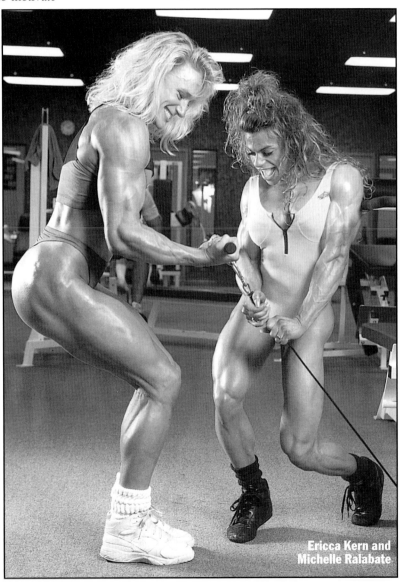

Ericca Kern and
Michelle Ralabate

I'm selective about the photographs I choose to have taken. I always remember that I'm a fitness professional first. I won't pose for a picture showing my rear end just to get in a magazine.

Mia Finnegan, *Oxygen* **columnist and fitness champion**

few weeks of training under your belt will quickly lead to physical exhaustion. You'll be a nervous wreck within a couple of weeks.

All of the previous may raise the question, can a guy make a good workout partner? The answer is yes, provided the aforementioned points are met. If there's an advantage to co-ed training it's the intensity levels generated by the battle of the sexes! As a final comment, some happy long-term relationships have started from such training, so give it a try.

TAKE PICTURES

One of the problems with looking at yourself every day is that you won't notice any major changes in your physical appearance. You're wearing smaller clothes, your strength levels have gone up, and friends comment on how good you look, but you don't see anything different when you look in the mirror. It's because the change from day to day is so gradual. It's like a plant growing. Observe it every day and you see nothing. But go away for a few weeks and the new growth will be obvious. The changes in your physique are just as hard to spot. It would be idiotic to try and not look in the mirror every day. A more practical solution is to take a couple of pictures and hide them away. After a couple of months take another set from the exact same angles and compare. The difference will be obvious.

Don't let some guy at the gym calling himself a "photographer" take your pictures without first doing a background check. Weight training, like most sports, has a few shady characters hanging around. There are many legitimate photographers, but you can't forget the "scum element." Who knows where your pictures may end up. If there's any doubt play it safe and have a trusted friend or relative take the shots.

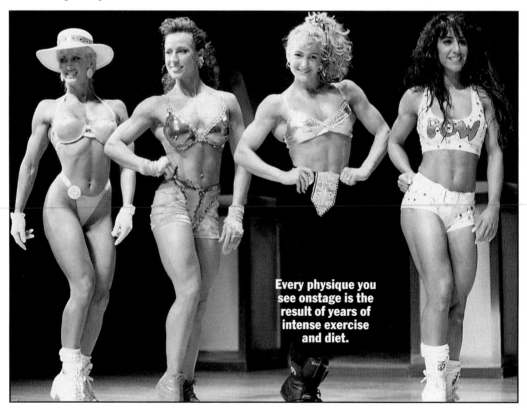

Every physique you see onstage is the result of years of intense exercise and diet.

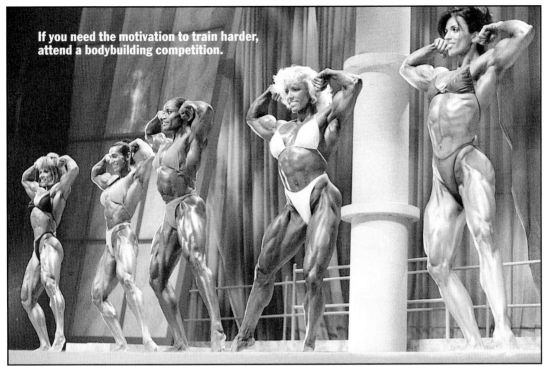

If you need the motivation to train harder, attend a bodybuilding competition.

GO TO A FITNESS OR BODYBUILDING CONTEST

There's nothing like observing great physiques to get your training spirits revved up. Competitions are a great way to see just how far the human body can be developed. And don't think the competitors were born that way. Every physique you see onstage is the result of years of intense exercise and diet. Besides looking at the competitors, you can strike up conversations with those around you. Body-building and fitness audiences are storehouses of information. Chances are you'll leave the venue and go straight to the gym for a workout.

KEEP A JOURNAL

Although not an absolute necessity, one of the best ways to know where you're going is to know where you've been. Keeping a daily record allows you to monitor your progress, and serves as a source of inspiration. Weights that were at one time lifted for heavy sets of six to eight reps are now used as warmup weights. See how far you've come. Besides work-out poundages, sets, and reps, record such information as nutrition, supple-ments taken, and even how you feel during the day. Little things often

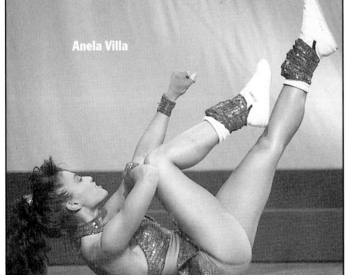

Anela Villa

make big differences to your training. Refer to it before your next workout. Try to use the same weight used in your previous workout for one extra rep, or do the same number of reps with five to 10 extra pounds. Either way you're increasing the intensity and quality of your workout.

I suggest keeping a log initially, so that you can determine when, how, and why you eat. You'll be a lot happier if you maintain a leaner look, and you'll be able to see the fruits of your efforts during each workout.

Dale Tomita, top fitness pro

MUSIC

You may think something as simple as music wouldn't make a difference but numerous psychological studies have suggested otherwise. Music can cheer us up, make us cry, even lift some people out of the depths of depression. The size of the recording industry should give you an idea of just how important music is to our lives. When you go hunting for a gym, check and see what type of music they play over the audio system. Most gyms play the top 40 as it adds life to the atmosphere. While there are exceptions, most members find it difficult to work out to classical music or slow music of any kind. If your gym has a lousy music selection switch gyms or invest in a portable stereo system. Put on the headset, crank up the volume, and away you go. Those sluggish workouts may be cured for the price of a few CDs.

CREATE A STRENGTH AND FITNESS LIBRARY

The fact that you bought this book means you've already started your library. There's nothing like pictures and training advice to get you over the training blues. Every month there's dozens of magazines that feature the latest in bodybuilding and nutritional information. Bookstores have large sections devoted exclusively to health and fitness publications. Every chance you get, buy a book or magazine and add it to your library. If your budget is tight, check a

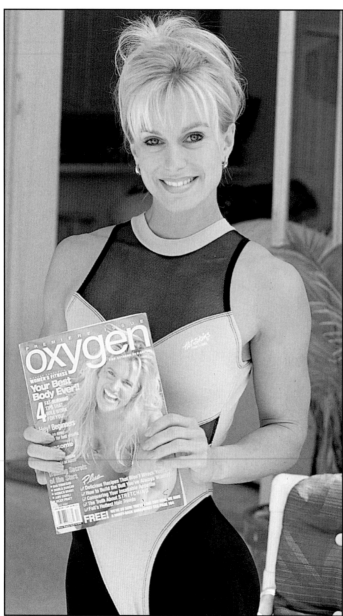

Magazines are a great source of training inspiration. – Brandi Carrier

used bookstore. Most have hundreds of back issues of heath magazines that can be purchased for mere pennies. On those days you lack motivation, flip through a magazine. Chances are within five to 10 minutes you'll be raring to get to the gym!

I get psyched for my workout by reading a training article about someone I admire. I then plan a workout based on the article for the bodypart I am to train that day.

Tonya Knight, former *MuscleMag* columnist and former pro bodybuilder

ONE LAST SUGGESTION – MAKE IT PART OF YOUR LIFE

Hopefully this suggestion will come naturally, and you won't have to force yourself to work out. Some readers may need to develop strategies that get them in the habit of working out. Many long-time fitness competitors and trainers report that the first couple of months were the hardest, and many would have given up had they not forced themselves to go to the gym when they really wanted to make excuses.

Working out will eventually became part of your daily routine – no different than going to work, sleeping, or eating. In fact many say that nothing relieves school- or work-related stress like a good workout. What we're trying to say is do whatever it takes to stay motivated. Once the bug bites your biggest problem won't be finding time to work out but trying to control the addiction.

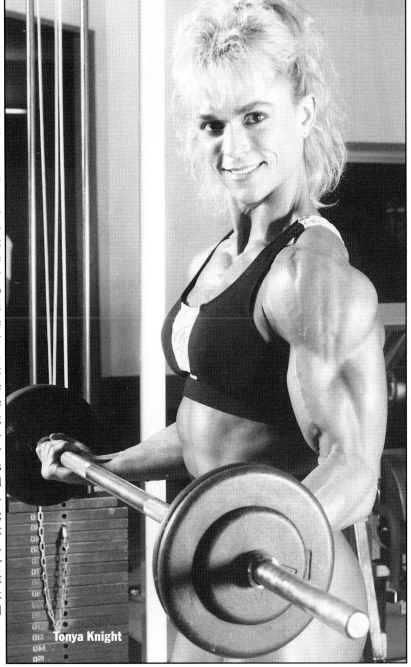
Tonya Knight

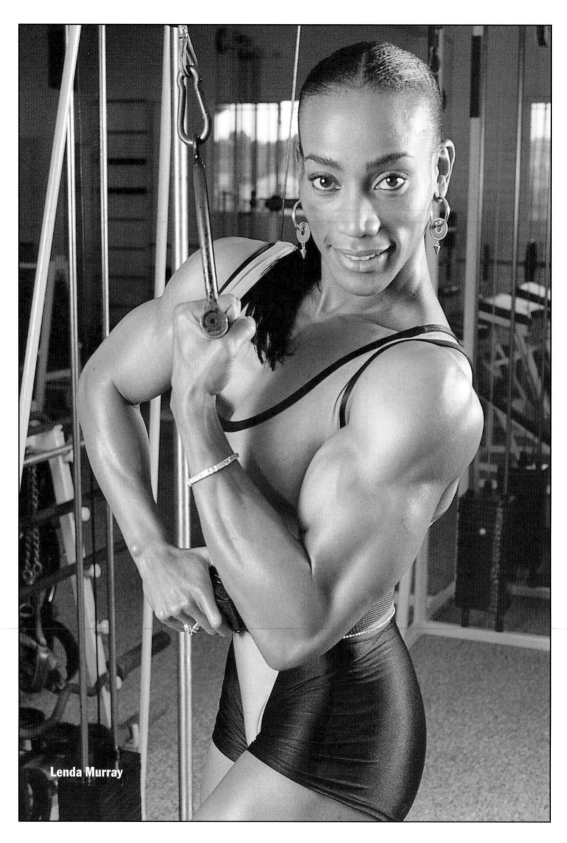

Lenda Murray

Book Three
Almost There!

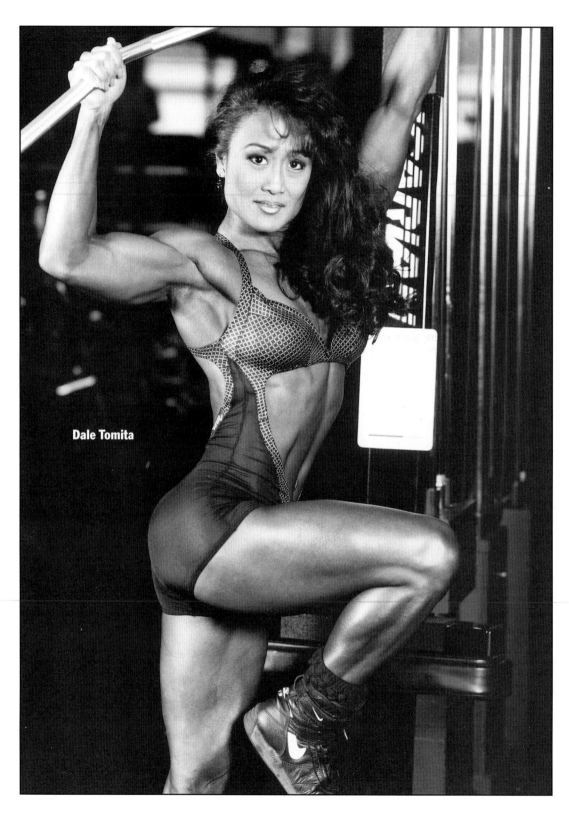

Dale Tomita

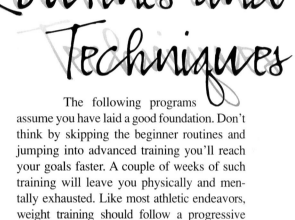

Chapter 11
Advanced Training Routines and Techniques

Congratulations and welcome to the advanced level of training. By now the gym should no longer intimidate you. We told you it wouldn't be long before training became an important part of your life. By now, chances are, beginners are coming to you for advice!

In the following chapter we're going to outline various techniques and routines that will shock your muscles into new growth. Beginner routines are fine but now you've reached the point where your muscles have become complacent. They're used to doing the same exercises week after week, month after month. It's time to employ strategies to catch them off guard.

The following programs assume you have laid a good foundation. Don't think by skipping the beginner routines and jumping into advanced training you'll reach your goals faster. A couple of weeks of such training will leave you physically and mentally exhausted. Like most athletic endeavors, weight training should follow a progressive and systematic format. First we crawl, then we walk, and then we run.

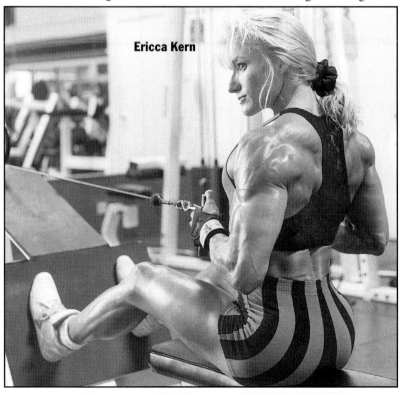

Ericca Kern

Everybody who has trained with weights for any period longer than a year knows that what worked on the first day, doesn't always produce the same results on the 365th day. By changing your exercise routine to accommodate what your body has become accustomed to, you may easily avoid or overcome a plateau.

Robert Kennedy, publisher and best-selling author

ADVANCED TRAINING TECHNIQUES
CHEAT REPS

Cheat reps are one of the first training techniques people learn to employ, but they're also one of the most abused. It may sound like a contradiction, but cheating can be constructive. For example, pick a weight for barbell curls that only allows 10 reps in good style. As soon as you fail on the tenth rep gently swing the weight up using the thighs and lower-back muscles. The key is to cheat just enough to keep the weight moving.

I want to shock the muscles. Your muscles get used to the same routines. When they do, you stop getting results. You have to hit them in different ways from different angles.

Mia Finnegan, 1995 Ms. Fitness Olympia and *Oxygen* columnist

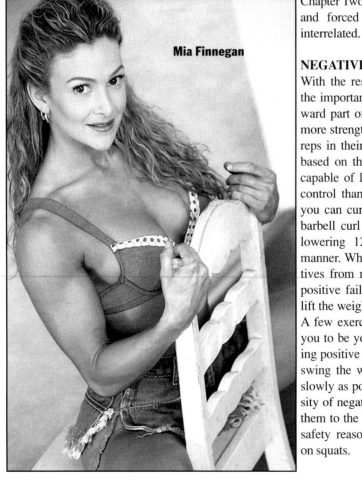

Mia Finnegan

Unfortunately, many abuse cheating and start swinging from the very first rep. You should be able to perform about 80 percent of your reps in strict style. Cheating right from the start defeats the purpose of the technique.

FORCED REPS

Forced reps are probably one of the simplest advanced training techniques one can learn. Many stumble onto it by accident. In the bench press, a forced rep is employed when your partner provides a couple of pounds of upward pressure, enabling you to compete a couple of extra reps after reaching positive failure. If the description sounds familiar it's because we touched on spotting in Chapter Two. Spotting and forced reps are interrelated.

You don't have to include forced reps in every workout, and many successful trainers never employ forced reps.

Robert Kennedy, *MuscleMag* founder and publisher

NEGATIVE REPS

With the research these days indicating the importance of the negative or downward part of a rep, you'll see more and more strength trainers including negative reps in their routines. Negative reps are based on the principle that a muscle is capable of lowering more weight under control than it can lift. For example, if you can curl 80 pounds in the standing barbell curl you're probably capable of lowering 120 to 140 in a controlled manner. While you can start doing negatives from rep one, most trainers go to positive failure and then have a partner lift the weight back up at the end of a set. A few exercises like barbell curls allow you to be your own spotter. After reaching positive failure use the upper body to swing the weight up and then lower as slowly as possible. Because of the intensity of negative reps we suggest limiting them to the last set of each exercise. For safety reasons, don't perform negatives on squats.

I believe in feeling the weight all the way up and all the way down. I believe in keeping tension on the muscle, so sometimes the weight isn't moved all the way up to lockout but close to it.

Sherilyn Godreau, fitness champion

PYRAMIDING

Pyramiding is the training technique where weight is added for the first couple of sets, and then decreased for the remaining sets. The following is a sample bench-press pyramid:

SET 1	50 lb x 15 reps
SET 2	75 lb x 12 reps
SET 3	100 lb x 8 reps
SET 4	75 lb x 12 reps
SET 5	50 lb x 15 reps

The reps decrease on the front slope of the pyramid, while on the back slope the weight decreases and the reps increase. Such a training style has two advantages. The high reps at the beginning serve to fully warm the muscle before the use of heavier weight. The high and low reps serve to hit the different fiber types.

Many weight trainers modify the previous and perform half-pyramids. For example:

FRONT-SLOPE PYRAMID

SET 1	60 lb x 15 reps
SET 2	80 lb x 12 reps
SET 3	100 lb x 10 reps
SET 4	120 lb x 8 reps
SET 5	150 lb x 6 reps

BACK-SLOPE PYRAMID

SET 1	85 lb x 8 reps
SET 2	60 lb x 10 reps
SET 3	45 lb x 12 reps
SET 4	25 lb x 15 reps

Of the two, the front slope is safer as you start with your lightest weight. If such training has a disadvantage it's that the muscle may tire out before you reach the heaviest weight. Back-slope pyramids allow you to start with your heaviest weight; however, the issue

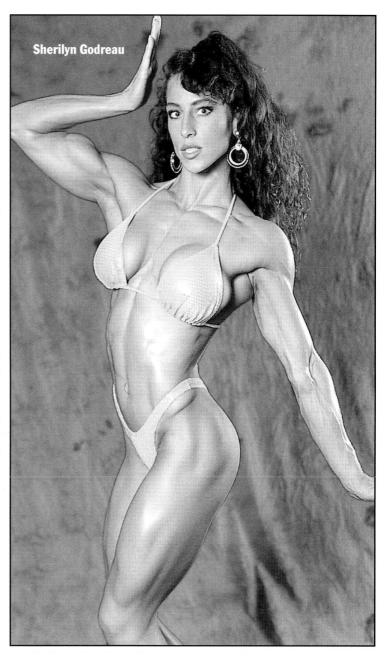

Sherilyn Godreau

of safety arises. Even if you want to start with heavy weight, we strongly recommend doing one or two light warmup sets just to get the blood into the muscles.

SUPERSETS

Supersets are a great way to increase the intensity of your workout without spending extra time in the gym. You can hit the muscles harder in a shorter time period. Supersetting is gym jargon for the alteration of two exercises

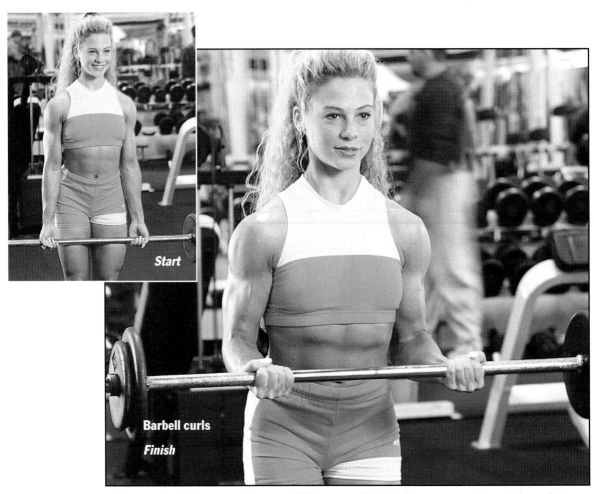

Start

Barbell curls

Finish

without resting in between. Supersets fall into two categories – those for the same muscles and those for opposing muscles. The following are examples of both:

I think they are great, but with conditions. I do not think they are appropriate for beginners. And I think supersets should not be done all the time, or at least not all the time for every muscle group.

Greg Zulak,
former *MuscleMag* editor
and columnist

SAME MUSCLES	
Chest	– Flat flyes
	– Incline presses
Back	– Wide pulldowns
	– Narrow pulldowns
Shoulders	– Lateral raises
	– Upright rows
Biceps	– Incline curls
	– Barbell curls
Triceps	– Pushdowns
	– Bench dips

OPPOSING MUSCLES	
Chest	– Bench presses
Back	– Chinups
Quads	– Leg extensions
Hams	– Leg curls
Biceps	– EZ-bar curls
Triceps	– Lying extensions

TRISETS

For variety and intensity nothing beats trisets. As the name implies, trisets involve performing three exercises back to back for the same muscle group. As with supersets try not to rest between exercises. This means you will have to drop the weight on the last two exercises, but you don't need to use the same weight to get the same effect. That's the beauty of trisets. Examples of trisets include:

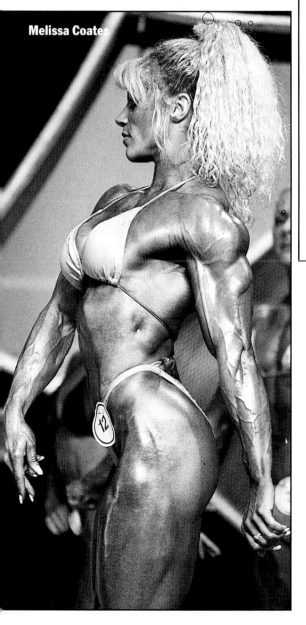

Melissa Coates

MUSCLE	TRISETS
Chest	Flat-bench barbell presses
	Incline flyes
	Pec-deks
Back	Lat pulldowns
	Seated rows
	Straight-arm pushdowns
Shoulders	Dumbell presses
	Lateral raises
	Upright rows
Quads	Squats
	Leg presses
	Leg extensions
Hams	Lying curls
	Stiff-leg deadlifts
	Hyperextensions
Biceps	Barbell curls
	Incline curls
	Narrow reverse chinups
Triceps	Pushdowns
	Lying extensions
	Bench dips
Abdominals	Crunches
	Reverse Crunches
	Leg raises

Regular trisets are done with light to moderate-light weight, with no rest between exercises and a minute or less between trisets.

Greg Zulak, *MuscleMag* columnist

GIANT SETS

Upping the level of intensity involves putting four or more exercises together. Not only are giant sets a great way to blast stubborn muscles but they give the cardio system a great workout as well. The intensity of giant sets is such that you should only include them in your training every third or fourth workout. Also, limit them to the larger muscles groups like the legs, chest, back, and shoulders. The latter is a great candidate for giant sets as you can do separate exercises for each of the three deltoid heads plus one for the trapezius.

REST PAUSE

Rest pause is based on the principle that an exercising muscle carried to positive failure can regain about 90 percent of its strength in about ten seconds. To perform a set of rest pause, carry the set to positive failure, and then wait ten seconds. Resume the exercise trying to force out as many additional reps as possible. The key is to use the same weight you performed the initial set with. The 10-second rest should allow for an additional three to five reps.

PRE-EXHAUST

First discussed by MuscleMag's own Bob Kennedy in the late 1960s, pre-exhaust is a great way to circumvent the various weak links that exist with many exercises. For example, when doing flat-bench presses it's usually the front shoulders and triceps that give out before the larger chest muscles. Pre-exhaust gets around this by tiring the chest muscles first with an isolation exercise like flat flyes. When you perform bench presses for the chest, the triceps and shoulders are no longer the weak links. The following are pre-exhaust combinations you can try:

By using the pre-exhaust principle you can force your lats to work harder than normal. I suggest you pre-exhaust the lats by performing either high-rep sets of barbell or dumbell pullovers or straight-arm pulldowns prior to every set of reverse rows.

Greg Zulak, former *MuscleMag* editor and columnist

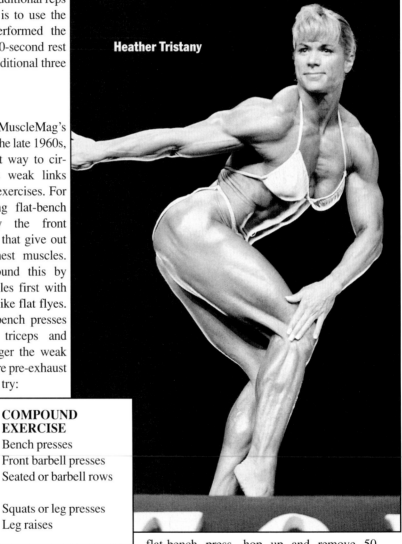

Heather Tristany

MUSCLE	ISOLATION EXERCISE	COMPOUND EXERCISE
Chest	Flat flyes	Bench presses
Shoulders	Lateral raises	Front barbell presses
Back	Straight-arm pushdowns	Seated or barbell rows
Quads	Leg extensions	Squats or leg presses
Abs	Crunches	Leg raises

DROP OR STRIP SETS

One of the easiest training techniques, drop or strip sets, involve dropping the weight after carrying a set to positive failure, and then performing an additional few reps. For example, after going to failure with 135 pounds on the flat-bench press, hop up and remove 50 pounds and then continue the set for a few additional reps. You can do the same with dumbells or machines. The term strip set applies to barbells and drop set applies to dumbells. Either term can apply to working out on a machine.

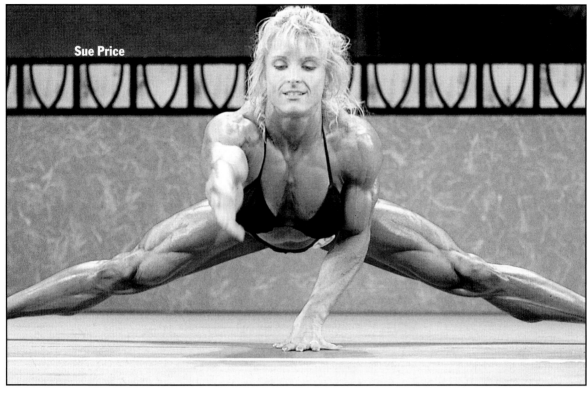
Sue Price

STAGGERED SETS

While staggered sets don't increase training intensity they do allow you to perform extra work for lagging muscle groups. Let's say your calves are lagging behind. While resting between sets for another muscle group, go over to the calf machine and bang out 15 to 20 reps. One of the nice things about calf training is while the little suckers hurt like the dickens, they don't take much out of you. Alternating calves with other muscles doesn't decrease your training intensity.

Besides the calves you can do staggered sets for the forearms. Just don't do them with a major upper-body muscle. Let's face it, most exercises require a strong grip and tiring the forearms will decrease your gripping power. We suggest staggering forearms with lower-body muscles.

TWENTY-ONE'S

This technique is one of the best ways to shock lagging muscles groups, particularly flexor muscles like the biceps and hamstrings.

To perform 21's start by curling a barbell from the thighs up to the halfway point. Do seven reps in this manner and on the seventh rep curl the weight all the way up and then lower to the halfway point seven additional times. To complete the set try to force out seven additional reps curling the barbell through the full range of motion. Because of the intensity of 21's you'll need to drop the weight (about 75 percent of what you'd normally use for straight curls). The number 21 is arbitrary and you can do 18's (3x6) or 24's (3x8).

EXTENDED SETS

Extended sets are another great way to carry a muscle past the point of positive failure. In simple terms extended sets are based on the principle that a muscle can be brought to failure by hitting it from one angle and still be capable of additional reps from another angle. For example, after reaching positive failure on lying triceps extensions, switch over and rep out on narrow presses. Not only are the triceps stronger in the pressing motion but the front delts and chest can assist the triceps as they become fatigued. The following are extended set combinations you can incorporate into your training. You'll notice that all the exercises involve using the same piece of equipment for both exercises. This way you can switch from one to the next in a matter of seconds.

MUSCLE	FIRST EXERCISE	SECOND EXERCISE
Chest	Dumbell flyes	Dumbell presses
Back	Wide chins	Narrow chins
Shoulders	Lateral raises	Dumbell presses
Legs	Barbell lunges	Squats
Biceps	Preacher curls	Standing barbell curls
Triceps	Lying EZ-bar extensions	Narrow presses
Abs	Crunches	Reverse crunches

I train six days a week, working one bodypart per day. On my day off from weights I'll do some form of cross-training.

Kiana Tom, of *Kiana's Flex Appeal*

ADVANCED ROUTINES

Perhaps the biggest disadvantage to training the whole body during one session is that by the time you reach the last couple of muscles you're too tired to do them justice. You could try switching things around and doing arms first but then your large torso muscles would suffer as the arms are involved in most torso exercises. The way to get around this is by splitting the body into sections and training different muscles on different days. By doing two or three workouts you only have to train two or three

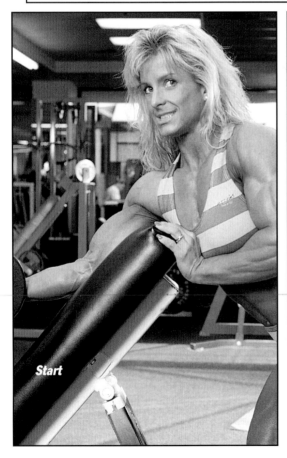

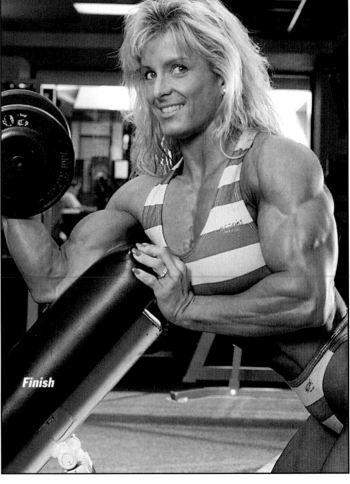

Sue Price demonstrates preacher curls.

Start

Finish

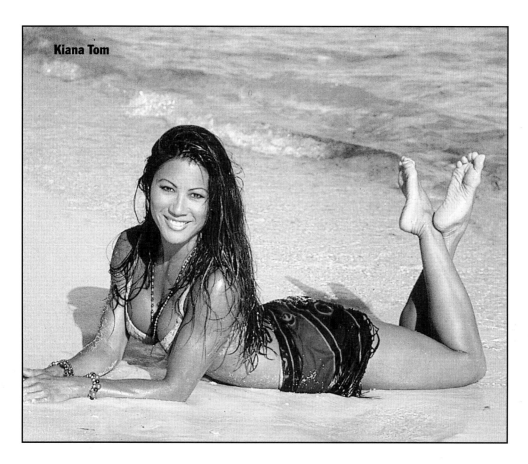

Kiana Tom

muscles per session. This means you can hit all the muscles with equal intensity. In the following section we'll present different split routines that can be followed to increase your workout intensity. For the first couple of weeks we suggest doing straight sets. Then start incorporating some of the advanced techniques outlined in the previous section.

FOUR-DAY SPLIT ROUTINES

The four-day split routine is the most common routine seen in gyms. It requires you to perform two different workouts on two different days. Its most common form is the two-on, one-off, two-on schedule. Another popular version is to workout Monday and Tuesday, take Wednesday off, repeat the routines on Thursday and Friday, and then take the weekend off. Although there's no magic way to combine muscle groups, try to train the same

number of muscle groups on both days. It wouldn't make sense to train legs, back, and chest on one day as these are the three largest muscle groups in the body. The following are examples of four-day split routines. We suggest alternating them every six to eight weeks. Depending on the equipment in your gym, you may have to modify the exercises.

ROUTINE 1

DAY 1 LEGS/ARMS

EXERCISE	SETS	REPS
Leg presses	3	10-12
Leg extensions	3	10-12
Leg curls	3	10-12
Adductions	3	10-12
Calf raises	3	15-20
Barbell curls	3	10-12
Incline curls	3	10-12
Triceps pushdowns	3	10-12
Lying dumbell extensions	3	10-12

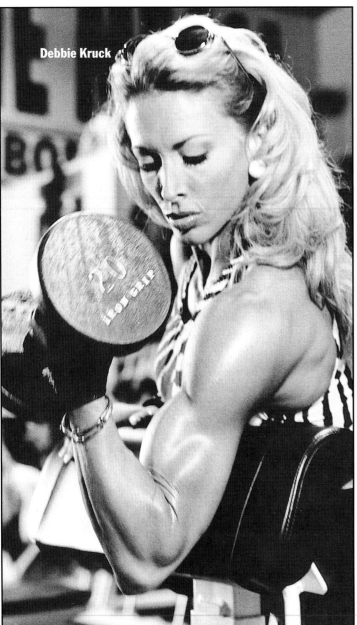
Debbie Kruck

ROUTINE 2

DAY 1 CHEST/BACK/BICEPS

EXERCISE	SETS	REPS
Incline barbell presses	3	10-12
Flat dumbell flyes	3	10-12
Barbell rows	3	10-12
Chins	3	10-12
Preacher curls	3	10-12
Concentration curls	3	10-12
Reverse crunches	3	20-30
Crunches	3	20-30

DAY 2 LEGS/SHOULDERS/TRICEPS

EXERCISE	SETS	REPS
Squats	3	10-12
Lunges	3	10-12
Stiff-leg deadlifts	3	10-12
Toe presses	3	15-20
Front machine presses	3	10-12
Cable lateral raises	3	10-12
Upright rows	3	10-12
Lying EZ-bar extensions	3	10-12
Kickbacks	3	10-12

ROUTINE 3

DAY 1 THIGHS/CHEST/SHOULDERS/TRICEPS

EXERCISE	SETS	REPS
Leg presses	3	10-12
Hack squats	3	10-12
Leg extensions	3	10-12
Incline barbell presses	3	10-12
Flat dumbell presses	3	10-12
Dumbell presses	3	10-12
Lateral raises	3	10-12
Shrugs	3	10-12

DAY 2 CHEST/BACK/SHOULDERS

EXERCISE	SETS	REPS
Flat barbell presses	3	10-12
Incline flyes	3	10-12
Wide front pulldowns	3	10-12
Seated rows	3	10-12
Dumbell presses	3	10-12
Lateral raises	3	10-12
Reverse pec-deks	3	10-12
Lying leg raises	3	20-30
Crunches	3	20-30

DAY 2 BACK/HAMSTRINGS/BICEPS/CALVES/ABS

EXERCISE	SETS	REPS
Narrow pulldowns	3	10-12
One-arm rows	3	10-12
Leg curls	3	10-12
Stiff-leg deadlifts	3	10-12
Barbell curls	3	10-12
Cable curls	3	10-12
Standing calf raises	3	15-20
Seated calf raises	3	15-20
Hanging leg raises	3	20-30
Machine crunches	3	20-30

SIX-DAY SPLIT ROUTINES

For those who become addicted to exercise the six-day split is for you. The main advantage of six-day training is that you only have to hit two muscles per workout. This enables you to do more for each muscle. Keep in mind that training six out of seven days is very taxing on the body's recovery system. Even the top pros only follow such training in the few months leading up to a contest. Our advice is to limit six-day training to four- to five-week stretches.

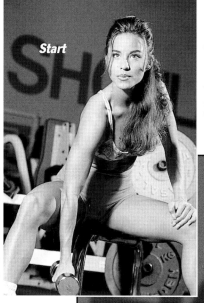
Start

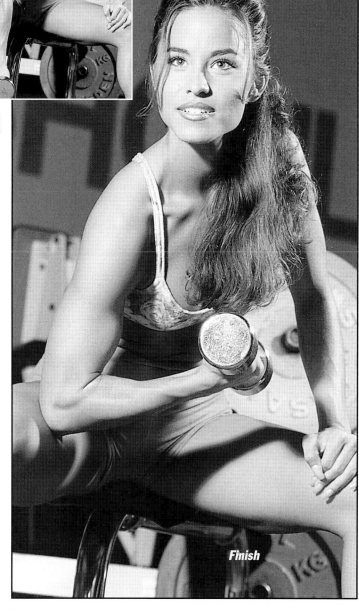

Choose a routine that fits into your weekly schedule. You'll be more likely to stick with it. – Angel Teves performs concentration curls.

Finish

ROUTINE 1

DAY 1 CHEST/BACK

EXERCISE	SETS	REPS
Flat barbell presses	3	10-12
Incline dumbell flyes	3	10-12
Cable crossovers	3	10-12
Barbell rows	3	10-12
Wide front pulldowns	3	10-12
One-arm rows	3	10-12

DAY 2 SHOULDERS/ARMS

Front machine presses	3	10-12
Side dumbell laterals	3	10-12
Reverse pec-deks	3	10-12
Lying EZ-bar extensions	3	10-12
Pushdowns	3	10-12
Barbell curls	3	10-12
Incline dumbell curls	3	10-12

DAY 3 LEGS/ABS

EXERCISE	SETS	REPS
Squats	3	10-12
Leg extensions	3	10-12
Leg curls	3	10-12
Adductions	3	10-12
Standing calf raises	3	10-12
Crunches	3	20-30
Reverse crunches	3	20-30
Leg raises	3	20-30

ROUTINE 2

DAY 1 CHEST/SHOULDERS

EXERCISE	SETS	REPS
Incline barbell presses	3	10-12
Flat flyes	3	10-12
Pec-deks	3	10-12
Smith presses	3	10-12
Cable lateral raises	3	10-12
Dumbell shrugs	3	10-12

DAY 2 THIGHS/TRICEPS

EXERCISE	SETS	REPS
Leg presses	3	10-12
Hack squats	3	10-12
Cable/machine adductions	3	10-12
Lying dumbell extensions	3	10-12
Bench dips	3	10-12

DAY 3 HAMSTRINGS/BICEPS/BACK

EXERCISE	SETS	REPS
Seated rows	3	10-12
Chins	3	10-12
Straight-arm pushdowns	3	10-12
Lying leg curls	3	10-12
Stiff-leg deadlifts	3	10-12
Preacher curls	3	10-12
Concentration curls	3	10-12

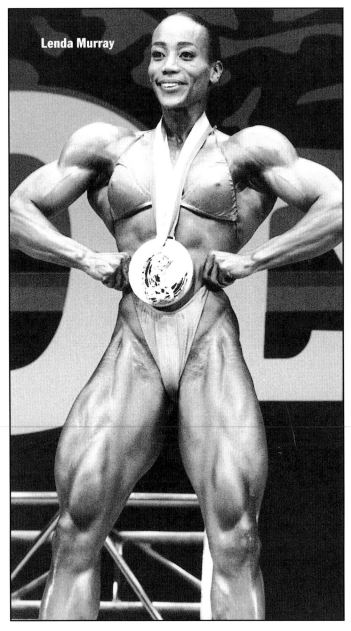

Lenda Murray

TWO-WEEK SPLIT ROUTINE

The two-week split is a variation of the four-day split. It's beneficial for those who want to split the body up, but can only make it to the gym three days a week. Instead of following a traditional seven-day week, you work the same muscles three times over two weeks. The following is an example.

WEEK 1

Monday	Chest, back, shoulders
Tuesday	Legs and arms
Friday	Chest, back, shoulders

WEEK 2

Monday	Legs and arms
Tuesday	Chest, back, shoulders
Friday	Legs and arms

During week one you hit one group of muscles twice, and the other group only once. The following week you reverse things around. If you are stuck for time, or feel overtrained after four workouts a week, a two-week split routine may be just what you need. During a 14-day cycle you only work out six times.

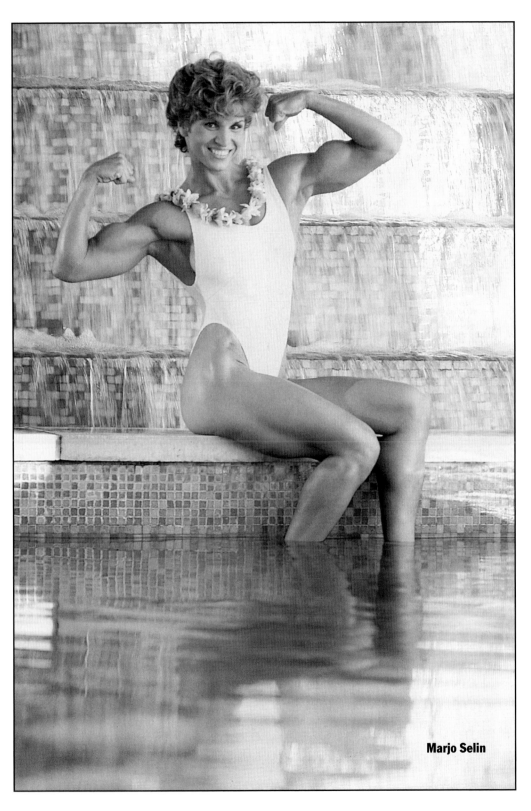

Marjo Selin

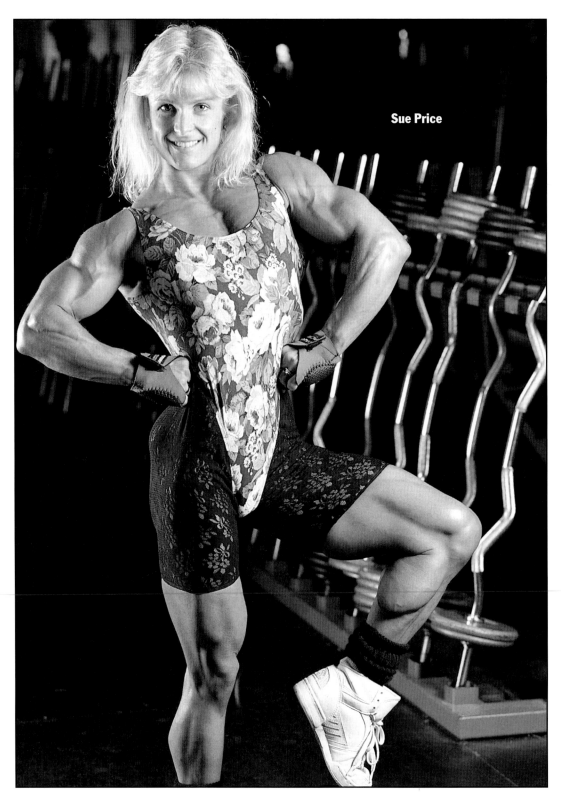

Sue Price

Chapter 12
High-Intensity Training

It's safe to say most weight trainers are their own worst enemies. They attempt to emulate their favorite fitness or bodybuilding stars by following routines only designed for the most genetically and pharmacologically enhanced. Unfortunately, they quickly become overtrained. But instead of reducing training volume, they increase it! This leads to further overtraining. The end result is a vicious circle leading to despair. One of the ways around this is to switch to high-intensity/low-volume training.

High-intensity training received its first big endorsement back in the late 1960s and early 1970s by Dr. Arthur Jones – best known as the inventor of the Nautilus line of training equipment. After careful observation and research, Dr. Jones came to the conclusion that most athletes, particularly bodybuilders, were in a constant state of overtraining. They were doing far more high-volume exercise than was needed. Not only were they not making progress but in many cases they were going backwards! Going against the accepted training principles of the time, Dr. Jones reasoned that workouts must be both intense and brief. The two concepts go together as an intense workout must be brief. Despite his best efforts, Dr. Jones never convinced many trainers of the soundness of his ideas and the concept moved to the background.

> *I read a lot by Mike Mentzer on heavy-duty training. I read a lot of stuff by Arthur Jones, who is the inventor of the Nautilus machines. I saw a lot of logic in that kind of training. I started with low sets and I noticed that when I increased the number of sets or frequency beyond a certain level, very quickly I would become overtrained.*
>
> **Dorian Yates, six-time Mr. Olympia**

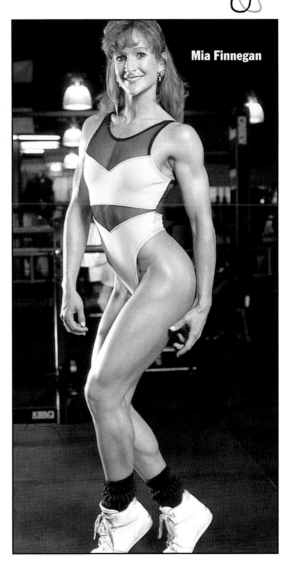

Mia Finnegan

In the late 1970s and early 1980s (and since revived in *Natural Muscular Development* magazine) high-intensity training received a second boost from former Mr. America and Mr. Universe, Mike Mentzer. Mike expanded on Dr. Jones' ideas and packaged them under the title Heavy Duty. Like Dr. Jones, Mike suggested that four to six days a week was far too much training for the average individual. Yet despite a regular col-

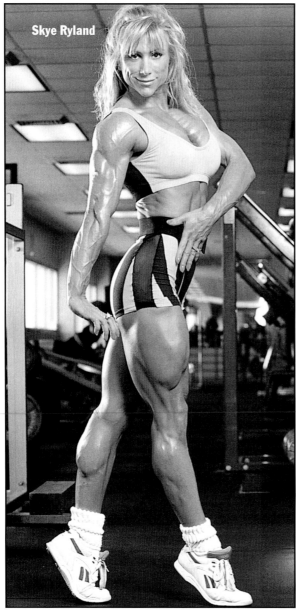

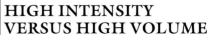
Skye Ryland

umn in *Muscle and Fitness* magazine, and numerous guest lectures and seminars, Mike's ideas never became mainstream. It is only in recent years that hardcore strength trainers have begun to take a closer look at Heavy Duty, and this is primarily due to the words of the current Mr. Olympia, Dorian Yates.

While never admitting his training style is based solely on Mike's ideas, Dorian nevertheless borrowed heavily from them. Where Mike suggests one to two sets total per muscle group, Dorian usually performs three to four high-intensity sets – a far cry from the 20 to 25 sets that was the norm back in the 1960s and 1970s. Other bodybuilders have followed Dorian's lead. If you go into any gym you'll see numerous weight trainers putting all their effort into 45- to 60-minute routines.

HIGH INTENSITY VERSUS HIGH VOLUME

Before outlining some high-intensity programs we thought it interesting to compare the two types of training styles. We should add that despite its growing popularity most weight trainers still follow the high-volume training method. It will be interesting to see if the same can be said 10 years from now.

The main advantage to high-intensity training is the decreased drain it places on the recovery system. For most individuals 45 to 60 minutes is the maximum the body can sustain intense exercise. After that you're mainly going through the motions and reducing the body's ability to recover for the next workout.

The second advantage to high-intensity training is the reduced time spent in the gym. Averaging 20 to 25 minutes a day, two to three days a week, you are left with a lot of extra time on your hands. Think of what you can accomplish with the time saved. There's no reason to be spending two to three hours, six to seven days a week working out.

A final advantage to high-intensity training concerns its effects on energy levels. Two-hour workouts often leave the individual physically drained and exhausted. On the other hand high-intensity/low-volume training will let you leave the gym with energy to spare – much of which will be used to speed up recovery between workouts.

One set per muscle group taken to failure does not maximize the tension in a muscle. Only multiple sets will do that.

Robert Kennedy, *MuscleMag* **founder and publisher**

Now that we've got you sold on high-intensity training, we should put forward a few reasons against it. Perhaps the biggest complaint against high intensity is it's not enough! Many top trainers, including Charles Poliquin, argue that there's no way the average individual can adequately stimulate a muscle with one or two sets. It takes multiple sets to recruit all the different muscle fibers in the muscle. And while 20 to 25 sets is far too many, switching to the other extreme does not make sense either.

The second supposed strike against high intensity is it's not much fun. This argument holds some merit. Let's face it, weightlifting is as much social as physical. A 20-minute workout does not leave much time for socializing. The one- to two-hour workout at the end of the day can be a great source of stress relief.

A third strike against high intensity is it doesn't do much to stimulate the cardiovascular system. This argument is valid as research suggests the higher-volume approach does more for the cardio system than originally thought. The high-intensity advocates counter that it's a matter of priorities, and the time saved on training allows time for extra cardio work if desired.

IS IT FOR ME?

Unlike some proponents of high intensity we are not going to say it's the only way to train. But we will admit nothing halts progress like overtraining. If your high-volume training is yielding little or no results, the answer may be less training, not more. The following routines

can be completed in 15 to 20 minutes, two to three times per week. In order to get the most from them, carry every set to positive failure. And resist the urge to add sets to the program. This defeats the purpose of high-intensity training. Save that extra energy for recovery.

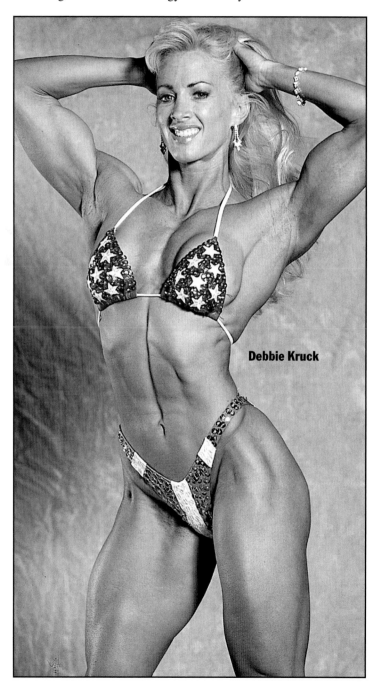

Debbie Kruck

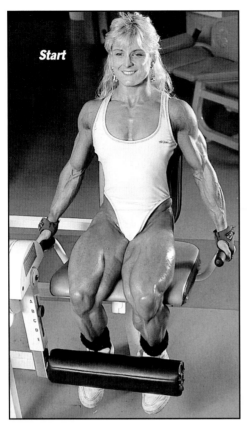

Start

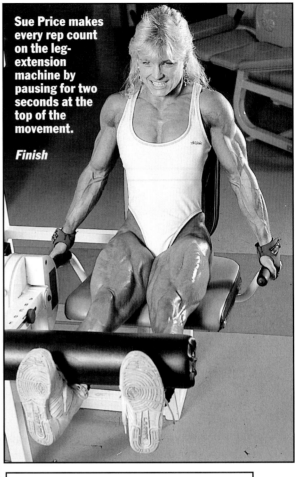

Sue Price makes every rep count on the leg-extension machine by pausing for two seconds at the top of the movement.

Finish

HIGH-INTENSITY ROUTINES

FULL-BODY WORKOUT

LEGS

EXERCISE	SETS	REPS
Leg extensions	1	10-12
Superset with:		
Leg presses or squats	1	10-12
Leg curls	1	10-12
Superset with:		
Stiff-leg deadlifts	1	10-12
Standing calf raises	1	15-20
+ two strip sets		

CHEST

Flat dumbell flyes	1	10-12
Superset with:		
Incline barbell presses	1	10-12

BACK

Chinups	1	10-12
Superset with:		
Seated rows	1	10-12

SHOULDERS

Lateral raises	1	10-12
Superset with:		
Dumbell presses	1	10-12

BICEPS

Barbell curls	1	10-12
+ rest pause set		

TRICEPS

Lying EZ-bar extensions	1	10-12
Superset with:		
Narrow presses	1	to failure

ABS

Crunches	1	20-30
Superset with:		
Reverse crunches	1	to failure

SPLIT ROUTINE – ONE DAY ON, ONE DAY OFF
DAY 1
LEGS

EXERCISE	SETS	REPS
Leg presses	1	10-12
+ rest pause set		
Leg extensions	1	10-12
+ 2 strip sets		
Leg curls	1 set of 21's	
Stiff-leg deadlifts	1	10-12
Seated calf raises	1	15-20
Superset with:		
Standing calf raises	1	15-20

BICEPS

Incline curls	1	10-12
Superset with:		
Preacher curls	1	10-12

TRICEPS

Pushdowns	1	10-12
Superset with:		
Bench dips	1	to failure

DAY 2
CHEST

EXERCISE	SETS	REPS
Incline flyes	1	10-12
Superset with:		
Flat barbell presses	1	10-12

BACK

Wide front pulldowns	1	10-12
Superset with:		
Narrow reverse pulldowns	1	10-12

SHOULDERS

Dumbell side laterals	1	10-12
Barbell front presses	1	10-12

Mia Finnegan shapes her shoulders with dumbell presses.

CONCLUSION

The purpose of so many supersets is to both save time and increase intensity. Besides supersets you can incorporate many of the other training techniques found in the advanced training chapter. With regards to the reps, we have chosen 10 to 12 as most readers are interested in muscle tone rather than building muscle size. If your goal is the latter, drop the reps to six to eight and increase the weight accordingly.

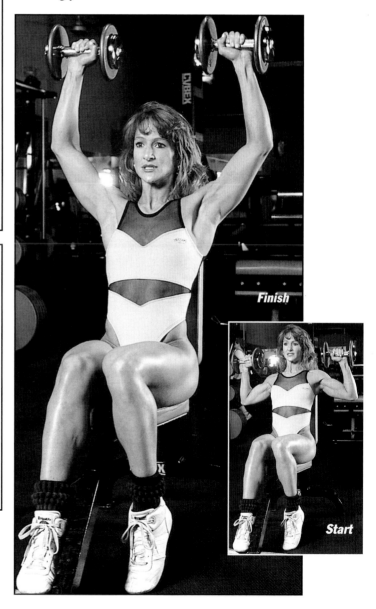

Finish

Start

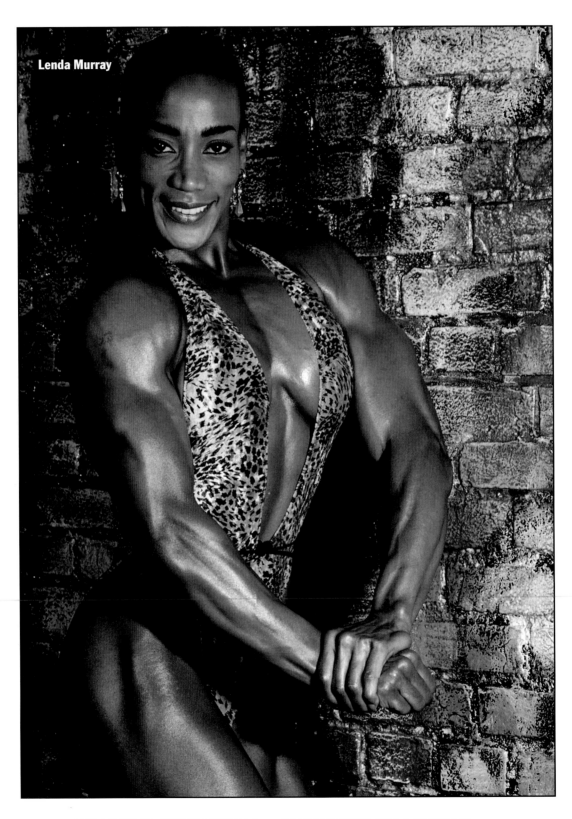

Lenda Murray

Chapter 13
Priority Training

SPECIALIZED PROGRAMS FOR STUBBORN MUSCLES

Although the programs outlined in this book have been designed to train the entire body, it will become apparent after a few months that some areas respond better than others. For females the inner thighs can be the source of much anguish. When a muscle group refuses to cooperate it's time to target it with a specialized training program. The following routines are not designed to be followed year-round. Instead, incorporate them into your routine for four to six weeks. At the same time cut back your training on muscles that have been quick to respond. As soon as the lagging muscle is brought up to par, you can switch back to your regular training routine. By this time another group will probably be lagging behind and you'll need to address it. For some, this constant body sculpting is what makes weight training such an exciting form of fitness.

It is normal to make quick gains, reach a point where gains stop for a while (plateau) and then with continued effort, the muscles start growing again. Unfortunately another plateau is eventually reached. Training more intensely and paying more attention to nutrition, rest, and recovery, will get you over that next hurdle.

Robert Kennedy, *Oxygen* publisher and best-selling author

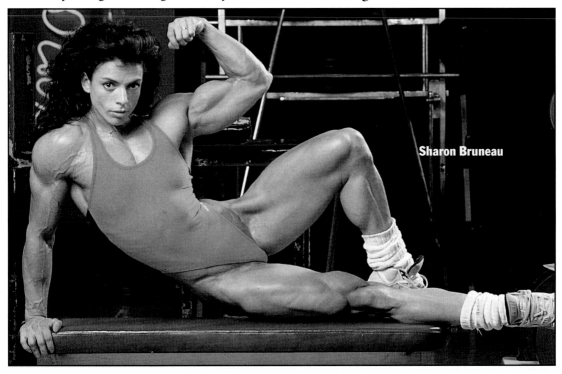

Sharon Bruneau

INNER THIGHS

ROUTINE A

EXERCISE	SETS	REPS
Leg adduction machine	3	12-15
Leg presses	3	12-15
(high and wide foot stance)		
Lunges	3	12-15

ROUTINE B

EXERCISE	SETS	REPS
Squats	3	12-15
(feet wide and pointed slightly outward)		
Cable adductions	3	12-15
Hack squats	3	12-15
(feet high and wide)		

ABS

ROUTINE A – TRISETS

Crunches
Reverse crunches
Ab machine
Perform two trisets with as little rest as possible between exercises. Try for 25 to 30 reps on each set.

ROUTINE B – GIANT SETS

Leg raises
Crunches
Reverse crunches
Hanging leg raises
Rope crunches
Perform 1 to 2 giant sets trying to average 25 to 30 reps per set.

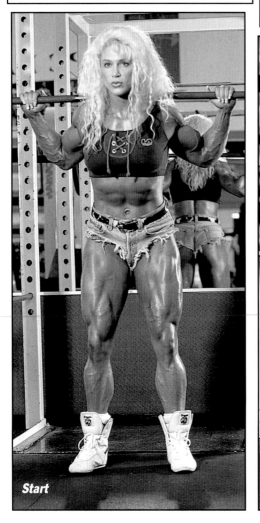

Start

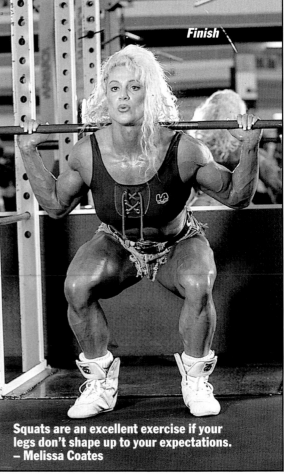

Finish

Squats are an excellent exercise if your legs don't shape up to your expectations. – Melissa Coates

CALVES
ROUTINE A

EXERCISE	SETS	REPS
Standing calf raises	3	15-20
Seated calf raises	3	15-20
Toe presses	3	15-20
Donkey calf raises	3	15-20

While the accepted rep range for calves is high (15 to 20), some individuals may respond better to heavier weight and lower reps (6 to 10).

ROUTINE B
Repeat the above exercises in a giant set.

TRICEPS
ROUTINE A

EXERCISE	SETS	REPS
Lying EZ-bar extensions	3	12-15
Pushdowns	3	12-15
Kickbacks	3	12-15

ROUTINE B

EXERCISE	SETS	REPS
Dumbell extensions	3	12-15
Dips	3	12-15
Narrow presses	3	12-15

SHOULDERS
ROUTINE A

EXERCISE	SETS	REPS
Shoulder rotations	3	12-15
Dumbell presses	3	12-15
Dumbell lateral raises	3	12-15
Reverse pec-deks	3	12-15
Dumbell shrugs	3	12-15

ROUTINE B

EXERCISE	SETS	REPS
Machine presses	3	12-15
Cable lateral raises	3	12-15
Bent-over lateral raises	3	12-15
Upright rows	3	12-15

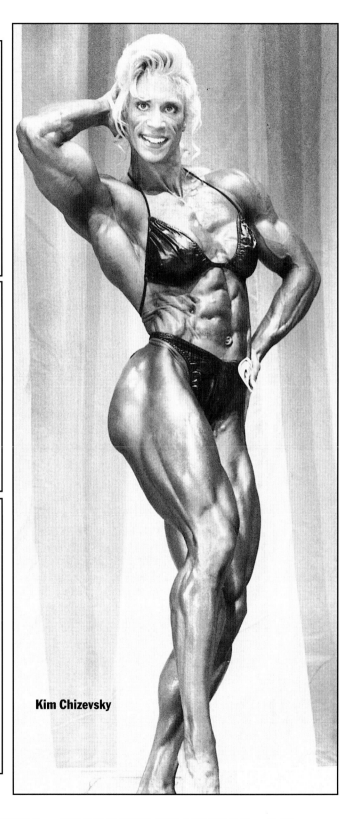

Kim Chizevsky

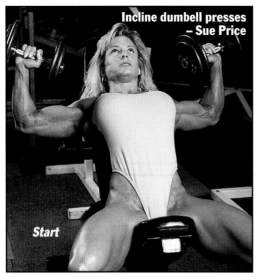

Incline dumbell presses
– Sue Price

Start

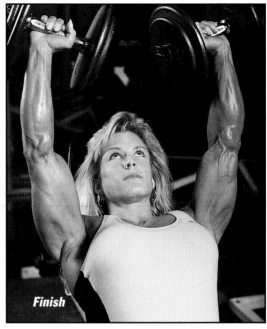

Finish

CHEST

ROUTINE A

EXERCISE	SETS	REPS
Barbell bench presses	3	12-15
Incline dumbell presses	3	12-15
Pec-deks	3	12-15
Pullovers	3	12-15

ROUTINE B

EXERCISE	SETS	REPS
Incline barbell presses	3	12-15
Flat dumbell flyes	3	12-15
Cable crossovers	3	12-15
Decline dumbell presses	3	12-15

BACK

ROUTINE A

EXERCISE	SETS	REPS
Lat pulldowns	3	12-15
Seated rows	3	12-15
T-Bar rows	3	12-15
Straight-arm pushdowns	3	12-15

ROUTINE B

EXERCISE	SETS	REPS
Barbell rows	3	12-15
Chinups	3	12-15
One-arm rows	3	12-15
Narrow pulldowns	3	12-15

HAMSTRINGS

ROUTINE A

EXERCISE	SETS	REPS
Lying leg curls	3	12-15
Stiff-leg deadlifts	3	12-15
Hyperextensions	3	12-15

ROUTINE B

EXERCISE	SETS	REPS
Standing leg curls	3	12-15
Stiff-leg deadlifts	3	12-15
Lying leg curl 21's	2	12-15

BICEPS

ROUTINE A

EXERCISE	SETS	REPS
Barbell curls	3	12-15
Incline dumbell curls	3	12-15
Concentration curls	3	12-15

ROUTINE B

EXERCISE	SETS	REPS
Preacher curls	3	12-15
Standing dumbell curls	3	12-15
Narrow reverse chin *	3	12-15

* As you'll be lifting your bodyweight on this exercise 12 to 15 reps may be optimistic. Perform as many reps as possible up to 15.

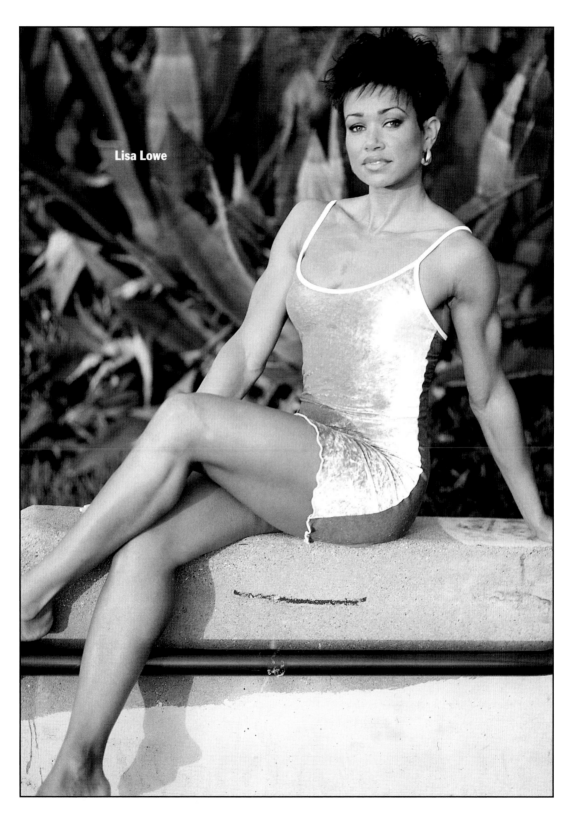

Lisa Lowe

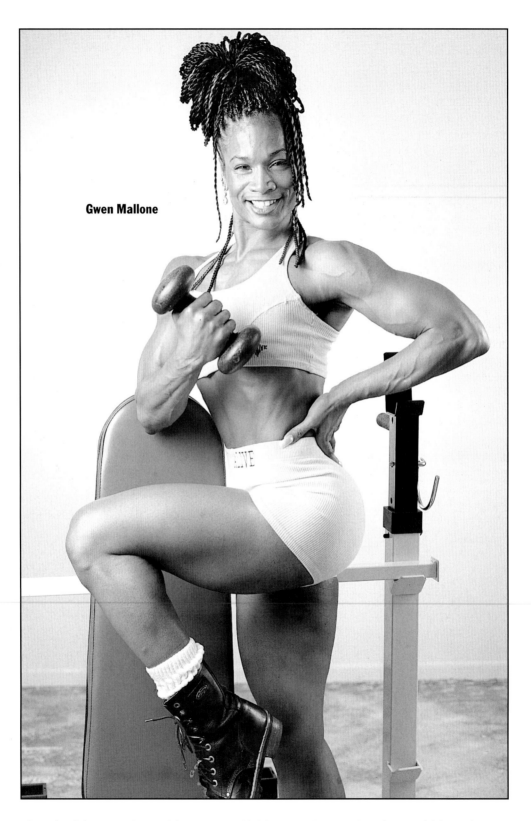

Gwen Mallone

Chapter 14

Staying In Shape At Home

While commercial gyms offer an almost unlimited variety of equipment, practical considerations (time, distance, finances, etc.) may necessitate training at home. But don't despair. You can develop a tremendous physique in the comfort of your own home. Some of the greatest fitness stars and bodybuilders got their start in home gyms. For the investment of a few hundred dollars (less if you hit the right flea market) you can set up a mini gym in your basement or spare room.

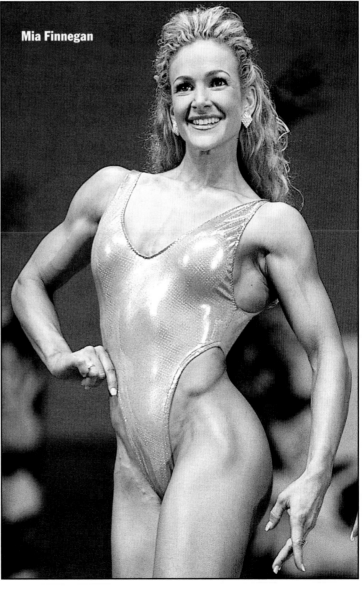

Mia Finnegan

WHAT TO BUY

The nucleus of any home gym is a barbell and dumbell set. Barbell plates designed for home use come in two general forms; solid iron plates and plastic weights. The latter are plastic weight-shaped containers filled with sand or cement. Plastic weights have an advantage in that they're usually much easier on carpet. Of course the purists argue that anything less than iron is sacrilegious! The primary disadvantage to plastic weights is their thickness – usually double that of iron plates. Two hundred to 225 pounds is about the maximum that will fit on a plastic barbell set. For most women this will suffice with the possible exception of squats and deadlifts.

Besides a barbell set you'll need a set of dumbells. You can choose between iron and plastic. If you have the space you can buy several pairs to work all the muscles, or use one pair of adjustable dumbells.

Two other pieces of equipment needed are flat and incline benches. Even better, buy an adjustable bench that goes from 0 to 90 degrees. This one bench will allow you to train most of the muscles of the upper body.

There are many fine exercises you can do at home without specialized equipment such as situps, leg raises, twists, pushups, triceps dips between chairs, lunges, free-hand squats, sissy squats, and calf raises.

Marjo Selin,
former *MuscleMag* columnist

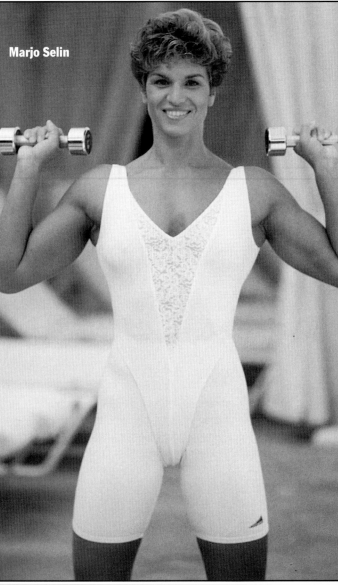

Marjo Selin

While the previous would suffice to work most of the body's muscles, a few additional pieces of equipment will complete your home gym. To give the legs a good workout invest in a squat rack. This will enable you to position the bar at shoulder height thus eliminating having to lift the bar from the floor and lay it on your shoulders. It won't be long before your legs are capable of squatting far more than you can lift from the floor.

You can easily save on the cost of a squat rack by getting someone handy with a blow torch to weld you one out of scrap iron. The authors have seen homemade squat racks that would rival any commercially bought racks.

To round out your home gym, pick up a weightlifting belt, and set of wrist straps. To save time going to the kitchen or bathroom, purchase a large water bottle.

THE ROUTINES

Now that you've set up your home gym, it's time to pump some iron! The programs outlined can be followed three, four, or six days a week. Don't skip the three-day routines in favor of the six thinking the latter will achieve your goals faster. If you don't lay a quality foundation, jumping to an advanced routine will probably burn you out in a few short weeks. It may even set you up for an injury – one of the classic outcomes of overtraining. Three-day routines are more than intense enough for those new to weight training.

THREE-DAY WORKOUTS

Three-day routines require you to hit the full body on three nonconsecutive days during the week. The most popular days being Monday, Wednesday, and Friday, but feel free to train Tuesday, Thursday, and Saturday, or Thursday, Saturday, and Monday.

If you don't lay a quality foundation, jumping to an advanced routine will probably burn you out in a few short weeks. – Kelly Ryan

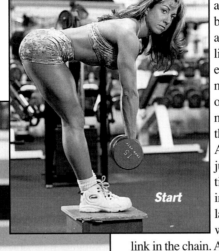

Start

Stiff-leg deadlifts
Finish

The following routines are designed to hit the entire body. They also require access to the equipment outlined earlier. You'll notice the exercises hit the largest muscles to the smallest. This only makes sense as it takes more energy to train the legs than the arms or abdominals. As the arms are required in just about every exercise, tiring them out first only interferes with training the larger muscle groups. In other words, they become the weak link in the chain. Always train the arms, as well as other smaller muscle groups, toward the end of your routine.

ROUTINE 1

LEGS

EXERCISE	SETS	REPS
Squats	3	12-15
Stiff-leg deadlifts	3	12-15
Dumbell calf raises	3	15-20

CHEST

Flat-bench barbell presses	3	12-15
Incline dumbell flyes	3	12-15

BACK

One-arm rows	3	12-15
Dumbell pullovers	3	12-15

SHOULDERS

Side lateral raises	3	12-15
Dumbell presses	3	12-15
Upright rows	3	12-15

BICEPS

Incline dumbell curls	3	12-15

TRICEPS

Kickbacks	3	12-15

ABDOMINALS

Abdominal crunches	3	20-30

ROUTINE 2

LEGS

EXERCISE	SETS	REPS
Lunges	3	12-15
Dumbell deadlifts	3	12-15
Dumbell calf raises	3	15-20

CHEST

Incline presses	3	12-15
Flat flyes	3	12-15

BACK

Two-arm rows	3	12-15
Barbell pullovers	3	12-15

SHOULDERS

Barbell presses	3	12-15
Lying laterals	3	12-15
Bent-over laterals	3	12-15

BICEPS

Barbell curls	3	12-15

TRICEPS

Lying dumbell extensions	3	12-15

ABDOMINALS

Reverse crunches	3	20-30

FOUR-DAY SPLITS

One of the disadvantages of training the whole body in one session is that by the time you reach the last couple of muscles you're too tired to do them justice. The way around this is to split the body over two days and train four times a week. Four-day split routines are probably the most common routines followed by weight trainers. They hit the muscles hard, but allow sufficient (three days) time for recovery. The following are examples of four-day split routines. We suggest changing the combinations every couple of months to keep the body guessing.

Brandi Carrier works her upper chest with incline dumbell presses.

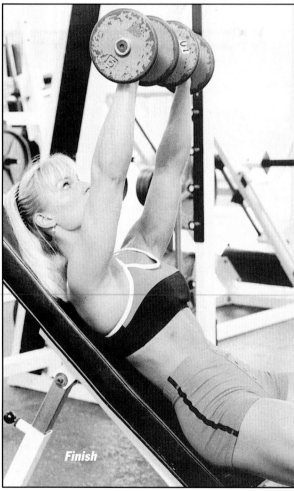

Finish

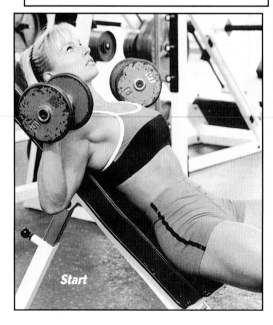

Start

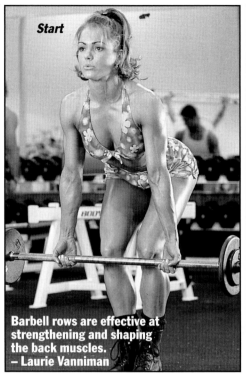

Start

Barbell rows are effective at strengthening and shaping the back muscles. – Laurie Vanniman

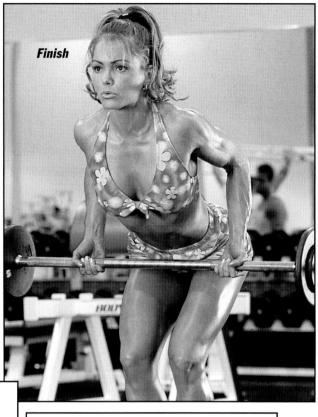

Finish

ROUTINE 1
DAY 1 LEGS/ARMS

EXERCISE	SETS	REPS
Squats	3	12-15
Lunges	3	12-15
Stiff-leg deadlifts	3	12-15
One-leg calf raises	3	12-15
Barbell curls	3	12-15
Incline curls	3	12-15
Kickbacks	3	12-15
One-arm extensions	3	12-15

DAY 2
CHEST/BACK/SHOULDERS/ABS

EXERCISE	SETS	REPS
Incline dumbell presses	3	12-15
Flat dumbell flyes	3	12-15
One-arm rows	3	12-15
Pullovers	3	12-15
Dumbell presses	3	12-15
Side lateral raises	3	12-15
Upright rows	3	12-15
Abdominal crunches	3	15-20
Reverse crunches	3	15-20

ROUTINE 2
DAY 1 CHEST/BACK/BICEPS

EXERCISE	SETS	REPS
Flat barbell presses	3	12-15
Incline dumbell flyes	3	12-15
Barbell rows	3	12-15
One-arm rows	3	12-15
Concentration curls	3	12-15
Standing dumbell curls	3	12-15

DAY 2 LEGS/SHOULDERS/TRICEPS/ABS

EXERCISE	SETS	REPS
Lunges	3	12-15
Stiff-leg deadlifts	3	12-15
Dumbell calf raises	3	15-20
Front dumbell presses	3	12-15
Lateral raises	3	12-15
Bent-over laterals	3	12-15
Lying dumbell extensions	3	12-15
Kickbacks	3	12-15
Abdominal crunches	3	15-20
Reverse crunches	3	15-20

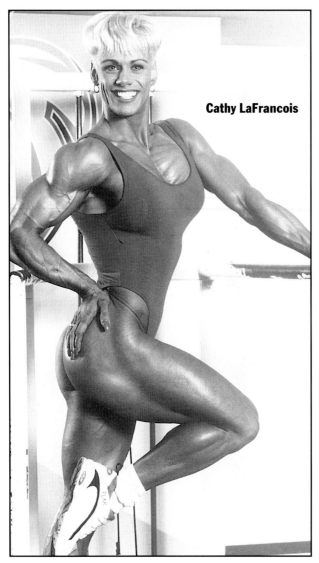

Cathy LaFrancois

If six-day splits have an advantage it's that you only have to hit two muscles per workout – 45 to 60 minutes and you're finished. For those with work and family responsibilities it means only having to find an hour a day to workout.

ROUTINE
DAY 1 LEGS

EXERCISE	SETS	REPS
Squats	3-4	10-12
Lunges	3-4	10-12
Stiff-leg deadlifts	3-4	10-12
One-leg calf raises	3-4	10-12

DAY 2 CHEST/BACK

Incline barbell presses	3-4	10-12
Flat dumbell flyes	3-4	10-12
Dumbell pullovers	3-4	10-12
Barbell rows	3-4	10-12
One-arm rows	3-4	10-12

DAY 3 SHOULDERS/ARMS

Dumbell presses	3-4	10-12
Side lateral raises	3-4	10-12
Upright rows	3-4	10-12
Barbell curls	3-4	10-12
Incline dumbell curls	3-4	10-12
Kickbacks	3-4	10-12
Lying dumbell extensions	3-4	10-12

SIX-DAY-A-WEEK TRAINING

Six-day splits are one of the most advanced forms of training, and, therefore, also one of the most taxing. You generally have two choices when it comes to six-day training. You can work out three days and take a day off, or work out six and take two off. Of the two we suggest the former as six days straight without a break can be too strenuous, except for the genetically blessed or pharmacologically enhanced. Even three on, one off will catch up with you after three to four weeks. We suggest saving six-day splits for precontest training.

The previous routine can be performed by anyone with a minimal amount of equipment. As time goes on, however, you might want to consider expanding. For the cost of $300 to $400 you can purchase multistations that are designed for home training. Most come with leg-curl, leg-extension, lat-pulldown, and shoulder-press attachments. The newer models now have pec-deks attached. For the price of a year's membership at a gym you can set up a complete training area in your basement. Who knows, word may get around and before you know it a new gym chain has started in your own home!

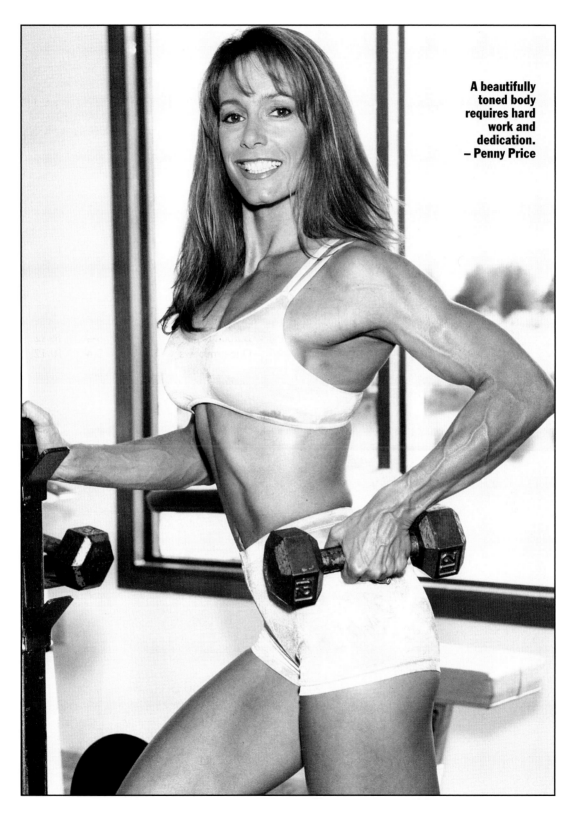

A beautifully toned body requires hard work and dedication.
– Penny Price

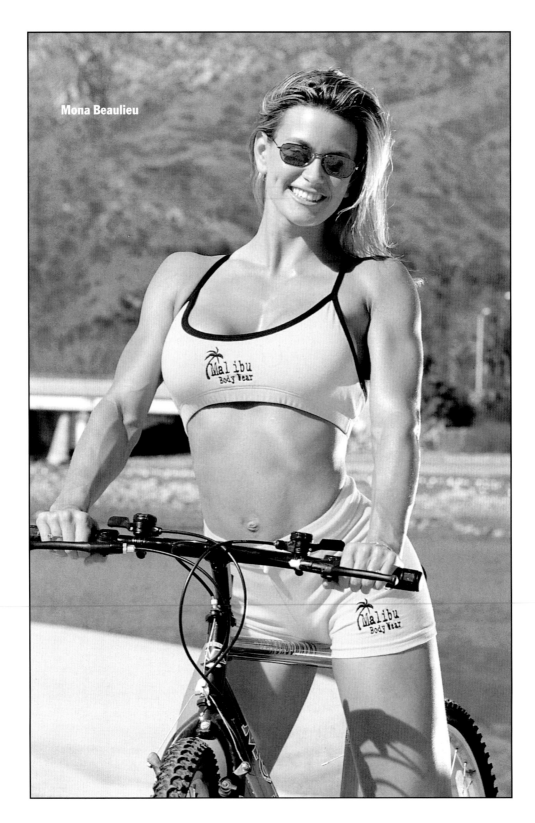

Mona Beaulieu

Book Four
Playing It Safe

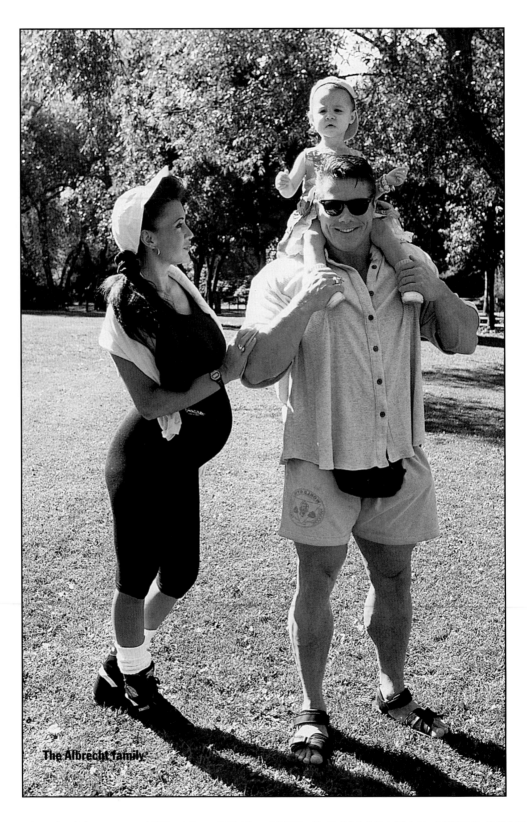

The Albrecht family

Chapter 15

Pre- and Post-Natal Exercise

Up until a few years ago, pregnancy signaled the end of a woman's exercise program. The belief nowadays is that exercise is not only safe during pregnancy but beneficial. Even women who have never exercised before can start exercising during pregnancy[1] provided they follow the guidelines set out in the following chapter. How things have changed!

Marla Duncan

The following chapter is a guide to pre- and post-natal exercise, but make sure you tell your physician that you are exercising. He or she knows much more about your state of health, and therefore, has the last word on advising against or for exercise.

RECOMMENDATIONS FOR PRE- AND POST-NATAL EXERCISE

Your primary goal during and immediately after pregnancy is maintenance. You are not out to set new goals. Those four- to six-day-a-week intense exercise programs will be replaced by two or three light workouts per week. We strongly suggest all competitive activities be discontinued. They are too strenuous.

Another suggestion is to avoid exercising in hot, humid weather. Your core body temperature will rise slightly with pregnancy anyway. It doesn't make sense to make things worse by dehydrating in hot weather or in a hot sticky gym.

Unless you have a special medical condition, or have had previous trouble carrying a baby to full term, there is no reason why you shouldn't continue with your training.

Vicky Pratt, *Oxygen* **columnist**

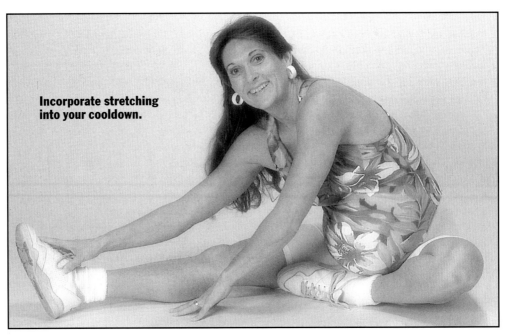

Incorporate stretching into your cooldown.

While you probably shouldn't be doing ballistic (bouncing) movements under normal circumstances, it is especially true during pregnancy. To ease strain on the joints and connective tissue, limit your exercise to wooden floors and carpet surfaces. This reduces shock and also provides better traction. Avoid pavement, concrete, and gravel surfaces.

Women who take multivitamins at the time of conception face half the risk of having a baby with a neurological birth defect. Women who take vitamins are also more likely to have better eating habits.

The late Bruce Page, *MuscleMag* **contributor**

Before starting your exercise program perform a minimum of five to ten minutes of light cardio training to get the muscles and cardiovascular system warmed up. You should be doing this year-round, but if you haven't, now's the time to start. Nothing fancy either. A slow to medium walk on the treadmill will suffice.

Closely related to the previous is the issue of a cooldown period. After exercise it doesn't make sense to quit cold turkey. Try to finish off with some light cardio and stretching exercises.

Finally, consume adequate amounts of liquid before, during, and after exercise. If drinking from the gym fountain turns you off, bring bottled water and have a sip every couple of minutes. Keep in mind the thirst mechanism doesn't kick in until after your body has become dehydrated.

CONSIDERATIONS DURING PREGNANCY

In addition to the previous recommendations, the following points should be heeded. At no time should your heart rate exceed 140 beats per minute. As a safety precaution you should learn how to take your pulse – either at the wrist or neck. A nurse, physician, or fitness instructor should be able to help in this regard. If at any time your heart rate goes above 140 beats per minute, stop exercising immediately. Wait for it to drop between 100 and 110 beats per minute and then resume at a lower-intensity level. If it climbs high again we suggest stopping exercise completely.

Besides heart rate, another consideration is duration. Early in the pregnancy limit intense exercise to 15 minutes or less. As the pregnancy progresses eliminate intense exercise completely.

After the first four to six months of pregnancy eliminate all supine (facing upward) movements from the program. The weight of the developing fetus may make this position very uncomfortable for the mother. There is also some evidence to suggest that the fetus may push down on the mother's inferior cava vein, thus reducing blood return to the heart. The primary symptom of this is dizziness upon standing.

Finally, increase your calorie intake to meet the demands of both the developing fetus and exercise. Those late night cravings are often a sign the body didn't receive adequate nutrition earlier in the day.

STRENGTH-TRAINING GUIDELINES

If a pregnant woman has never worked out before, the best time to start is during the second trimester. The various hormonal changes that begin during the first semester often lead to nausea. A first-time exercise program is challenging enough without having to work out during morning sickness.[2]

Although the second trimester is the best time to start exercising it too has its disadvantages. The weight of the developing fetus will soon reach the point where lying in the supine position is both uncomfortable and dangerous. This means modifying the program to avoid supine movements. For example, substitute incline movements for chest training instead of flat. In place of lying leg curls do standing or seated curls.

Another concern is hyperextension at the joints because of increased levels of the hormone relaxin. This hormone allows the hip joints to become more flexible thus allowing delivery of the baby. Unfortunately the hormone is not specific to the hip joints. Every joint is affected to a degree. In the months leading up to delivery such elasticity puts the mother at risk for overstretching the connective tissue around her joints.[2]

As the pregnancy progresses it is strongly recommended you eliminate all exercises that greatly increase blood pressure. While all movements do this to some extent, squats, bent-over rows, and deadlifts boost it considerably (these exercises are also hard on the lower back which is under enough stress as it is). Besides these isotonic exercises, eliminate all isometrics from your program (a poor method to exercise under any circumstances). Pushing against a stationary object like a wall is a great way to drive your blood pressure sky high.

WHEN TO STOP

Although there's general agreement as to when pregnant women should start exercising, there's less concensus as to when to stop. Many women have continued to exercise up until a couple of days before delivery. Others find by the sixth or seventh month a combination of fatigue and lower-back stress necessitates they stop exercising. If your physician sees no problem, and you feel up to it, continue exercising.[1] Just pay close attention to any warning signals your body may give.

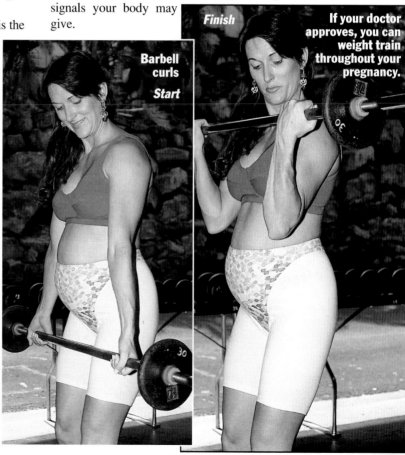

Barbell curls
Start

Finish

If your doctor approves, you can weight train throughout your pregnancy.

SUMMARY POINTS

AVOID:
1) ballistic movements
2) stretches that stress the lower back
3) exercises that risk hyperextension of the joints
4) exercises with the legs locked straight
5) hyperextension of the spine
6) exercises in the supine position

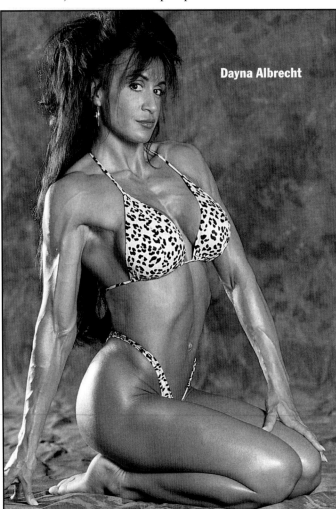

Dayna Albrecht

The second the baby was born I asked my doctor when I could go to the gym, she laughed 'well not today, but you can start light exercise in about two weeks, and weight training in four weeks.'

Dayna Albrecht, *MuscleMag* contributor

POST-NATAL CONSIDERATIONS

Note – before resuming exercise following delivery, get clearance from your physician.

1) As the hormone relaxin is still in the body up to nine months after delivery or nine months after cessation of nursing, the connective tissue surrounding the joints is still overly flexible. It sounds great in theory but it's an artificial condition. Make sure your exercise program takes this into account. Perform all movements in a slow and controlled manner.

2) Keep your heart rate below the target heart rate for your age group. At the very least keep it in the lower half of the target zone. Your goal is to ease back into training. Don't think you can pick up where you left off. Pregnancy places an incredible demand on the human body. It's going to take a minimum of a couple of months to get the body back to peak efficiency.

3) For the first couple of months weight train within 60 to 70 percent of your maximum poundages – no heavy singles, doubles, or triples. Light dumbell and machine exercises are preferable to heavy barbell movements.

PRE- AND POST-NATAL PRECAUTIONS

At the first sign of any of the following conditions stop exercising and see your physician.

Fainting – If you faint the body has made the decision to stop exercising for you. Rarely do people faint without a prior warning. Usually the first sign is light headedness followed by dizziness. At the first sign of any of these symptoms stop exercising and sit down with your head tilted slightly forward to increase circulation. It's probably better to lie down and elevate the legs.

As any number of things can cause fainting, the safe course of action is to seek medical attention. It could be dehydration, or something far more serious.

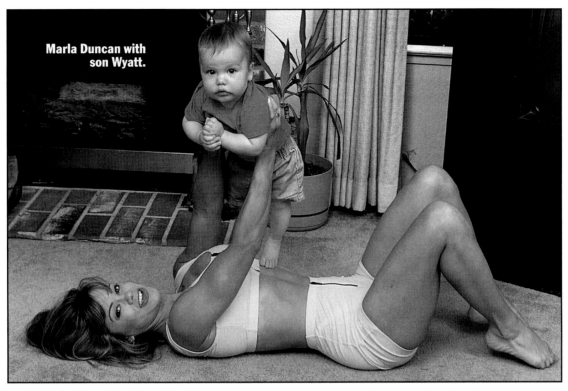

Marla Duncan with son Wyatt.

Vaginal bleeding – This is one symptom that must not be ignored. Seek immediate medical attention.

Nausea – As most women experience varying degrees of sickness while pregnant, it often becomes a judgement call as to whether or not to seek medical aid. We should add that morning sickness usually strikes during the first trimester. If after delivery the symptoms remain, check with your physician.

Temperature fluctuations – If you experience temperature variations – hot to cold to hot – stop exercising. While these symptoms are indicative of the flu and dehydration, if there's any doubt check with your physician.

Headaches and blurred vision – These are two additional symptoms that must not be taken lightly, especially the latter. Blurred vision is not a normal day-to-day occurrence. At the first sign of visual problems seek medical attention. With regards to headaches, it becomes a judgement call. If the headaches are longer in duration or more intense than normal, play it safe and see your doctor.[3]

HORMONAL CHANGES DURING PREGNANCY

HORMONE	ACTIONS
Estrogen	Breast and uterus enlargement. Increases cardiac output. Initiates labor.
Progesterone	Breast and uterus enlargement. Increases breathing depth and volume. May cause depression.
Relaxin	Relaxes ligaments, making them more pliable.
Human Chorionic Gonadotropin (HCG)	May increase resting heart rate during early pregnancy.

CARDIOVASCULAR AND RESPIRATORY CHANGES DURING PREGNANCY

1) Increase in heart rate.
2) Increase oxygen intake by 25 to 30 percent.
3) Increase blood volume by as much as 50 percent.
4) Increase in cardiac output and stroke volume.

THE MOM-TO-BE'S WORKOUT PROGRAM

NOTE – We strongly advise checking with your physician before beginning the following exercise program. Perform the following program two to three times per week on nonconsecutive days.

LEG EXTENSIONS – Sit down in the chair with your back placed firmly against the machine's back pad. Set the leg roller just above the feet (in the curve where the lower leg and feet meet). Extend your legs just short of locking out. Pause for a split second and then lower (just short of letting the plates touch at the bottom). Perform 2 to 3 sets of 12 to 15 reps.

Comments – Leg extensions are a much safer lower-body exercise to perform while pregnant because they don't produce the same blood pressure build-up. And unlike leg presses or squats (a no-no at this stage), leg extensions don't put stress on the lower abdomen.

SEATED LEG CURLS – Sit in the chair with your heels resting on the roller. Curl or push your legs back as far as you can trying to feel the contraction in your hamstrings. Return to the starting position. Perform 2 to 3 sets of 12 to 15 reps.

Comments – The advantage of the seated leg curl is you can use it right up until you stop training. Lying leg curls will quickly become uncomfortable as the baby grows. In fact it's safer (and more comfortable) to skip leg curls altogether if you don't have access to the seated version.

PULLDOWNS – Grab the overhead bar or handles and sit down with your thighs resting comfortably under the two support pads. Pull the bar down to your collarbone and then return to the starting position. Perform 2 to 3 sets of 12 to 15 reps.

Comments – We strongly advise against pulling the bar behind the head. This puts considerable stress on the rotator cuffs (the collection of small muscles connected to the shoulder blades).

INCLINE CHEST PRESSES – Sit down in the machine's chair and grab the handles with a slightly wider than shoulder-width grip. Push upward until the arms are almost locked out. Lower back to the starting position until the plates are almost touching. Perform 2 to 3 sets of 12 to 15 reps.

Comments – We suggest the incline press over flat presses as it puts less pressure on the developing fetus. Even the incline bench may become difficult as time goes on, so use the vertical press machine if your gym has one.

SHOULDER PRESSES – Sit down in the chair with your back placed firmly against the back brace. Grab the handles and push upward (just short of a locked position). Return to the starting position. Perform 2 to 3 sets of 12 to 15 reps.

Comments – You can substitute dumbells in place of the machine for variety. Just make sure you have your back braced securely against an upright pad.

TRICEPS PUSHDOWNS – Stand in front of a cable machine and with your palms facing downward grab the bar about two to three inches from the middle. Keep your elbows tucked in by your sides and push downward until the arms are straight. Return to the starting position with your hands about chest high (producing a 45-degree angle between your upper and lower arms). Perform 2 to 3 sets of 12 to 15 reps.

Comments – Late in your pregnancy this exercise may become difficult as the baby's size may make pushing the bar down awkward. In this case you can substitute behind-the-head dumbell extensions or machine triceps extensions.

SEATED DUMBELL

CURLS – Sit down in a chair and holding a dumbell in each hand curl upward. Lower the dumbells until your arms are straight. Perform 2 to 3 sets of 12 to 15 reps.

Comments – You can perform this exercise standing, but it won't be long before the extra weight will put stress on your lower back. We suggest sitting in a chair – preferably one with a back brace.

There you have it, seven easy exercises that will help keep your muscles toned and strengthened during your pregnancy. Please remember the key here is maintenance, not setting new records. Always keep your physician up to date on what you are doing. And at the first sign of any warning signal stop training and see your doctor for advice. And one other thing – CONGRATULATIONS!

References
1. M. Mottola, seminar, (Toronto, ON: Can Fit Pro Conference, September 1997).
2. The YMCA Strength and Conditioning Leader's Manual, Pre- and Post-Natal Exercise (Canada, 1994).
3. L.A. Wolfe and others, "Prescription of Aerobic Exercise During Pregnancy," *Sports Medicine*, 8:5 (1989), 273-301.

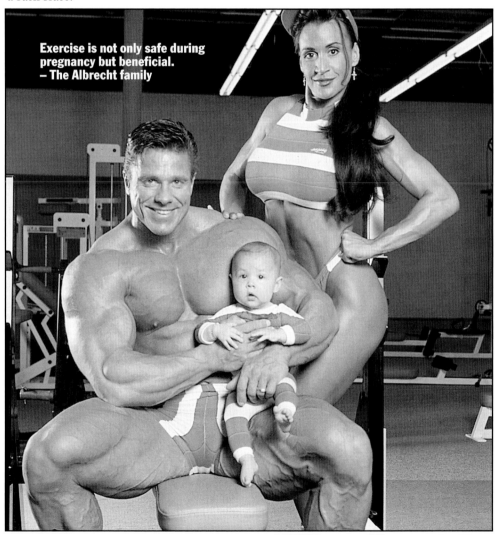

Exercise is not only safe during pregnancy but beneficial.
– The Albrecht family

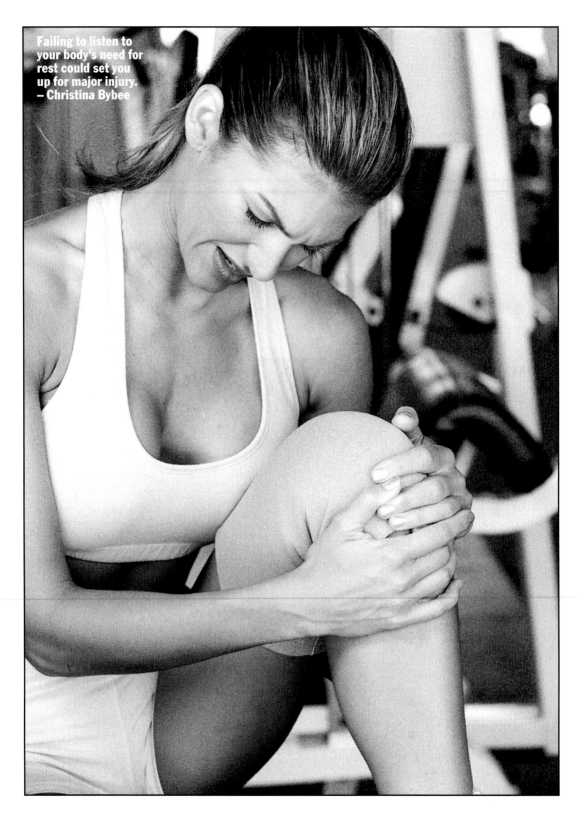

Failing to listen to your body's need for rest could set you up for major injury.
– Christina Bybee

Chapter 16
Injuries

No matter how strict your exercise technique, sooner or later you're bound to sustain an injury. Few serious weightlifters go through their careers without pulling or straining something. In the vast majority of cases the injury is minor and after a few days rest, normal training can resume. Occasionally, however, the damage is such that medical intervention is warranted.

In the following chapter we'll look at the most common injuries and their causes. Keep in mind the information outlined is not meant to be used as a self-diagnostic tool. At the first sign of an injury consult your physician.

COMMON CAUSES OF INJURY
TOO MUCH WEIGHT

Although this one applies more to the guys (remember those male egos!), occasionally women try to hoist that extra pound or two. As long as your technique is good, you can use the extra weight. But on no account should you sacrifice form to put more weight on the bar.

First, you should always have your injury checked out by a doctor to make sure it isn't more serious than you thought. You want to make sure you didn't fracture anything.

Kendra Arthur,
Oxygen **contributor**

OVERTRAINING

Like any machine the human body has its limits. Tax it to the extreme and it will cease to work properly. Overtraining occurs when you place more stress on the body than it can endure. If you demand more of the body than it can provide, sooner or later one of its parts will give out. Three-hour workouts, six days a week will eventually catch up to you in the form of physical exhaustion or injury, both of which necessitates taking time off.

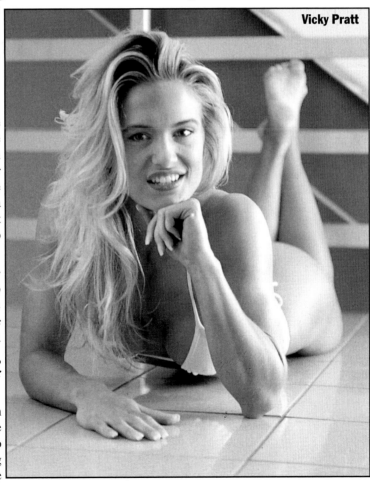

Vicky Pratt

NO WARMUP

As we reviewed in the stretching chapter, muscles are more pliable and flexible when warm. Failing to warm up is a sure way to rip or tear something. While warming up doesn't guarantee safety, the five to ten minutes it takes is well worth the investment.

POOR EQUIPMENT

If you're working out at a large commercial gym this is probably not an issue. The threat of lawsuits usually ensures owners keep old equipment up to date, and most modern equipment lines are well designed, at least from the safety point of view. Unfortunately the same cannot be said of basement gyms. While having a welder put your equipment together is a great way to save money, it does have its disadvantages. Unless the individual has a background in weight training, he or she probably doesn't know much about kinesiology. You can't just slap a few pieces of iron together and call it a leg press. The machine must mimic the biomechanics of the human body. If not, the risk of a serious injury increases tremendously. If you're unsure of a particular piece of equipment's design, avoid it.

POOR EXERCISE TECHNIQUE

Although this one is closely related to how much weight you're using (too much weight usually means poor technique), it is possible to injure yourself with "light" weight. As stressed throughout the text, always lift and lower the weight in a slow and controlled manner. Dropping the weight suddenly jerks and jolts the muscles, tendons, and associated connective tissues. Sooner or later something's got to give. Even though the weight may be light, the force it exerts on the muscle at the top and bottom of the movement is increased.

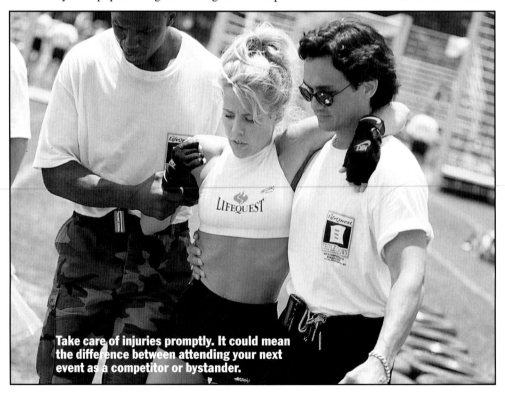

Take care of injuries promptly. It could mean the difference between attending your next event as a competitor or bystander.

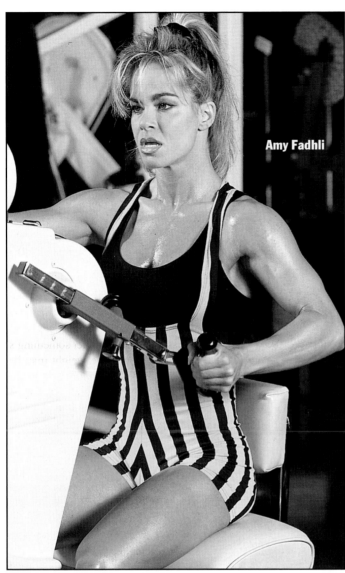

Amy Fadhli

twinge in the lower back during squats is often indicative of muscle or ligament damage. Likewise during chest training. Shoulder tenderness could be a warning of an impending rotator tear. We are not saying that every minor ache or pain is a major injury waiting to happen, but it may be the first sign. If you find yourself saying "that just didn't feel right" after an exercise, play it safe and give the area an extra days rest.

CATEGORIES OF INJURIES

With the human body containing over 600 muscles, not to mention all the associated tendons, ligaments, cartilage, etc., there's an infinite number of potential injury sites. For convenience we are going to put them into eleven categories. If you have symptoms that match any of the following, please see your physician.

Tendonitis – Probably the most common weight-training injury, it involves an inflammation of the tendon. It is caused when collagen-like protein material sticks to the outer covering of the tendon interfering with nerve conduction.

LACK OF CONCENTRATION
While we're not suggesting you be antisocial during your workouts, you should be mentally focused during your sets. Carrying on a conversation in the middle of a set of bench presses is a sure way to tear a pec or shoulder muscle. If you want to talk, it's best to do so between sets.

FAILURE TO LISTEN TO YOUR BODY
Believe it or not, the body usually gives warning signals before an injury occurs. Rarely does an injury occur right out of the blue. A slight

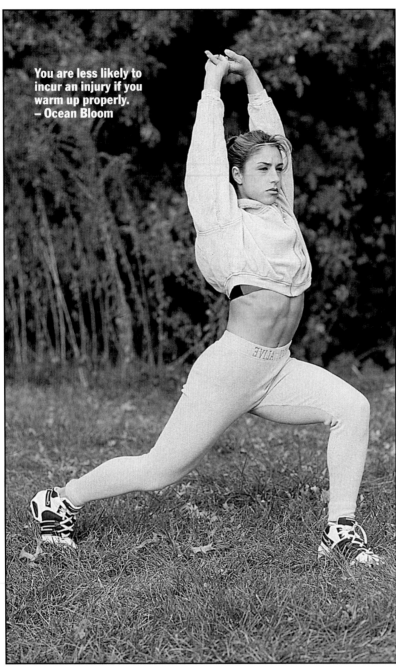

You are less likely to incur an injury if you warm up properly.
– Ocean Bloom

Sprains – Another common injury, a sprain is damage to ligaments caused by a sudden jerking or overstretching motion. Unlike most muscle strains, sprains often take weeks if not months to heal.

Strains – A strain is similar to a sprain except the injury site is the muscle or muscle-tendon attachment. Most minor strains heal within a few days but resting the area for a week or two is the best course of action.

Tears – Tears are one of the most painful weight-training injuries. As the name implies, tears involve a tearing or ripping of the tendon, muscle, or ligament. In most cases surgery is required to completely fix the injury. The most common sites for tears (due to weightlifting) are the biceps and pectorals.

Dislocation – Dislocation involves one bone coming out of its associated socket on the next bone. Dislocation injuries are rare in weightlifting. The shoulders and hips are the sites of most dislocations.

Spasms – A spasm is an uncontrollable muscle contraction that usually lasts for a few minutes but occasionally lasts for hours. As the latter case may be indicative of nervous system impairment, immediately see your physician.

Bursitis – Bursa are fluid-filled sacks that surround joints giving protection and lubrication. Like tendonitis, bursitis involves a chronic inflammation of the region. While heat helps most injuries it seems to worsen bursitis. The best course of action is to apply ice and elevate the area to help drain away fluid.

Cramps – A cramp is an intense spasm. At the first sign of repeated cramping (lasting more than a few minutes), see your physician.

Hernia – A hernia is said to occur when an internal organ begins protruding through its protective sheath covering. As a rip or tear in the covering marks the condition, immediate medical attention is required.

Shin splints – Although more common with runners, weight lifters occasionally develop the condition. Shin splints occur when repetitive flexing of the lower-leg muscles starts rubbing or chafing the underlying leg bones, particularly the larger tibia. Eventually the area becomes inflamed. If not addressed, shin splints can lead to a weakening of the bone, leading to fractures.

Fractures – The partial or full breakage of a bone is called a fracture. Fractures are extremely rare in weightlifting as the muscle or tendon usually tears before the bone breaks.

Slipped Disks – Although they don't really "slip" the intervertebral disks in the lower spine may rupture. The result is the gelatinous material inside protrudes outward, and presses on spinal nerves.

The most important piece of advice we can give is to listen to your body. It won't take long before you can distinguish between muscle soreness due to exercise and pain due to an injury. If you find yourself thinking 'that just didn't feel right,' chances are something's happened. While a minor muscle strain will heal in a few days, more serious injuries need weeks of rest. If in doubt see your physician.

As a final comment, no matter what the injury, the following steps should be followed:

1) Stop training and apply ice to the injury site.
2) See a physician immediately.
3) Apply heat if necessary.
4) Avoid the gym until given medical clearance.
5) After medical clearance try to rehabilitate the area with light exercise and stretching.

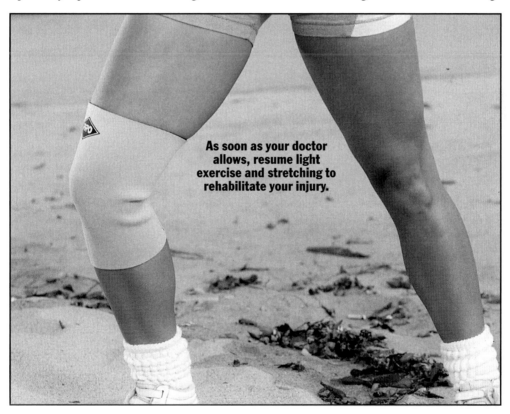

As soon as your doctor allows, resume light exercise and stretching to rehabilitate your injury.

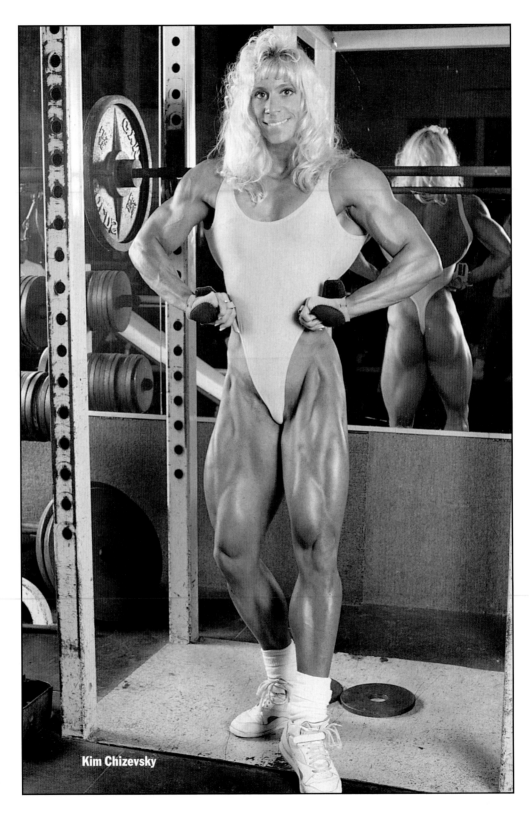

Kim Chizevsky

Chapter 17

Good Exercises, But...

No matter how strict your technique, there are a few exercises that may cause unwanted grief. We're not convinced the following movements are dangerous, but we'll readily admit they don't allow as much room for error as other exercises. However, the culprit is usually bad technique not the exercise itself. As a word of caution, if your physician advises you to avoid any of the following, please follow his or her recommendations.

SQUATS

Few exercises get as much bad press as squats. They're called everything from butt builders to back wreckers. In our opinion squats are the best exercise for the legs. No other leg exercise stresses as much muscle mass, but you have to do them correctly for them to be effective and safe. Unfortunately, even with correct form some individuals still find them too stressful on the knees and lower back.

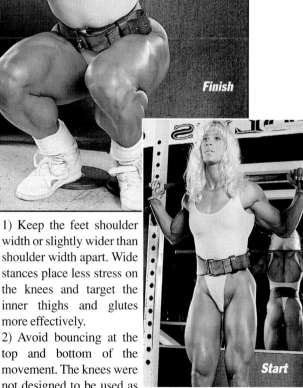

The use of a weightlifting belt with heavy poundages helps increase intra-abdominal pressure, which helps stabilize the lower back.
— Kim Chizevsky

Finish

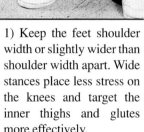

Start

Squats are one of the most effective exercises for the lower body. They work all of the muscles in the legs and butt, therefore they should be included in every fitness program.

Jacqui Elder,
Oxygen **contributor**

If you have a knee or lower-back injury, avoid squats. But for those with no pre-existing problems, squats won't cause them. Regular squats will help strengthen the knees and lower back, helping prevent injuries to those areas. The following points will make your squatting safe and effective:

1) Keep the feet shoulder width or slightly wider than shoulder width apart. Wide stances place less stress on the knees and target the inner thighs and glutes more effectively.

2) Avoid bouncing at the top and bottom of the movement. The knees were not designed to be used as

elastic bands. Bouncing at the bottom may enable you to lift more weight, but at what cost? As for bouncing at the top of the exercise, many do this to readjust the weight on their shoulders. Either position and hold the bar correctly from the beginning or put the weight back on the rack to reposition it. Bouncing to readjust the bar puts incredible stress on the lower back.

3) Descend until the thighs are parallel with the floor. Some experts advise you to "go to the floor" but this can only be obtained at the risk of tearing knee ligaments or injuring the lower back. Parallel squats will give you good thigh development without damaging the knees or lower back.

4) The use of a weightlifting belt with heavy poundages helps increase intra-abdominal pressure, which helps to stabilize the lower back.

HYPEREXTENSIONS

One of the ironic problems of training the lower-back muscles (spinal erectors) is you also put stress on the spinal column, particularly the lower-back (lumbar) disks. Our advice on lower-back training is to ease into it by lying down on the floor and doing back extensions. After a few weeks you can try hyperextensions on a good hyperextension machine. We say good because many gyms have inferior designs that do more harm than good. The name hyperextension is itself misleading as you don't really hyperextend the back. The more excessive the back arch the more compression on the lower spinal disks. The goal is to arch enough to work the spinal erectors without overstressing the disks.

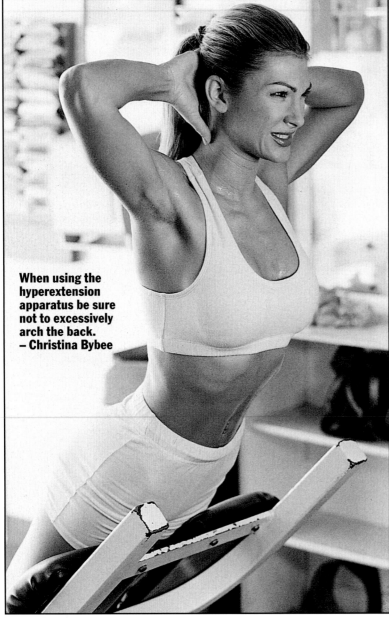

When using the hyperextension apparatus be sure not to excessively arch the back.
– Christina Bybee

DIPS

Although one of the best exercises for the chest and triceps, dips place a tremendous amount of stress on the shoulders. We suggest thoroughly warming up the shoulders with a few light sets of lateral rotations before doing dips. Don't lock out at the top as this puts the entire weight of the body on the shoulders. With all exercises, don't bounce at the bottom of the movement.

STIFF-LEG DEADLIFTS

Stiff-leg deadlifts are a great way to strengthen the lower back, glutes, hamstrings, and trapezius. Unfortunately, like hyperextensions, they put considerable stress on the lower-back disks. When performing deadlifts, always keep the back in proper alignment (slightly curved), abdominals tight, and knees slightly bent.

Performed correctly, in a slow and controlled manner, stiff-leg deadlifts can be a safe and effective addition to your weight-training routine.
– Laurie Donnelly

GOOD MORNINGS

Good mornings are probably the one exercise we suggest avoiding altogether. For a limited amount of spinal-erector stimulation, the exercise places excessive stress on the lower-back disks. We suggest doing back extensions on the floor or on a machine instead of good mornings.

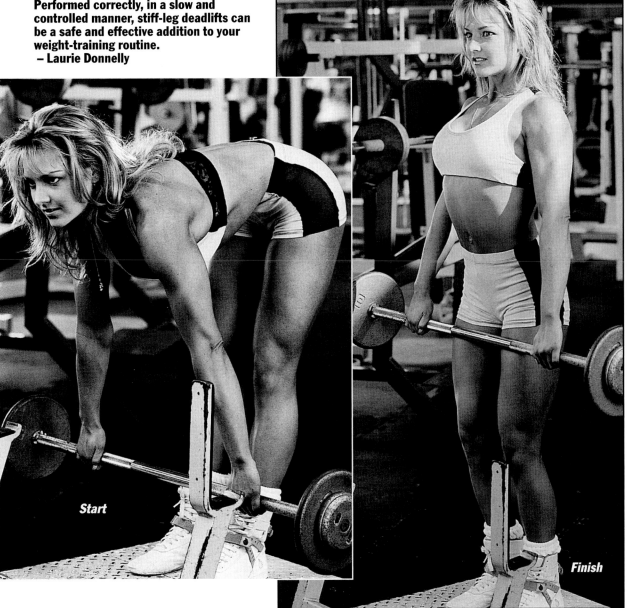

Start

Finish

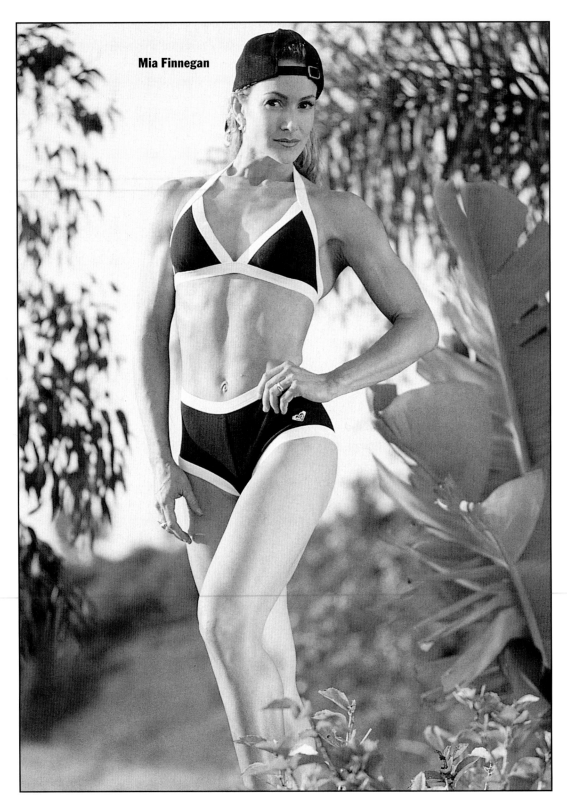

Mia Finnegan

Chapter 18
Special Issues

ANEMIA

Numerous studies have shown that up to 30 percent of adult women and 40 percent of adolescent girls are anemic. Women involved in strenuous exercise may be at special risk. Most studies involving female athletes show the percentages to be even higher.[1]

Anemia is caused by a deficiency of iron. Iron enables oxygen to bind to red blood cells for transport in the blood. It is iron's color that gives blood its characteristic red color. If iron levels drop, the cardiovascular system is unable to transport adequate levels of oxygen to the body's cells for respiration. The symptoms of iron deficiency include chronic fatigue, nausea, and persistent muscle cramping and soreness.

Without adequate iron, the oxygen delivery system won't work, nor will oxygen be bound properly inside the cells. Clearly iron has a central position in producing energy.

**John Parrillo,
exercise and nutrition expert**

CAUSES OF IRON DEFICIENCY

Low or negative iron balance can be due to many factors. In athletes inadequate intake of iron is the primary cause of deficiency. The RDA for women is 15 milligrams per day. Unfortunately studies have shown the average intake for US women to be in the five- to seven-milligram range.

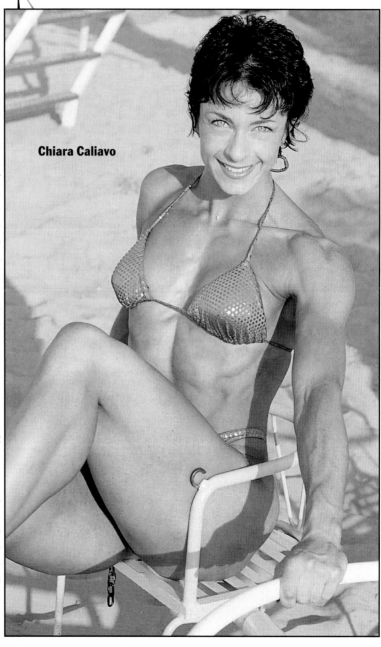

Chiara Caliavo

The primary cause of iron loss is menstruation. Menstrual blood loss varies from female to female, ranging from 1.5 to 200 milliliters per cycle. Studies show that women who lose more than 60 milliliters per cycle are more susceptible to iron deficiency. Women who use hormone-regulating contraceptives may have their menstrual blood loss cut by 50 percent, while those using intrauterine devices may double the amount lost.

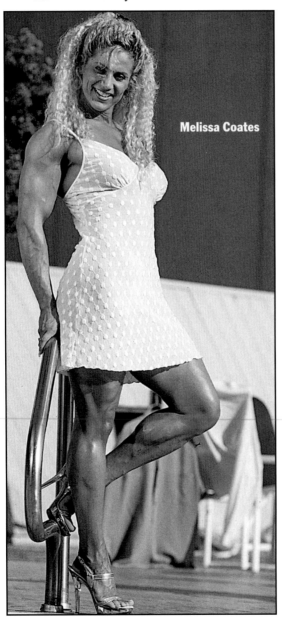

Melissa Coates

Another cause of iron-deficiency anemia is bleeding of the digestive tract. Although uncommon among weight lifters, studies with marathoners and triathletes suggest long-term exercise causes bleeding from the large intestine and bowel. The problem is compounded in women who take aspirin or ASA-like NSAIDS (nonsteroidal anti-inflammatory drugs) because prolonged usage can cause gastrointestinal bleeding.[7]

A final reason for iron deficiency is reduced iron absorption. The individual may be consuming adequate levels in the diet but for some unknown reason much of it is poorly utilized by the body.

TREATMENT AND PREVENTIVE MEDICINE

As women are at a greater risk for iron deficiency than men – especially those that exercise regularly – they should take steps to address the situation. One suggestion is to make an analysis of the diet. This will give a rough idea of how much iron is being consumed daily. Another suggestion is to consult a dietician for a more accurate assessment.

As the body utilizes iron from meat sources better than plant sources, vegetarians will need to take special steps to insure adequate iron levels. The best plant sources of iron are dried fruit, green vegetables, and beans.

To increase the absorption of iron, add a vitamin-C supplement to your diet. Research has shown that vitamin C increases the body's ability to use iron. Conversely, avoid taking iron-rich foods or supplements with foods that inhibit iron absorption. Examples include tea, antacids, and milk products.

BIRTH CONTROL PILLS

For those women deciding to compete, birth control pills may raise concerns. Besides their contraceptive properties, they may cause water retention. Year-round this may not make much difference, but come contest time it has its disadvantages. With few exceptions the competitors winning shows these days are the

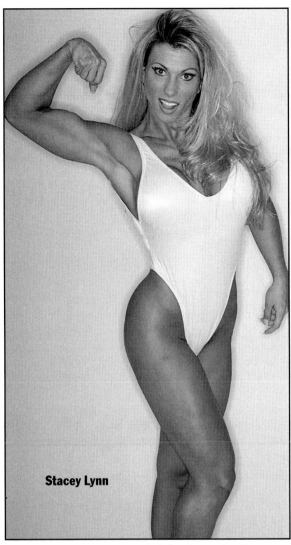

Stacey Lynn

active ingredient may give you a positive test for the anabolic steroid nandrolone (Deca-Durabolan). And while new tests can probably distinguish between the two, the risk is there. If in doubt, switch brands or use another form of birth control.

MUSCLE CRAMPS

You don't have to be an athlete to experience muscle cramping, but this group seems to suffer the most. A cramp is an involuntary contraction of the muscle fibers. Unlike voluntary contractions, which you have control over, cramps are random spasms. Although they can occur in any muscle, the legs, and in particular the calves, are the most common site.

To be honest, no one knows exactly what causes a muscle cramp. Many researchers believe cramps are the result of numerous variables that occur simultaneously.

DEHYDRATION

While humans have long since abandoned the seas, we're still dependant on water. The human body is over 90 percent water by composition. Water is so important to human survival that we've developed mechanisms to conserve its loss.

The first mechanism of water prevention is a case of preventative medicine. As soon as cellular water levels fall, the brain sends out signals which register as feelings of thirst. If there is a disadvantage to this it's that the body is usually dehydrated before you start feeling thirsty. This is why you should sip water regularly throughout the day regardless of whether you feel thirsty or not.

The second mechanism of water retention is pure biochemistry. Our bodies have a special hormone called aldosterone, the primary function of which is to conserve water. Aldosterone works by stimulating special parts of the kidneys to reabsorb electolytes and water from the circulatory system. The result is less water lost in the urine. (One of the ways athletes shed water for contests is to take aldosterone blockers which interfere with the hormone's actions.)

ones displaying well-defined muscles. From a competitive point of view it makes sense to discontinue the pill a few weeks before competition. Of course this raises the contraceptive issue and you'll need to put backups in place.

A second issue involves the pill's effects on muscle tissue. As most pills have estrogen and progesterone as their active ingredients, they may increase the rate at which the body catabolizes muscle tissue. Once bodyfat drops below a certain level, the body may begin to use muscle tissue as a fuel source. Birth control pills may compound this.

A third issue involves drug testing. Those brands that contain norethindrone as an

ELECTROLYTE IMBALANCE

Closely related to the previous is the issue of electrolyte imbalance. Electrolytes are electrically charged particles called ions that, among other things, aid in muscle contraction and relaxation. As ion balance is heavily dependant on the body's water levels, dehydration is especially dangerous for athletes. The most important ions are calcium, sodium, potassium, and magnesium. Consuming too little water, heavy sweating, or failing to obtain adequate amounts in the diet, are all factors that contribute to electrolyte imbalance leading to muscle cramping.

OTHER UNDERLYING CONDITIONS OF MUSCLE CRAMPS

Muscle cramps may also be due to an underlying disease. We know this sounds vague but a person can experience muscle cramps despite having adequate electrolyte and water levels. Diseases such as diabetes and atheroscerlosis can also lead to muscle cramps. Diabetes disrupts muscle glycogen levels, and atheroscerlosis interferes with blood flow to the muscles. Both conditions are marked by muscle cramps.

TREATMENT

Whatever the underlying cause, treatment for cramps is the same. For immediate relief, gently stretch the muscle. The degree of stretching may be limited by the intensity of the cramp. The theory behind stretching is it tricks the brain into relaxing the muscle. Located within the muscle are stretch receptors that when stimulated to a certain point, cause a neurofeedback mechanism to kick in and shut muscle contraction down. This is a safety feature that prevents the muscle contraction from becoming severe enough to damage the muscle, tendon, or surrounding tissues. In addition to stretching, application of ice may be necessary. If nothing else the ice will help numb the pain associated with the cramp.

PREVENTION

Although stretching may provide temporary relief after a cramp occurs, your primary goal is to avoid cramps in the first place. As the human body may lose up to two quarts of water per hour during exercise, consume as much water as you can before, during, and after exercise. A good rule of thumb is to weigh yourself before and after exercise. Virtually all lost bodyweight is water. Drink one pint of water for every pound lost.

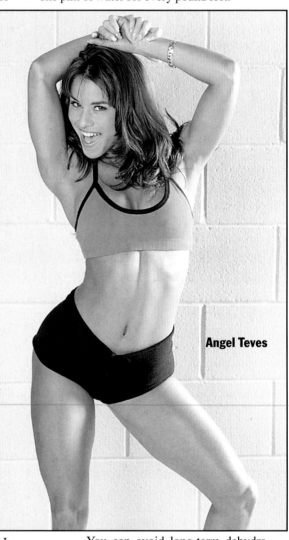

Angel Teves

You can avoid long-term dehydration by drinking six to eight glasses of water daily. As well, other liquids such as juice and skin milk contain large amounts of water.

Besides water, eat foods high in potassium such as oranges and bananas. Also, for those not concerned about a bit of extra sugar, electrolyte drinks may be a viable option.

A lesser-known method for avoiding cramping is to modify your wardrobe. During cold weather put on an extra layer or two to keep the muscles warm. Cramping tends to occur more in cold muscles than warm – due to reduced circulation.

Finally, avoid wearing tight-fitting clothes for extended periods of time. The reduced blood flow to the extremities may lead to cramping. The same holds true for elastic wraps or bandages. If you use such aids during your workouts be sure to slacken the tension periodically to allow for proper blood flow.

If you still experience muscle cramps despite the previous measures, see your physician. The cramping may be indicative of some other cause.

LOWER-BACK PAIN

Numerous theories have been put forward to explain the prevalence of lower-back pain in the general population – everything from overuse to unsuitable evolution. And unlike most injuries, lower-back pain is often difficult, if not impossible, to pinpoint. It's quite possible to go through a battery of tests only to be told nothing is wrong; however, your back knows differently.

The number of promising careers cut short by back problems runs into the tens of thousands. If you follow the weight-training instructions in this book you should never experience a lower-back injury (not to say you won't experience a lower-back injury from some other activity). Still the risk is there. Like any injury, your primary step in treatment is to contact your physician.

My first tip for you and anyone else who experiences back pain during exercise would be to get a doctor's diagnosis. Knowing the cause of the pain will allow you to work around your injury or encourage you to take time off to let it heal. Pain during training should not be ignored since it can lead to further problems.

Marla Duncan, *Oxygen* **columnist**

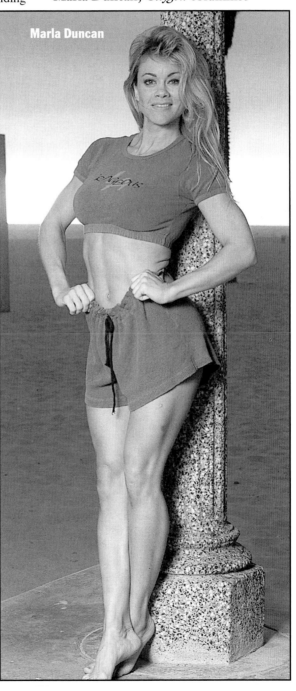

Marla Duncan

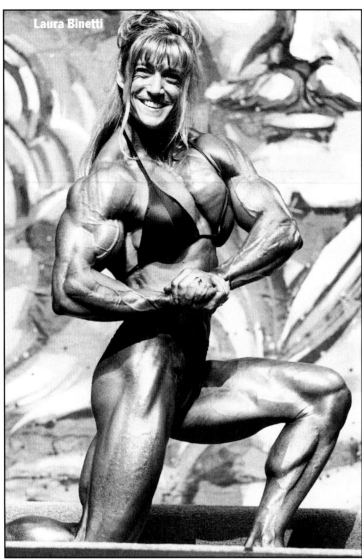
Laura Binetti

Besides structural injuries, the lower back can suffer damage to the soft tissue such as ligaments and muscles. Of the two, spinal-erector damage heals the quickest and a few days rest should get you back in the gym. Ligament damage on the other hand may take months if not years to fully recover. Even then there may be residual effects for life.

One cause of lower-back pain deserves special mention. The longest nerve in the human body is the sciatic. It is formed by the joining of several nerves on each side of the lower spinal chord. Starting at the hips, the nerve works its way down each leg to the foot. Any irritation of the nerve is called sciatica. In most cases the cause is pressure on the nerve near the spine. The culprit is usually a bit of cartilage protruding from between an intervertebral disk. The term slipped disk is often used, but the disk hasn't really slipped. The medical profession uses the term herniated disk as some of the disk's inner tissue has bulged out. Pain is not usually experienced until the individual bends forward causing the protruding material to press against the sciatic nerve. In extreme cases something as simple as a sneeze can send the individual into extreme pain.

SYMPTOMS

Although the symptoms for lower-back injuries vary among individuals, there are common characteristics. The most classic symptom is pain. The pain can range from a dull irritation to a sharp pain radiating down one or both legs. If the pressure is great enough, nerve conduction may be impeded and part or all of the leg may go numb. This is an extreme condition and must be immediately addressed by health-care professionals.

Another common symptom is a tightening of the lower-back muscles (spinal erectors) and hamstrings. In most cases this happens as these muscles work overtime to compensate for the injury.

CAUSES OF LOWER-BACK PAIN

When identifiable, lower-back pain in athletes can have numerous causes. In sports that produce quick jolts to the lower spine, or those requiring repeated flexing and extending of the spine, the posterior arches on the vertebrae may become injured.

In other cases, the vertebrae remain unharmed but the intervertebral disks may become injured. The disks are like cushions that keep the vertebrae from rubbing against one another as the spine bends. Depending on the nature of the injury, they may compress, move out of place, or in extreme cases, rupture.

A third symptom is less prevalent among the general population but common among athletes. Because the muscles of the lower back are overtaxed, they tend to fatigue quicker in response to prolonged exercise.

TREATMENT

If at any time you experience lower-back pain during training, immediately stop exercising and consult your physician. A battery of tests should pinpoint the cause. We say should because millions of North Americans suffer through back pain that has no diagnosable cause.

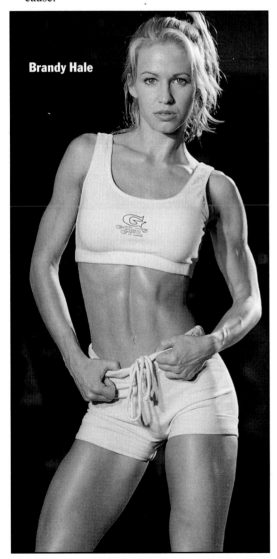

Brandy Hale

If there's one consolation, the vast majority of lower-back injuries caused by weightlifting are muscular in nature. A week or two of rest should put things right. The exercises that are linked to the most back problems are deadlifts, squats, bent-over rows, and hyperextensions. Ironically these exercises are also the best ones for strengthening the lower back!

Less frequent but more serious in nature, ligament injuries take longer to heal, in some cases months if not years. If you incur lower-back ligament damage you may have to radically modify your training. Still, this is better than no training at all.

Finally, structural damage to the lower back often necessitates surgery. You may have to cease training altogether.

PREVENTION

The following are a few tips that increase the odds you'll never have problems with your lower back:

1) Always use proper form on all exercises, especially those that put direct stress on the lower back.
2) Use a weightlifting belt when appropriate.
3) Include regular lower-back stretching in your routine. The more flexible the lower back the less chance of injuries.
4) Strengthen the spinal-erector and abdominal muscles with proper exercises.
5) Adopt proper posture when sitting.
6) If necessary apply heat to relax the lower-back muscles.
7) Make sure your bed offers proper support. For most, waterbeds only decrease back health.
8) See your physician if all else fails.

EATING DISORDERS

It's ironic that activities designed to improve one's health can be taken to the extreme and be life threatening. Millions of women the world over have taken dieting and physical activity to the limit, subjecting their bodies to more stress than if they had never got caught up in the fitness craze in the first place.

Unfortunately, female athletes are receiving mixed signals. On one hand they're expected to be tough, strong competitors, while on the other hand society expects them to exemplify the slender female form. The result is millions of teenage girls trying to blend the two, but falling short as they fall victim to eating disorders.

Keep your fat content around 15 to 20 percent of total calorie intake. The exact amount depends on your body type, metabolism, and exercise agenda. Do not get crazy and try to exorcise every gram of fat from your diet. Some fat is needed by the body for optimum health and also for muscle growth.

Kathleen Engel,
Oxygen **contributor**

In some cases parents and coaches must share the blame because they're the ones putting excessive pressure on young girls. Some teenage females feel the only aspect of their lives they have control over is their bodies. And one of the ways they fight back is by restricting food intake and losing weight. Making a weight class for an athletic event is one thing, but many go too far, reducing themselves to nothing more than skin and bones.

We should add that teenage females do not have a monopoly on eating disorders. Women of all ages fall victim, and the number of males who suffer is probably higher than reported.

EATING DISORDERS AND THEIR EFFECTS

The spectrum of eating disorders can range from minor restriction of food to almost total starvation. Food ingestion followed by voluntary vomiting is called bulimia. Depending on the study consulted, anywhere from 15 to 60 percent of female athletes have eating disorders. The sports that influence eating disorders the most are gymnastics, ballet, figure skating, and dance. These sports are scored subjectively and female appearance and attractiveness play a major role.

The main symptoms of anorexia are distorted body image, reduced estrogen levels, fear of fatness, refusal to maintain the weight normal for a person's height and frame, thinning scalp hair, and amenorrhea (loss of

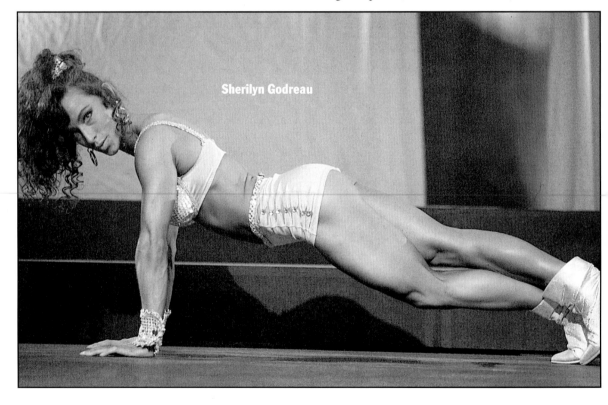

Sherilyn Godreau

menstrual periods). When taken to the extreme, anorexia nervosa can leave the individual emaciated.

Closely associated with anorexia is bulimia – the consumption of large quantities of food immediately followed by induced vomiting. In addition to vomiting, anorexic sufferers often take diuretics and laxatives to shed a few extra pounds. If there's a difference between the two, bulimics don't seem to have the same degree of body distortion as anorexic people. Based on the *Diagnostic and Statistical Manual of Mental Disorders (DSM-4)* a girl is said to be suffering from primary amenorrhea if she reaches the age of 16 without menstruating. Secondary amenorrhea is said to be present if a patient with previously normal periods starts having fewer than six to nine periods annually.

Some people get so obsessed with being thin, that they vomit everything they eat. Or they grovel in self-doubt and anxiety. They even may withdraw from people.

Dr. John Tristany, clinical psychologist

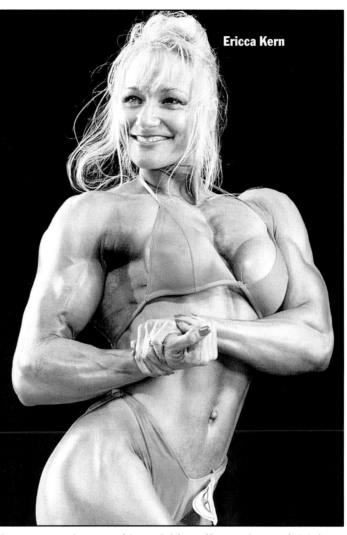

Ericca Kern

It was more of a control issue. I felt really out of control. Right before I started university my parents divorced. I ended up finishing high school living with friends. Your learn how to adapt to the new environment and circumstances but it was a very tough situation. Eating was the only thing I felt I could control.

Ericca Kern, pro bodybuilder

Besides menstrual irregularities eating disorders have been linked to osteoporosis – the loss of bone mass. There are two primary causes of this condition. It may be due to insufficient mineral deposition during the growth years, or calcium and other minerals may be leached from healthy bones in response to restricted diets. While little or no research has been conducted on food restriction in female bodybuilders, studies with marathon and triathlete women show a correlation between reduced caloric intake, osteoporosis, and low estrogen levels.

RECOGNITION

Before treatment can start, the problem needs to be identified. This can be difficult as anorexic sufferers may be very secretive about their behaviors. They may appear to be eating regularly, but secretly vomit. Loose fitting clothes can easily disguise weight loss. And laxatives and diuretics can be taken at almost

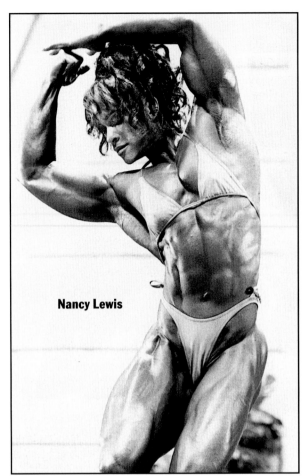

Nancy Lewis

A NOTE TO FEMALE BODYBUILDERS AND FITNESS COMPETITORS

The purpose of the previous was not to frighten readers but to make them aware of the dangers of eating disorders. As many former sufferers recall, the condition doesn't happen overnight but occurs gradually over a couple of months.

Current judging standards for fitness and bodybuilding shows almost encourage improper eating. Decreasing bodyfat percentages to eight to 12 percent requires drastic cuts to the diet and increased amounts of cardio exercise. By definition, a female in top competitive shape is probably suffering many of the symptoms of anorexia. However, the most important symptom, distorted body image, is usually missing. Further, female bodybuilders and fitness contestants only maintain such a condition for a few weeks before and after the contest. Only if they try to hold on to such condition year-round would there be cause for alarm.

Women's menstrual cycles are peculiar! I know some pro women who never miss a period, and others who can predict exactly how many they'll miss when dieting. I've also seen nonathletes who have plenty of bodyfat who get periods sporadically if at all.

Tonya Knight, former *MuscleMag* columnist

EXERCISE – A WAY TO MINIMIZE PMS?

Premenstrual syndrome (PMS) was first described over fifty years ago by a physician who claimed the condition was caused by monthly fluctuations in hormones. Despite such insight, a combination of media obliviousness and social morals kept the topic under wraps for most of the century.

The exact cause of PMS is still unknown. The most common theories for PMS – the physical and psychological symptoms experienced in the week leading up to menstruation – are hormone fluctuations, water retention, low blood sugar, and neurotransmitter imbalances. Current research suggests PMS is probably caused by a combination of all the previous.

any time. Many anorexics, despite their condition, are capable of high-level athletic performance. They rationalize that they can't be "sick" as they're still at the top of their sport. Even when malnutrition finally catches up with them they'll argue that they need to be thinner and train harder to regain their previous level. All of the previous means the identification of eating disorders requires a team effort by friends, parents, coaches, and family physicians.

TREATMENT

Once an athlete has been identified with an eating disorder, the next step is treatment. Everyone involved in the identification process can play a role in treatment. In most cases, a combination of proper eating, reduced exercise, and psychological counseling is sufficient to reverse the condition. If physical damage occurred during the suffering period, hormone treatment may be necessary.

The lack of agreement on the cause of PMS has led to much debate on treatment. Everything from drugs and vitamins to psychotherapy has been suggested. One area that is only now being considered is exercise. The importance of exercise is probably overplayed, but the anecdotal evidence looks promising.

We should point out that the number of scientific studies examining the issue are limited. Still many women who exercise regularly report their PMS symptoms are reduced. The few studies that have been conducted suggest that aerobics offers the most benefit, with the optimum schedule being three times a week for 25 to 30 minutes.[3]

The one area of contention with such conclusions is whether exercise is directly responsible for reducing PMS symptoms or whether the improved level of health produced by exercise is an indirect contributor. As of yet no one knows, but the evidence that regular physical activity may play a role in helping women deal with PMS is mounting.

In addition to the previous, columnist Marla Duncan (*Oxygen* #2) offers the following advice to PMS sufferers.

1) Starting about one week before your period stay away from foods high in salt, sugar, and caffeine. Such additives only make symptoms worse.
2) Eat plenty of fibrous foods for digestion and removal of wastes.
3) If you can resist, stay away from chocolate as the caffeine will stimulate the adrenal gland, possibly causing cramping.
4) Try eating soy products as they've been known to help alleviate PMS symptoms by modulating estrogen levels.
5) Finally, try experimenting with different herbs that have been known to ease PMS symptoms. Check your local health-food store for additional information.

AMENORRHEA

The temporary or permanent cessation of menstrual periods is called amenorrhea. Many women in the bodybuilding and fitness realms experience this condition. It occurs in the quest for a lean appearance. As women reach low bodyfat levels, they alter their hormone levels, setting themselves up for hypothalmic dysfunction. This can stop ovulation and lead to amenorrhea. No period! Wow! But wait. Amenorrhea is not such a desirable condition. It can lead to uterine hyperplasia (abnormal thickening of the uterus because the lining isn't shed through regular menstruation), which can, lead to uterine cancer.

If you experience amenorrhea (have missed three or more periods) due to exercise and low bodyfat levels it's time to see your doctor. One medical option that may be advised is to medically induce a period with progesterone administration.

References
1. Expert Scientific Working Group, "Summary of a Report on Assessment of the Iron Nutritional Status of the United States Population," *American Journal of Clinical Nutrition*, 42:6 (1985), 1318-1330.
2. E.R. Eichner, "Gastrointestinal Bleeding in Athletes," *The Physician and Sports Medicine*, 17:5 (1989), 128-140.
3. V. Cowart, "Can Exercise Help Women With PMS?" *The Physician and Sports Medicine*, 17:4 (1989), 168-178.

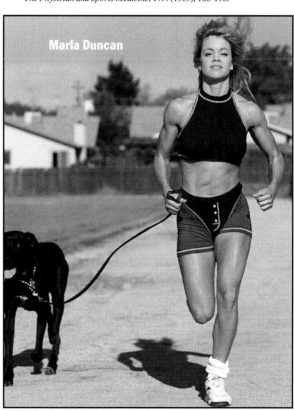

Marla Duncan

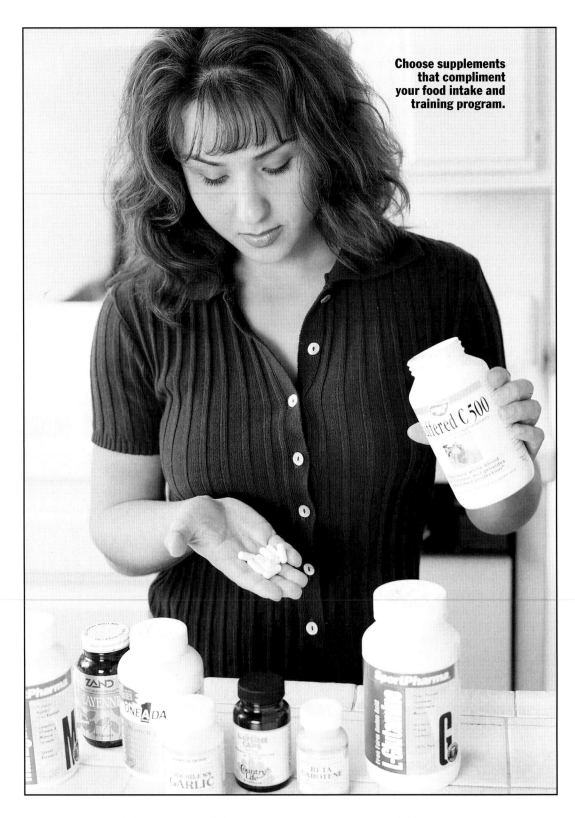

Choose supplements
that compliment
your food intake and
training program.

Chapter 19

Supplements

Few athletic endeavours are as associated with supplements as weight training. The relationship goes back to the early days of California's Muscle Beach when physique stars couldn't be seen without their tins of protein powder. The old concoctions have given way to today's state-of-the-art supplements, but one question still arises. Are they really needed?

Immediately after you work out there is a small but definite window of nutritional opportunity – a time when your body can best utilize certain nutrients for certain supplements, especially protein and carbohydrate.

Greg Zulak, former *MuscleMag* **editor**

CATEGORIES OF FOOD SUPPLEMENTS

Food supplements can be broken down into two broad categories: food replacers, and ergogenic aids. Food replacers are nothing more than nutrients found in foods. "Replacers" is a misleading term as no food supplement can replace food. They serve to supplement the calories and nutrients obtained in your daily diet. The most common food supplements are vitamins, minerals, and protein. If you are receiving adequate amounts in the diet, despite what manufacturers tell you, you don't need food supplements. The exception is when an individual is not eating properly. Skipping breakfast, eating a small sandwich for lunch, and stuffing yourself for supper is not eating properly! But we bet it sounds familiar. If you're not eating properly out of habit, we suggest modifying your schedule. Your body will thank you for it. On the other hand, if you work rotating shifts, have long commutes to work, or for any other reason cannot consume good food regularly, consider food supplements.

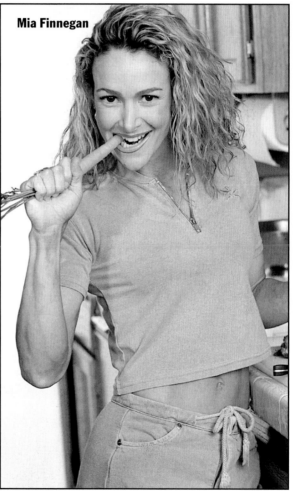

Mia Finnegan

Intense workouts that involve weight training and aerobics increase your nutritional requirements. That is why supplementation with vitamins is critical. However, vitamin and mineral supplements should not replace food. You should be eating properly . . . and then add supplements.

John Parrillo, exercise and nutrition expert

The world of supplements – bodybuilding supplements especially – is a strange mixture of rumor, research, gym gossip, fantasy, and marketing. We are left to our own devices to figure it all out as we attempt to swim through the sea of information which often distorts the truth.

Will Brink, *MuscleMag* **columnist and published author**

The second category of food supplements have seen the biggest leap forward in recent years. Ergogenesis can be defined as using supplementation to boost athletic performance. While the debate rages as to whether vitamins, minerals, protein, etc., boost performance, new supplements such as creatine, ephedrine, and HMB have a proven track record. In fact, ephedrine is a banned substance by the International Olympic Committee (IOC).

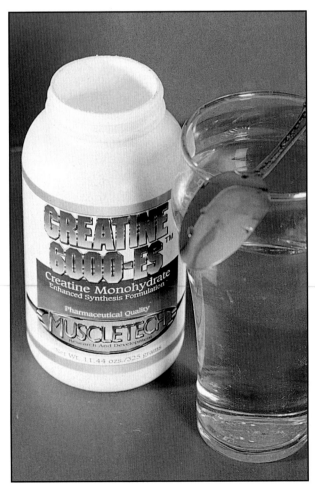

In the following chapter we'll outline some of the more popular athletic supplements. For a more detailed discussion on the topic see *MuscleMag International's Anabolic Primer*.

CREATINE

As supplements go, creatine seems to have everything going for it – effectiveness, safety, and legality. It is one of the few over-the-counter supplements that actually delivers.

Creatine is the common name for creatine monohydrate, which comes as a white crystalline powder. The color and texture is a good way to determine the quality of creatine supplements. Inferior products are more like the color of an off-white protein powder than the pure white crystals of better brands.

To fully understand the value of creatine supplements an understanding of energy production in the human body is required. The primary source of energy in the human body is adenosine triphosphate (ATP). During cellular respiration ATP is broken down into adenosine diphosphate (ADP) and one phosphate (P). It is the breaking of the phosphate bonds that supplies energy. The reformation of ATP from ADP + P recharges the batteries so to speak. Now this is where creatine comes in. Creatine binds with the free phosphate to form creatine phosphate. This complex, in turn, donates the phosphate back to ADP to reform ATP. The more creatine present the faster ATP is formed. Comparison studies have proven that athletes who supplement with creatine have much higher energy levels and faster recovery times than those who don't use creatine.

Remember, however, that the cheapest creatine supplement is not necessarily the best. As I have often stated, there are many poor quality and counterfeit creatine products flooding the market.

Greg Zulak, former *MuscleMag* editor

Besides energy production, creatine seems to play a role in protein synthesis. For weight trainers this translates into more lean muscle tissue. Almost everyone who uses creatine notices increases in strength, stamina, and muscle size within the first few weeks.

Finally, there is limited anecdotal evidence to suggest creatine may help relieve the symptoms of arthritis and tendonitis. The exact mechanism of action is unknown but one theory is that by boosting the body's recovery system, creatine may indirectly facilitate joint healing by reducing inflammation. As of yet no medical studies have been conducted to support the argument but firsthand reports from users looks promising.

Creatine supplementation generally follows two phases – loading and maintenance. Loading consists of taking 20 to 30 grams of creatine for five to seven days. This works out to four to six teaspoons daily (five grams per teaspoon). The purpose of loading is to force as much creatine into the muscles as possible. The next phase is called maintenance and involves taking five to 10 grams of creatine per day. This seems to be enough to keep creatine levels high. As a word of advice, don't take your daily dose all at once. Many users who have done so report gastric irregularities (diarrhea and nausea).

If creatine has a disadvantage it's cost. A one-month supply (about 300 grams) will set you back $50 to $60 US. You have to ask yourself if it is worth the investment. On the other side of the coin many drinkers and smokers spend that much money per week in supporting their habits. When you look at it from a health perspective creatine is a worthwhile investment. We are not claiming it has drug-like effects, but we're confident it will make a difference in your training.

HYDROXY METHYLBUTYRATE – HMB

HMB or hydroxy methylbutyrate is probably the hottest supplement around next to creatine. HMB is a metabolite or breakdown product of the amino acid leucine. HMB got its first big endorsement from Bill Phillips, editor and

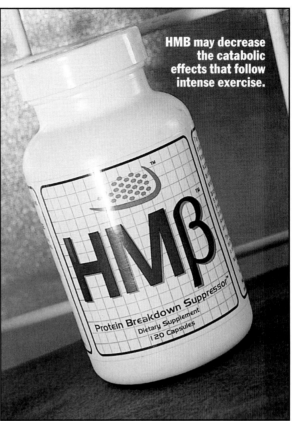

HMB may decrease the catabolic effects that follow intense exercise.

publisher of *Muscle Media*. Other writers were quick to criticize Bill for endorsing a product that had little scientific backing at the time, but most have now jumped on the bandwagon and market their own HMB supplements.

HMB is a perfect example of a supplement that was first hypothesized to work and later backed up by science. Although its exact mechanism of action is unknown, the best guess is that it decreases the catabolic effects that follow intense exercise. Instead of being anabolic (building up) it prevents muscle-tissue breakdown. Unlike creatine which produces its effects rather quickly (in the first few weeks) and then tapers off, HMB seems to take longer to kick in, but lasts longer.

Like creatine, HMB hasn't been linked to any health issues as of yet. Unfortunately, it's also one of the more expensive supplements to use, costing between $80 to $100 per month. HMB is also one of the more popular supplements to fake; therefore, buy a reputable brand like EAS or TWINLAB.

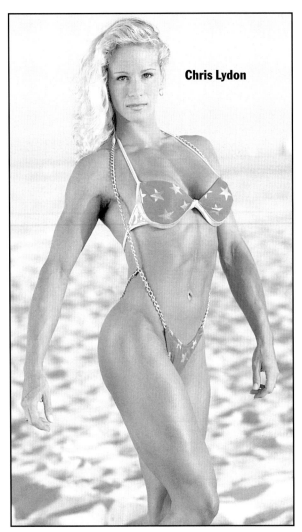

Chris Lydon

FAT-LOSS SUPPLEMENTS

EPHEDRINE

Without sounding like an advertisement for the manufacturers, ephedrine is probably the safest, cheapest, and most effective over-the-counter supplement there is. Despite the occasional media story suggesting otherwise, ephedrine is reasonably safe provided it's not abused, combined with other drugs, or used by those with pre-existing health problems.

Ephedrine is the active ingredient found in the common Chinese herb ephedra. Athletes use ephedrine as both a stimulant and fat-loss agent. The stimulant properties are due to ephedrine's effects on the sympathetic nervous system. Most users report a slight increase in blood pressure and heart rate as well as other common side effects of sympathetic stimulation. It is for these reasons ephedrine has been blamed for a couple of deaths. What the media failed to emphasize was most of the victims were teenagers using the substance as a party drug, combining it with copious amounts of alcohol and other drugs. It was not so much the ephedrine but the combination of drugs that caused problems. The few other cases involved users with a history of heart problems. They should never have been using ephedrine in the first place – no matter how slight its stimulant properties. The final comment about ephedrine's stimulant effects concerns competitive sports. Most athletic federations have banned ephedrine. Even common cold medications are banned as many contain trace amounts of ephedrine (used to combat the drowsiness effects of other ingredients and to act as a minor bronchial dilator). If you compete in competitive sports please check with your governing body for further details.

The primary use of ephedrine by women concerns its fat-loss properties. Ephedrine is what biochemists call a thermogenic drug as it increases the temperature of stored bodyfat allowing it to be mobilized and burned as a fuel source. The popular practice these days is to stack (combine) ephedrine with caffeine and aspirin. Caffeine itself is a thermogenic drug, and produces a synergistic effect when combined with ephedrine. While no one is sure why the aspirin adds to the effects, it's probably because aspirin is a vasodilator, and by thinning the blood the other two substances are carried throughout the body faster and more efficiently.

The standard stack consists of 25 milligrams of ephedrine, 200 milligrams of caffeine (one cup of coffee) and one aspirin.

For optimal fat burning and ergogenic effects, most sources recommend a maximum dose of 25 milligrams of ephedrine a day for two days followed by at least one day off. Continuous use leads to the development of tolerance.

Dr. Christine Lydon, *Oxygen* **consultant**

Those who find aspirin hard on the stomach can leave it out. We caution that those with cardiovascular problems should check with their physician before using ephedrine.

HYDROXYCITRIC ACID – HCA

HCA is a substance obtained from the rinds of the Garcinia fruit. Unlike ephedrine, which speeds up the loss of existing fat, HCA helps prevent the storage of new fat. It does this in two ways. First, it has appetite suppressing abilities, thus reducing the number of calories eaten. Second, it seems to inhibit the actions of the carbohydrate-storing enzyme ATP-citrate lyase.

If HCA has a strike against it, it's that most of the research so far involves animals. At the same time there have been no reported side effects. HCA is also relatively cheap ($40 to $60 for a four- to six-week supply).

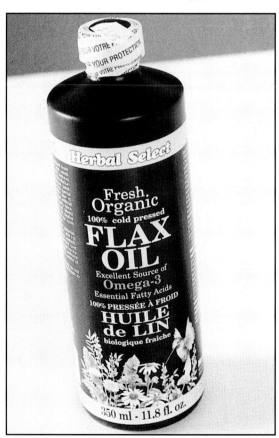

FLAXSEED OIL

Flaxseed oil got its first big endorsement from popular bodybuilding and supplement guru Dan Duchaine. Flaxseed oil is a rich source of essential fatty acids (EFAs). Like essential amino acids, the body cannot make its own essential fatty acids. They have to be included in the diet. Research has shown that EFAs can increase fatty acid oxidation (fat burning), increase resting metabolic rate, lower cholesterol levels, reduce fat storage, and even improve insulin sensitivity.

Another role of EFAs is in the production of hormone-like chemicals called prostaglandins. These vital substances do everything from regulating blood pressure, to boosting the immune system, and increasing insulin sensitivity.

For women, flaxseed oil's greatest benefit concerns its effect on fat stores. Although the evidence is limited, it seems EFAs trick the body into giving up its fat stores to be burned as a fuel source. Further, it's theorized that once the body detects EFAs it stores less fat for future use. Both biochemical effects on fat mean reduced bodyfat levels. Numerous women athletes who couldn't shed those last few pounds of fat report doing so in a matter of weeks after adding flaxseed oil to their diet.

Flaxseed oil comes in three forms: seeds, liquid and capsule. From a financial perspective the liquid form gives you more for your dollar. A $10 bottle of capsules only lasts a week to 10 days, while the same investment for liquid lasts about a month. Which ever form you use, be sure to keep it refrigerated as flaxseed oil will quickly go rancid at room temperature. And buy only enough for two to three weeks, as the shelf life is usually less than a month, refrigerated or not. The recommended dose is one to two teaspoons a day.

> *What's amazing about this stuff is that it has the ability to somehow increase the activity of fat-burning enzymes in the body, making the conversion of excess carbohydrates to bodyfat more difficult.*
>
> **Jon Simmons,**
> *MuscleMag* contributor

> *I don't think it is particularly healthy to cut out all dietary fat, which is why I take flaxseed oil. This oil is great for keeping your skin and hair soft.*
>
> **Brandi Carrier,
> top fitness competitor**

Sure. Put it in your protein shakes or meal-replacement drinks. That's what I do. Oil doesn't mix well with water or milk, but if you put the blender on high, the flaxseed oil will be put in a state of dispersion, allowing you to drink it down.

Greg Zulak, former *MuscleMag* editor and columnist

PROTEIN

Although creatine and HMB receive more attention, protein is probably the most used supplement. It certainly has the longest history going back 40 to 50 years to the early days of California's Muscle Beach.

The first protein supplements were soy derivatives from plants. Although cheap and easy to use, soy sources are not fully utilized by the body and often produce gastric irregularities.

The next step up in protein quality are milk and egg sources. These staple foods are among the best sources of protein. For $25 to $30 you get about a month's supply of good-quality protein. If milk and egg sources have a disadvantage it's that you need a blender to mix them properly. Stirring with a spoon only causes the powder to clump together. And for those with lactose intolerance you'll either have to add digestive enzymes or skip milk protein altogether. Given their price, quality, and availability, milk and egg sources are a great buy.

Your best sources of amino acids are whey protein concentrate and egg white protein which provide 100 percent of the amino acid mixture your body needs to function.

Elle Anderson, *Oxygen* contributor

At the top of the hierarchy we have the Cadillac of protein – whey protein. Whey is derived from milk serum and is the soluble part of milk protein. Whey has many advantages over other protein sources. First it is easy to mix. Throw one or two heaping tablespoons in a glass, add milk, and stir with a spoon. It's that easy. No clumping or having to use a blender. Second, studies have shown that whey protein helps keep the immune system in top form. Given that many weight trainers overtax their immune systems with intense workouts, adding an immune booster makes perfect sense. Third, whey protein has the highest concentration of the amino acid

glutamine. Glutamine is recognized as one of the most important amino acids. Studies suggest supplementing the diet with glutamine may provide an ergogenic effect. A fourth selling point to whey protein concerns it's ease on the digestive system. The bloating and cramping often seen with milk, egg and plant proteins doesn't seem to occur with whey sources.

I always include high protein in my diet as the staple of all foods. I eat about 40 to 50 percent of my calories in protein form. I include 30 to 40 percent carbs in my diet, and 10 to 20 percent fat.

Mia Finnegan, *Oxygen* columnist and top fitness competitor

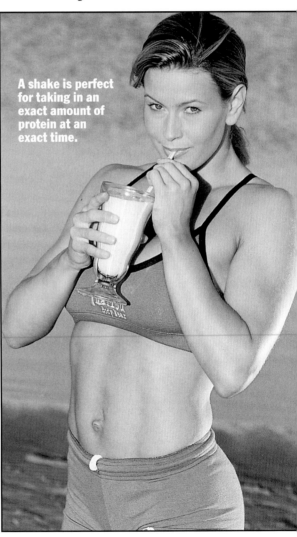

A shake is perfect for taking in an exact amount of protein at an exact time.

A final advantage to whey protein is taste. Most milk and egg proteins taste bland, where as whey proteins can taste as good as any Dairy Queen milkshake.

If whey protein has one disadvantage it's cost. A month's supply will set you back about $40. This is more expensive than other protein sources but given its quality, we give whey protein our number-one recommendation.

SPORTS DRINKS

There are basically three types of sports drinks. The first and most popular are electrolyte replacers. Such drinks replace the valuable ions lost through sweat during intense exercise. These charged particles control everything from heart rate and nerve conduction to fluid balance and muscle contraction. While those engaged in short workouts probably don't need them, those engaged in marathon (more than one hour) activities or those training in hot climates may want to add them to their supplement arsenal.

The second category of sports drinks are carbohydrate replacers. Carbohydrates are the single most important nutrient in the diet because they are the predominant source of energy for exercising muscles. Athletes need carbohydrates for both supplying energy during exercise and speeding recovery after exercise. Supplement manufacturers have cashed in on this by offering drinks that can be sipped before, during, and after exercise.

The first carbohydrate drink that received any amount of publicity was Gatorade – developed at the University of Florida by Dr. Robert Cade in 1967. Even to this day Gatorade is well known and few sporting matches are seen without the familiar green container.

Liquid carbohydrate drinks come in two forms. Those that are ready to drink, and those in concentrate form that must be diluted

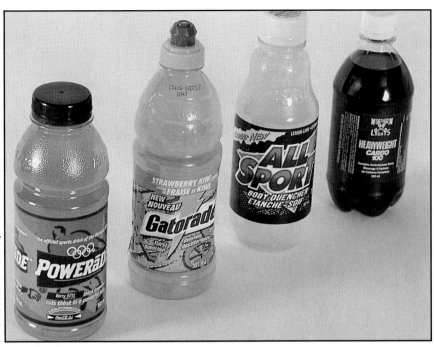

For sports of short duration there is enough carbohydrate stored in muscle to provide energy, but once this is used up, it is useful to have a source of energy that will fuel the work ahead.

Susan Davis, registered dietician

with water. Virtually all forms contain varying amounts of sucrose, glucose, and fructose. The general recommendation is to consume at least 50 grams of carbohydrate immediately after exercise. This will replenish glycogen supplies for the next day's session of exercise.[1]

Those training for short periods of time probably don't need them as their carbohydrate reserves are sufficient. Keep in mind carbohydrate is sugar and in the case of carb drinks, usually simple sugar, so any excess will be stored as fat. Those with diabetes or diabetes-like symptoms should get clearance from their physician before consuming carbohydrate drinks.

The final category of sports drinks are meal replacers. These supplements usually have copious amounts of protein, carbohydrate, and in some cases fat. Meal-replacer

A good carb drink has a manageable sugar level. A solution containing up to five percent simple glucose hardly inhibits stomach emptying at all, yet provides a boost to your blood-sugar level.

Oxygen staff columnist, offering advice on choosing a carb drink

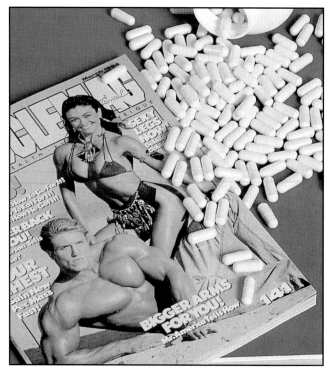

one of the body's most powerful anabolic compounds. Insulin speeds up the absorption and utilization of amino acids. These building blocks of life can then be used for protein synthesis. As chromium mimics the actions of insulin it is believed to have the potential of increasing muscle-tissue synthesis. We should add that little or no scientific evidence support these claims. Still those using chromium report a fuller feeling in the muscles. The recommended dosage is 200 to 400 micrograms per day.

HERBS

There are a multitude of herbs presently on the market. They are generally safer than pharmaceutical drugs (because herbs are usually weaker), but problems arise when the wrong plant is gathered and put on the shelves. In one case, a woman in England was hospitalized after using a herbal remedy that accidentally contained a deadly herb called NightShade.

Herbs are also difficult to standardize because the amount of active ingredients can vary. If the weather conditions were not ideal for growing, the harvested herb might be completely lacking in the active ingredient. If you opt for a herbal supplement, we suggest you buy those imported from Germany. In Europe, the medical establishment has long accepted herbal remedies, and the German government rigorously enforces standards of quality. Look for the DIN (drug identification number) on the bottle.

ANTIOXIDANTS

With all the attention given to creatine, HMB, and whey protein, it's ironic that the one class of supplements that may contribute the most to long-term health often gets overlooked. It doesn't help matters that the group of supplements called antioxidants don't produce observable benefits. Even if they add ten or twenty years to your life you'll never know!

If exercise has one disadvantage (and it's about the only one), it is that it increases the amount of oxidation in the body. Oxidation is the biochemical term used to describe the loss

drinks are nothing more than premixed versions of the popular powdered forms. Use them as a meal supplement not a meal replacer. And read the labels. Some brands are loaded with extra calories you just don't need.

CHROMIUM

Chromium is one of the new supplements that may or may not boost athletic performance. The substance got its first big break from research conducted in the field of diabetes. Some studies have found that regular supplementation with chromium may help the body regulate carbohydrates more efficiently. By itself chromium is poorly absorbed, but combined with picolinate the resulting complex is readily used by the body.

Like any trace element, chromium is toxic when administered in extremely high doses. However, the recommended chromium intake is several hundred times below levels which are known to cause toxic effects.

Dr. Christine Lydon,
Oxygen **columnist**

Bodybuilders and other athletes take chromium not so much for its effects on sugar but in the belief it may increase amino-acid uptake. Insulin regulates sugar, but it is also of electrons by atoms or molecules to produce free radicals. Free radicals are not something left over from the late 1960s, but molecules containing unpaired electrons. Such entities don't like to exist on their own so they go around looking for other molecules with unpaired electrons. Unfortunately they attack everything in sight, including cell membranes and tissues. Such free-radical damage, called oxidation, is one of the theories put forward to explain the decline in health that accompanies old age.

Many factors accelerate the body's production of free-radicals – cigarette smoke, pollutants, exercise, sunlight, certain drugs and stress, to name just a few. Even exercise can generate free radicals.

John Parrillo, exercise and nutrition expert

Antioxidants are substances that give free radicals something to react with. The resulting complex is then rendered inert (biochemically inactive). Many common vitamins and minerals are powerful antioxidants and given their low cost and availability, we suggest adding them to your diet.

VITAMIN A
Vitamin A is a fat-soluble vitamin. It is important for normal vision, keeps the skin healthy, and reduces oxidation damage in lung tissue.

VITAMIN C
Probably the most well-known vitamin, vitamin C is water based and cannot be stored to any degree in the body. Vitamin C is necessary for normal immune responses to infection and wound healing.

Vitamin C is a powerful antioxidant.

First off, vitamin C is a very potent antioxidant and is effective at maintaining high glutathione levels. It is also good for preventing colds from coming on, and is excellent for the immune system.

Greg Zulak, former *MuscleMag* editor

VITAMIN E
Vitamin E is fat-soluble vitamin and hence stored by the body. While deficiencies are rare, the vitamin's importance in preventing cellular membrane oxidation suggests taking it in supplemental form.

GLUTATHIONE
Glutathione is what's called a tripeptide, composed of the amino acids glutamic acid, glycine, and cysteine. Glutathione seems to play an important role in neutralizing free-radical damage formed from peroxides.

SELENIUM
The latest research suggests selenium works with vitamin E to increase the effectiveness of enzymes that help destroy free radicals.

Reference
1. E. Coyle, "Carbohydrates That Speed Recovery From Training," *The Physician and Sports Medicine*, 21:2 (1993), 111-123.

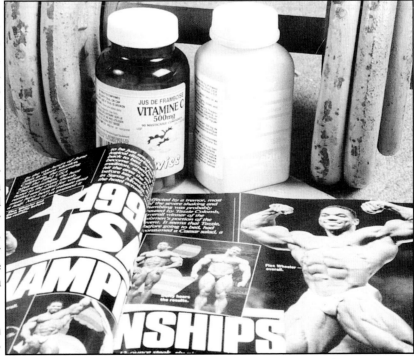

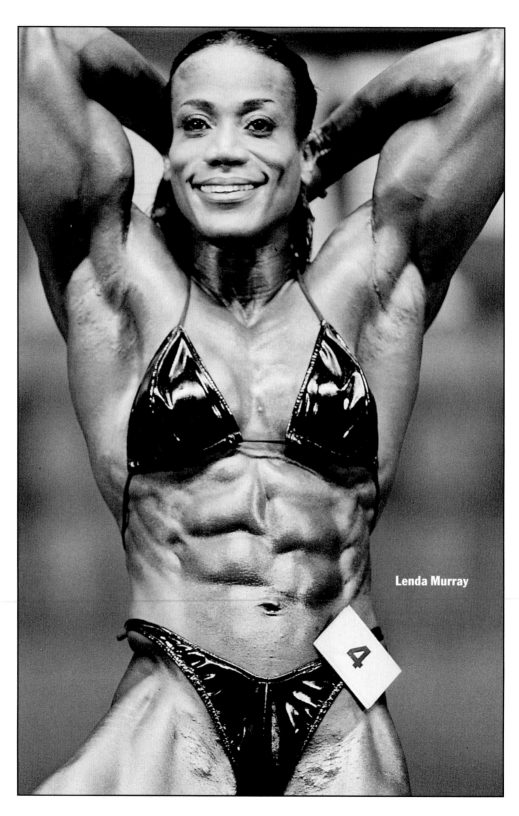

Lenda Murray

Book Five

Competitive Bodybuilding and Fitness

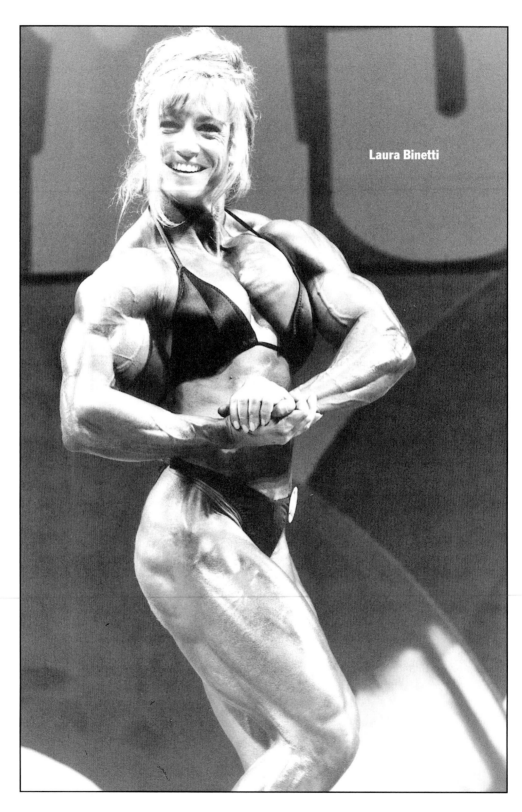

Laura Binetti

Chapter 20
Contest Time!

Although many readers have no intention of ever competing, a few of you may decide to venture into the realms of competitive bodybuilding or fitness. For the rest of you, maybe the following chapter will convince you to change your mind. If you do get hooked, additional information can be found in *MuscleMag International's Encyclopedia of Bodybuilding*.

WHY COMPETE?

Competing is fun! The authors have yet to interview one female who didn't find the competitive experience exhilarating. They have found the affair worth every rep and reduced calorie. And while some were disappointed with their placings, none condemned the whole competition.

Another reason for competing is that preparing for competition will get you in the best shape of your life. The months leading up to the contest will be a blockbuster time for losing bodyfat and improving muscle tone. Many women have said that their training had reached a point of stagnation until they began training for a contest. Sometimes the change of pace is all it takes to shock the body into new areas of physical perfection.

A third reason for competing concerns the acquisition of knowledge. Few but the most genetically gifted individuals attain the physique they want without knowing a thing or two. It's safe to say you'll double if not triple your weightlifting knowledge while preparing for a bodybuilding contest.

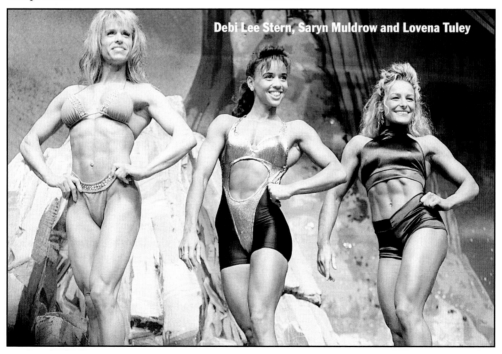

Debi Lee Stern, Saryn Muldrow and Lovena Tuley

A fourth reason to compete is that it's a great place to meet people. Without sounding like a newspaper personal ad, bodybuilding and fitness competitions bring together people from all walks of life that share one passion – physical fitness and bodybuilding. From the competitors themselves to the audience members and vendor operators outside, all come together to talk. Few sports have such devoted fans. You're surrounded by people who love bodybuilding and more important love to talk about it. Odds are, you'll be chatting away with everyone around you within a couple of minutes. Previous strangers often become lifelong friends.

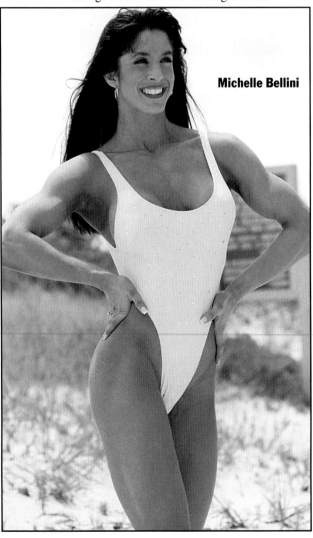

Michelle Bellini

CHOOSING A CONTEST

You've decided to compete. The first order of business is to decide which contest to compete in. If you're a beginner you'll have to enter a local show such as a city championship. Those in smaller states or provinces may be able to jump directly to this level but check with your local federation first. Bodybuilding and fitness competitions are like most sports in that you have to first qualify at a lower level before moving up. Placing in the top three will earn you your ticket but it all depends on the federation you affiliate with. It's possible only the winner in each weight class moves on.

Women's shows correspond to their male counterparts. You work from city to state or province to country and then on to the world championships. Another route is to win your state or provincial championship and then compete in a regional show such as the Midwest, Atlantic, Southern, etc. If you happen to win the nationals or other such qualifying show (the North American Championships) you earn your pro card. The top female bodybuilding contest is the Ms. Olympia, first held in 1980 and won by Rachel McLish. Other women's shows include the Jan Tana and Ms. International.

If you don't follow a nutritious diet, train well and have strict discipline, it shows. You'll look smooth as a baby onstage under the bright lights. The audience can tell the difference.

Michelle Bellini, fitness pro

For those who decide to go the fitness route, the contests are structured very similar to their bodybuilding counterparts. The popularity of fitness contests over the last few years has led to an explosion of new contests. Every year dozens, if not hundreds, of new shows are promoted. Check the local gyms in your area for updates.

Like bodybuilding, fitness competitors have top shows to strive for. Among the biggest are the Ms. Fitness Olympia, the Galaxy Fitness Championship, The Pro World Fitness, the Ms. Fitness USA, and the Ms. Fitness World. Unlike bodybuilding shows (where appearance is almost everything), fitness shows are scored on a combination of appearance and athletic ability.

I recommend that you first observe some local shows. Find out what the judges are looking for. The focus may be on facial beauty, symmetry, leanness, or overall presentation.

Mia Finnegan,
Oxygen columnist

If you don't believe us check out coverage on ESPN. Anyone who thinks such contests are nothing more than glossed up beauty contests better take a second look. The contestants in such shows are among the fittest in the world.

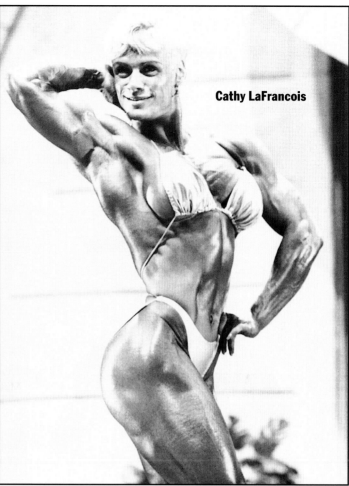

Cathy LaFrancois

YOUR FIRST CONTEST

This may come as a shock to you but your first contest should not be the one you enter. Few people can compete in a sport if they've never even witnessed it from the spectator's box. Our advice is to attend a minimum of at least one show before venturing onstage as a contestant. The perspective from the audience will pay big dividends when you finally decide to compete.

A WEIGHTY MATTER

Like many sports, bodybuilding competitions require the contestants to be divided into weight divisions. Because of the wide range in men's sizes – from 100 to 120, to 250-plus pounds, men's shows contain more divisions. Women's shows usually have two or three divisions. It often comes down to numbers and some shows have only one weight class. Your show will either be divided into light, medium, and heavyweight, or over and under 100 pounds. As different organizations have different cutoff weights for the classes we strongly suggest making contact with a representative from the federation you intend to compete in. As most weigh-ins are Friday night, you'll have to be within a pound or two of your target weight. If you go over, many organizations will give you an hour to lose the weight. A couple of minutes in the sauna, a brief run, even using the bathroom, is usually all it takes to shed the extra pound. As

a generally rule, bodybuilders try to come in at the top of their weight division (provided they're in shape of course).

THE PRECONTEST DIET

Few athletes endure what competitive bodybuilders and fitness women go through in the months leading up to a contest. Not only is training frequency increased, but it has to be tolerated while on an ultra-strict diet. You have to take in enough nutrients to sustain energy requirements and maintain muscle mass, while at the same time encouraging the body to burn stored fat. To give you an idea of what's involved we're going to present sample diets from the top female bodybuilders and fitness stars. At the same time, we're going to advise you not to follow them. We don't like these diets, neither did the proof-readers or nutrition experts we consulted. They are nothing more than *starvation* diets! No one is going to argue that a protein drink and a cup of coffee for a meal is healthy. A good thing about *MuscleMag* publications is that a diversity of opinions is accepted. Well, we're expressing ours. Women are constantly bombarded with the idea that they all must look like supermodels. Since these same role models are often walking coatracks, this is unhealthy.

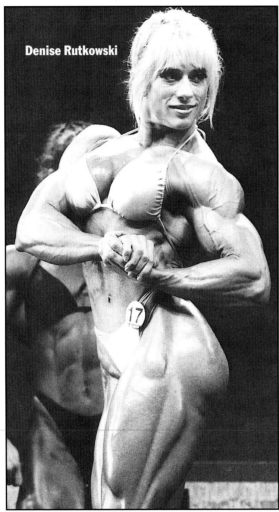

Denise Rutkowski

The top fitness stars and female bodybuilders have expert nutritional guidance, medical supervision, and top supplements. Even so, we've never been comfortable with precontest dieting because it encourages binge eating and excessive weight gain/loss. This can only be harmful in the long run. By eating

sensibly year-round, one can keep one's body-fat levels at a reasonable level. And for those judges who still believe that a woman's body-fat level should be so low that she stops menstruating and her breasts disappear, we have three words, Get Over It!

Please be sensible, speak to your physician, see a dietician, and strive for dietary goals that are both realistic and healthy. Uncomfortable as we are with this, here are the diets as reported by the stars.

EATING PLANS OF THE STARS

PRECONTEST DIET OF DENISE RUTKOWSKI
MEAL 1 – 10 egg whites,
   3 servings of cream of rice
MEAL 2 – 1 can tuna, 1/2 cup rice
MEAL 3 – same as meal 2
MEAL 4 – 1/2 pound swordfish, 1/2 cup rice
MEAL 5 – 1/2 pound swordfish, 2 cups rice
MEAL 6 – 10 egg whites

AMY FADHLI'S RECIPES FOR SUCCESS

BREAKFAST SCRAMBLE
6 egg whites
1 egg yolk
3 mushrooms
1/2 small tomato
2 thin slices turkey breast
1/2 cup shredded fat-free cheese
1 serving cream of wheat, oatmeal,
   or cream of rice
All the ingredients are scrambled together in a hot skillet.

AM CHOCOLATE SPECIAL
6 egg whites, 1 egg yolk
1 serving cooked oatmeal, cream of wheat,
   or cream of rice
2 packets sweetener
2 tbsp of sugar-free chocolate Nestle's Quik
Mix all the ingredients together and heat through.

MEAL REPLACEMENT

1 serving MET-RX protein powder
1 sliced banana
2 tbsp sugar-free chocolate Nestle's Quik
Mix all the ingredients with ice water until a pudding texture is reached.

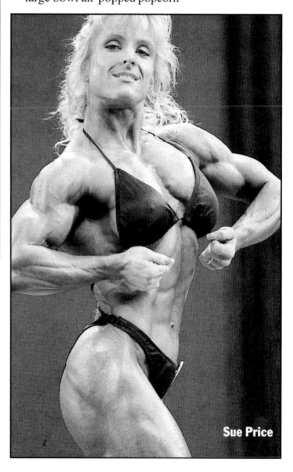

Amy Fadhli

CURRIED CHICKEN DINNER

1 can fat-free vegetable soup
1 tbsp mild curry powder
1/2 tsp onion powder
1/2 tsp garlic powder
3/4 lb skinless, boneless chicken breast, cooked and diced
3/4 cup frozen peas
2 tsp honey
1/3 cup raisins
Combine the soup, curry, onion, and garlic powders in a blender. Place the soup mixture in a one-quart saucepan and bring to a boil. Add chicken and simmer for five minutes. Add honey, peas, and raisins, then cook for an additional five minutes. Serve over brown or white rice.
Calories per serving (not including the rice) – 253
Fat – 3.5 g
Fat percentage – 12%
Sodium – 236 mg
Fiber – 3.7 g

SUE PRICE'S DIET

MEAL 1 – 8 egg whites, 2 oz oatmeal, coffee
MEAL 2 – large salad plus water
MEAL 3 – 8 oz chicken breast, bag frozen broccoli, 1/2 baked potato
MEAL 4 – protein shake, coffee
MEAL 5 – 10 egg whites, 3 oz green beans, large bowl air-popped popcorn

Sue Price

TRISH STRATUS' DIET

MEAL 1 – 6 to 8 egg whites, 1/2 melon or
    two packs of cream of wheat or oatmeal
    topped with sweetener or raisins
MEAL 2 – 1 can of tuna mixed with
    1 tbsp ultra-light miracle whip, 4 rice cakes
MEAL 3 – 120 g of poultry,
    150 g of baked potato
MEAL 4 – 120 g of poultry, 1 cup rice,
    1 serving of vegetables
MEAL 5 – 6 to 8 egg white omelette plus
    mushroom or cauliflower filling
SNACKS – raw vegetables or fruit,
    air-popped popcorn

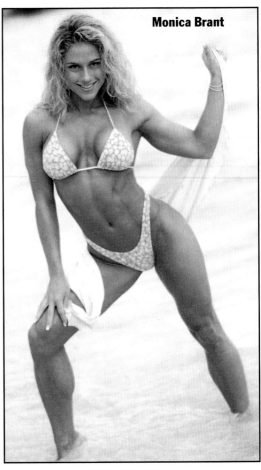

Monica Brant

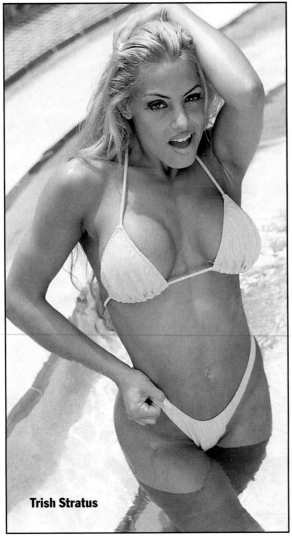

Trish Stratus

MONICA BRANT'S DIET

MEAL 1 – Whey protein shake and
    Dura Carb carbohydrate supplement
    (low glycemic)
MEAL 2 – powder pancake (blend and
    then cook the following ingredients
    like a pancake):
    5 egg whites
    1 egg yolk
    1/2 cup cottage cheese
    one serving raw oatmeal
    cinnamon and nutmeg to taste
MEAL 3 – whey protein shake and
    Dura Carb supplement
MEAL 4 – 6 oz chicken, mixed vegetables,
    potato or rice
MEAL 5 – egg whites, turkey or tuna
MEAL 6 – fibrous carbs (veggies) with
    egg whites, chicken or tuna

MIA FINNEGAN'S DIET

MEAL 1 – 3 egg whites plus 1 yolk
1 to 2 oz lite cheese, bowl of Bran Buds
with 2% milk, 4 to 6 oz orange juice
1 slice rye toast, 1 cup of coffee

MID MORNING SNACK –
8 Triscuit crackers, 1/2 cup cottage cheese

MEAL 2 – 1/2 turkey sandwich, (made with
turkey, lettuce and tomato on rye bread),
1/2 cup soup, 1 glass Crystal Lite

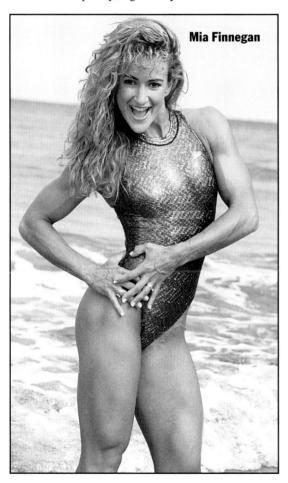

Mia Finnegan

MID AFTERNOON SNACK – 1/2 turkey
sandwich (the remaining half)

MEAL 3 – 1/2 cup yogurt (plain) with low
or no-sugar granola mixed in for crunch

MEAL 4 – 4 to 6 oz chicken, fish, beef
or pork, giant salad (made with 4 or
5 kinds of lettuce, various vegetables,
avocado and oil and vinegar dressing),
stir-fry vegetables or brocc-slaw
(broccoli cole slaw)

BEDTIME SNACK – 2 boiled eggs
(only 1 yolk), 4 to 6 oz orange juice

KELLY RYAN'S DIET

SUPPLEMENTS (6:00 am) – branched
chain amino acids

MEAL 1 (7:00 am) – AMP whey protein,
cream of rice

SNACK (9:00 am) – AMP whey protein

SNACK (10:00 am) – potatoes

MEAL 2 (1:00 pm) – roasted chicken breast,
corn tortilla

SNACK (4:30 pm) – cream of rice

MEAL 3 (6:00 pm) – 5 oz turkey breast,
green beans, Romaine lettuce

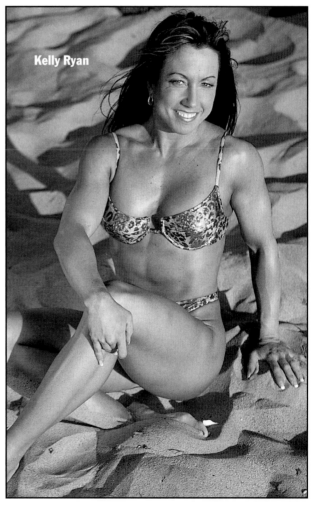

Kelly Ryan

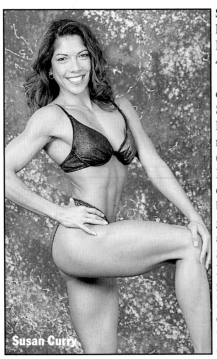

Susan Curry

SUSAN CURRY'S DIET

MEAL 1 –
4 to 6 boiled eggs,
1/2 cup oatmeal or
cream of wheat
SNACK –
Lean Body meal-
replacement shake
(by Lee Labrada)
MEAL 2 –
chicken salad (lettuce,
bean mixture – kidney,
garbonzo – with olive oil
and Balsamic vinaigrette)
SNACK –
Lean Body meal-
replacement shake
MEAL 3 –
chicken, lean beef or eggs,
veggies on the side
(cooked in olive oil)
OTHER SNACKS – peanuts or peanut butter
(what else would a Georgia girl eat?)

ROUND ROUND WE GO

Hockey games have three periods, baseball games have nine innings, and fitness and body-building competitions have three or more rounds respectively. In order to win or even place in the show you must impress the judges in all rounds. Few competitors blow a round and still place high. The competition is usually too tight. The following is a brief description of the rounds found in bodybuilding compe-tition and the rounds and/or events found in fitness competition.

BODYBUILDING ROUNDS

ROUND ONE –
COMPULSORY RELAXED

In this round you'll be asked to display your physique from four different angles – front, back, and left and right sides. The round starts with all competitors facing the audience. The judges are seated in the front row, just below the stage. The MC or head judge then asks the competitors to make a quarter turn so the left

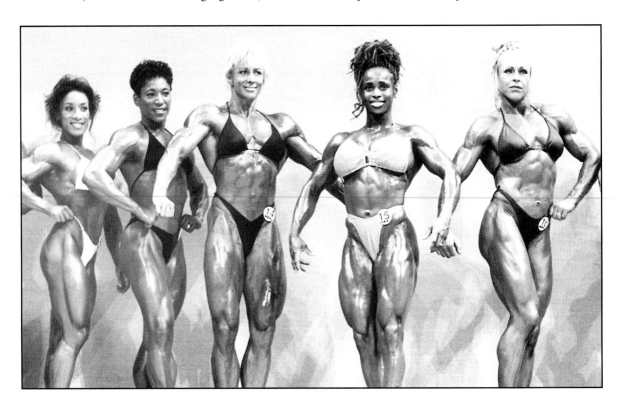

side of the body is facing the audience. Another quarter turn has the competitors back on. The final two turns bring the competitors to the right side and back to the front.

Although this is called the relaxed round you're never fully relaxed. The legs are kept flexed, abdominals tight, and the lats partially flared under the arms. The main purpose of this round is to compare your symmetry with the other competitors. Many individuals have one side slightly larger than the other. Usually the disparity is so small that only a contest judge can pick up on it. Occasionally, however, the difference is very noticeable. Muscle injuries are usually at the root of the problem. Tear a biceps tendon in the months leading up to a contest and symmetry goes out the window. No matter how hard you train the injured side will lag behind the uninjured side. And while the injury may not be your fault, the judges have no choice but to mark you down. (At least this is what's suppose to happen.) The authors have seen contests where less than symmetrical contestants have beaten out individuals who appeared flawless.

ROUND TWO –
COMPULSORY COMPARISON
Round two is similar to round one but this time the contestants are asked to hit the familiar bodybuilding poses. Men's contests require seven compulsory poses, while women's usually require five. The key word is "usually." The authors have attended contests where the judges made the women perform each one. Given this, we are going to describe all seven poses.

FRONT DOUBLE BICEPS
The most familiar bodybuilding pose, the front double biceps, does more than show the upper arm muscles, it gives the judges a look at just about the whole physique. With the possible exception of the central back, almost every major muscle in the body is put on display. When hitting this pose the first muscles to set are the legs. Make a slight V with the feet to show the calves and inner

thighs. Push down on the floor with your heels and balls of the feet. This brings a few extra degrees of tension to the leg muscles. Next, open the fingers and bring the hands together in front of the body about waist height. Pause for a second and start raising the arms to the familiar front double biceps pose. Twist the torso slightly to the left and right to make sure all the judges get a front view of your physique.

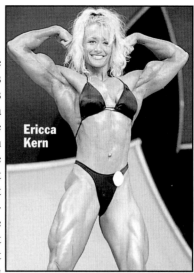

Ericca Kern

FRONT LAT SPREAD
Position the legs as in the previous pose. Place the thumbs on the lower rib cage, with the elbows bent. Push the arms forward until the elbows are about 10 to 20 degrees in front of the torso.

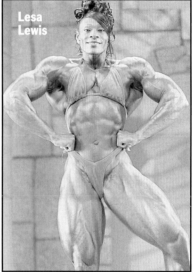

Lesa Lewis

SIDE TRICEPS
If given the choice you can turn your best side to the judges and draw the front leg forward and pivot on the toes to flex the calves and hamstrings. Hold the facing arm straight to the side and reach behind with the other arm and grab the wrist or hand of the flexing arm. We should add that some contests require all the contestants to hit the pose from the same side.

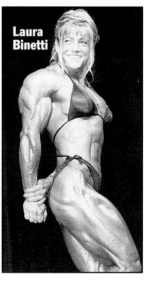

Laura Binetti

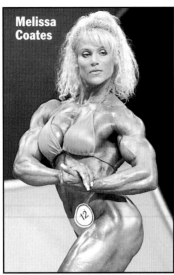
Melissa
Coates

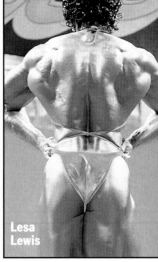
Lesa
Lewis

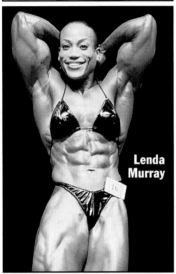
Lenda
Murray

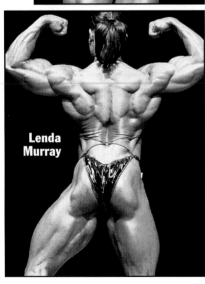
Lenda
Murray

SIDE CHEST

With the legs in the same position as the previous pose, clasp the hands in front and down by the lower rib cage. As the pose is as much an arm shot as chest, keep the palm of the lower arm facing upward (supinated). This brings out the separation of the arm muscles.

FRONT ABS

With one leg placed forward and pivoting on the toes, place both hands behind the head with the elbows pointed upward. Blow out most of the air in the lungs and flex the abs, intercostals, and thighs.

BACK BICEPS

This pose is very similar to the front version with the exception of having one leg placed back showing the calves and hamstrings.

BACK LAT SPREAD

With the thumbs on the lower rib cage, elbows bent, and arms back as far as possible, draw the arms forward spreading out the lat muscles.

ROUND THREE

While the first two rounds are restrictive, rounds three and four allow you to express yourself. Called the free posing round, round three is where a less than perfect physique can make up lost ground.

Creative posing is an art form and few bodybuilders are naturals. The best posers usually spend as much time posing as training in the months leading up to a contest.

The first step in designing a posing routine is to make a detailed analysis of your physique. We suggest doing this in two ways. First take a series of photos. Nothing fancy, just the basic compulsory poses. Sit down and examine the pictures, classifying them from good to bad. Rank your bodyparts in the same way. Your goal is to highlight your strong points and minimize your weak areas. During the compulsories there's not much you can do to hide weak areas, but during the free posing you can do a bit of camouflaging.

The second thing to do is obtain the advice of a trusted friend. While you may flatter yourself, your friend can be brutally honest. As a word of advice get someone who knows a thing or two about bodybuilding. Your boyfriend or husband is probably not the best person to consult. They probably think you're the greatest. And besides, do you really want your other half criticizing you? Remember how much fun it was learning to drive with mom or dad? The same thing applies here. Get someone from the gym that knows bodybuilding. They can give you an honest evaluation. Don't take things personal either. If you can't take constructive criticism you're in the wrong sport. The best bodybuilders use it to improve their physiques. You must do the same.

Remember, we only produce great output if we get great input. Even the best of the best need someone to assess their strengths and weaknesses in order to help improve in their particular sport.

Mia Finnegan, 1995 Ms. Fitness Olympia and *Oxygen* columnist

MUSIC SELECTION

Once you've evaluated your physique the next step is to design a posing routine that highlights it to your best advantage. This leads to music selection.

Choosing the appropriate music is not as easy as it sounds. Your favorite song may not be applicable for a posing routine. Most bodybuilders choose something from the top 40. Not only is such music upbeat, but it usually gets the audience into the swing of things. There's nothing like a shouting and clapping audience to make a favorable impression on the judges. Conversely, a selection of opera or classical music may put most of the audience and judges to sleep. Unless you have an overwhelming physique that's way ahead of the other competitors we strongly suggest sticking to something upbeat.

During your everyday travels, whether you're at work, the gym, the movies, the mall, or at a night club, pay attention to the music around you. You will likely hear something that jumps out and grabs you. If not, go to a music store that allows you to listen to various compact disks. Find music that inspires you, then decide if it will be exciting, exhilarating and fit your routine.

Mia Finnegan,
1995 Ms. Fitness Olympia
and *Oxygen* columnist

Once you have your music selected the next thing is to design your posing routine. Most contests limit you to 90 seconds onstage. This means that with each pose lasting about 5 seconds, you have time to hit 18 to 20 shots. Start with one of your best poses and go from there. Try to end with a bang, combining two or three good poses so as to leave a good impression on the judges.

As you set the poses to music, time it so the held poses match the high points of the music, and the transition movements correspond to the low points of the music. As you move from pose to pose, keep the hands open and appear graceful. Clench the fists together as you hold the pose. Above all, practice, practice, practice! Most bodybuilders will admit that posing is as strenuous as training.

To help with program design we suggest renting or borrowing a video camera. Hitting poses in the mirror is one thing but you can't really keep an eye on yourself as you move from pose to pose. The video camera allows you to get a judges perspective of your routine. Chances are you'll see areas where you need improvement.

An overall hard body with low bodyfat is preferred, but each show is judged differently. Given the same set of competitors and a different panel of judges you would probably have two different winners.

Marla Duncan,
***Oxygen* columnist**

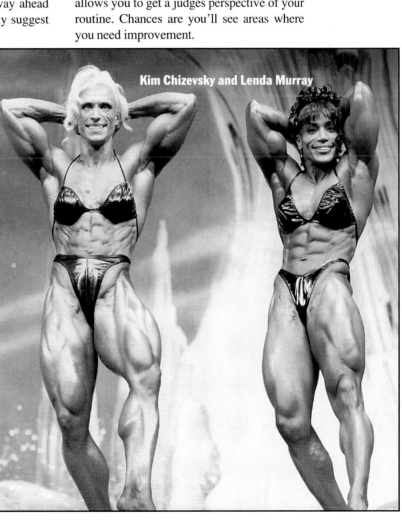

Kim Chizevsky and Lenda Murray

Another suggestion is to obtain the advice of someone who has a background in ballet or dance. Many of the top bodybuilders in the world hire professional choreographers to help with their routines. The time is well spent as the best posers look like poetry in motion.

ROUND FOUR

The final round is called the posedown. The top competitors in each class line up onstage, and at the judges' cue, launch into a posing free-for-all. If one of the competitors is the favorite the others will jockey for position trying to go for direct comparisons. Although it looks haphazard, there is strategy involved in posedowns. If the person next to you has better arms don't try to match them in arm poses. Hit poses that show your best bodyparts. Conversely, if you have a better bodypart than your rivals do, let the judges see it at every opportunity. Your competitors are doing the same and this is what makes a posedown so exciting.

SHOWTIME

Now that you've got your posing routine worked out, it's time to prepare for the big day. Most contests are divided into two parts – prejudging and an evening show. The prejudging usually starts around 10 Saturday morning, while the evening show usually starts between 7 and 8 at night. Competitors are required to be at the contest venue about one hour before both shows. As most promoters allow you to bring an assistant backstage, pick someone who is familiar with the sport of bodybuilding.

From the competitors point of view the prejudging is where the most points are earned and a good judging panel will usually have the placings decided by the end of the prejudging.

ONSTAGE

Once the judges are ready for your weight division, they'll send someone backstage to notify you. If there's one thing to remember onstage it's that there will always be someone watching you. Always keep your muscles partially tensed and maintain good body posture. Always smile and don't slouch or let the stomach hang out. Keep the abs tight. And pay attention to the individual giving directions. From here it's a case of giving it your best shot and then exiting the stage.

After the prejudging the rest of the afternoon is yours. Try not to do anything strenuous. In all the excitement you probably received little sleep the night before. Have a nap. Just make sure you have an alarm clock or trusted friend wake you up in time for the evening show. Unless the judges haven't decided on the placings the evening show should mirror the prejudging.

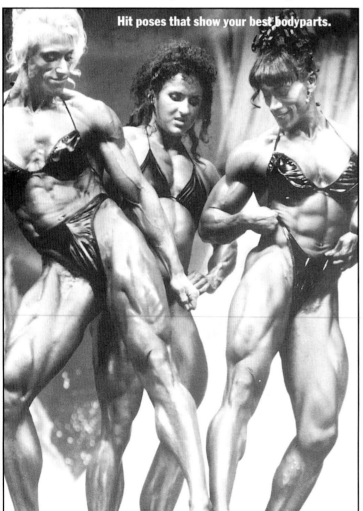

Hit poses that show your best bodyparts.

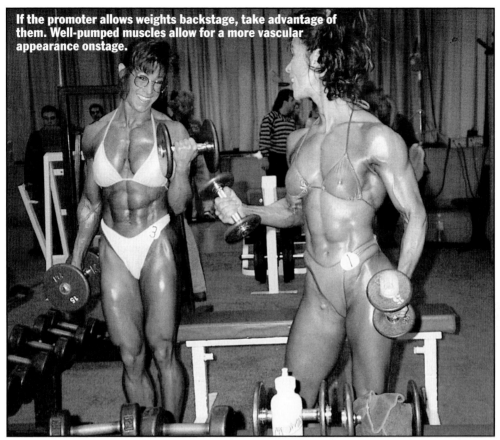

If the promoter allows weights backstage, take advantage of them. Well-pumped muscles allow for a more vascular appearance onstage.

In most contests the men's bantam and lightweight classes go on first followed by the women's divisions, and ending with the men's middleweight, light heavyweight, and heavyweight classes. If your show has a guest poser – usually a pro or top amateur – he or she will probably go on just before the men's light heavy or heavyweight classes. In some cases the promoter will put the guest poser on before the overall posedown.

The purpose of telling you all this is so you can budget your time wisely. As it takes around 15 to 20 minutes to judge each class, you will have about half an hour before going onstage once the judging commences. This is just enough time to apply oil and perform the backstage "pump up."

THE GREAT PUMP UP

Before oiling down most bodybuilding competitors prepare for the stage by pumping their muscles. You want to get enough blood in the muscles to increase their size slightly, but without tiring them out, or causing them to cramp. A well-pumped muscle not only looks large but the increased blood causes the veins to stand out, giving a more vascular appearance.

Many promoters still don't allow weights backstage as they may damage the venue's hardwood floors. This means you need to be creative to pump up those prize-winning muscles of yours. Try the following freeweight exercises.

CHEST – Alternate a couple of high-rep (15+) sets of wide and narrow pushups. To target the upper and lower chest elevate the legs on a chair or bench. The bottom steps of a staircase also work well.

TRICEPS – In addition to pushups you can target the triceps by performing dips between two chairs.

BACK AND BICEPS – Although you probably won't have access to a chinup bar, many venues (particularly the older ones) have exposed overhead pipes. Grab hold and perform a couple of sets of wide and narrow underhand chins. Another popular exercise is towel pulls. Have your partner hold one end of a towel while you grab the other. Pull the towel into the lower rib cage and then stretch forward as far as possible. Have your partner provide as much tension as possible.

QUADS – Grab hold of something for support and lean back and perform sissy squats. A couple of high-rep sets should do the trick.

CALVES – Try one-leg calf raises standing on the edge of a step, or have another person assistant you with donkey calf raises.

ABS – A few sets of crunches or reverse crunches wouldn't hurt, but the abs are one muscle group you don't want to appear fuller. Most bodybuilders find it difficult to control the abs once pumped up. Usually all it takes is a few practice poses to get the abs primed for the stage.

OILING UP

After you finish pumping up the final order of business is to apply posing oil. The purpose of poising oil is to help offset the bright stage lights. Such lighting, while necessary to the judges, can "wash" the muscles out making you appear flat and smooth. Posing oil helps to highlight the muscles by producing contrasts in the body's valleys and peaks.

Posing oil comes in many forms. Mineral and vegetable oils are the most common. We advise against mineral oil as it doesn't sink into the skin but tends to remain on the surface.

Pools of oil on the skin distract from the physique. Vegetable oil on the other hand will be absorbed by the skin giving the muscles a nice sheen.

FITNESS COMPETITION

Fitness competitions are expanding tremendously. There are competitions showcasing gymnastic, aerobics, and obstacle course talents, as well as those that focus strictly on the physique. For example, the Galaxy is known for its obstacle course component, while the Ms. Figure competitions place emphasis on an award-winning body, not athletic ability. For further information on specific contests and dates, pick up a recent copy of *Oxygen* or *MuscleMag International*. The following "rounds" are examples of how competitors are judged and how their athletic skills are put to the test in a number of different ways.

Not at all. I don't have any gymnastics background. Sure it he to know gymnastics bu it is by no means a prerequisite. I always like to tell girls that yo don't have to have formal training. You can make do with wha you know.

Monica Brant, 1998 Ms. Fitness Olympia

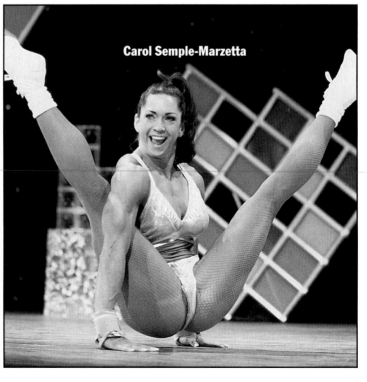

Carol Semple-Marzetta

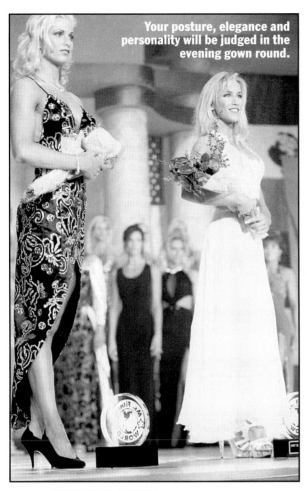

Your posture, elegance and personality will be judged in the evening gown round.

ONE-PIECE/TWO-PIECE SWIMWEAR

You will be required to wear a one-piece and/or a two-piece swimsuit and compared to the other contestants. As with round one in a bodybuilding contest you will be required to perform a series of quarter turns while onstage. Some muscularity is important but the judges' primary interest is overall symmetry and muscle separation and definition. Make frequent eye contact with the judges and audience, and while easy for us to say, try to appear calm and relaxed!

FITNESS ROUTINE

During your 90-second routine you will be judged on flexibility, endurance, and strength. You can combine aerobics, gymnastics, and dance. The best fitness stars hire professional choreographers to help put award-winning routines together. A choreographer can help make the most of your talents.

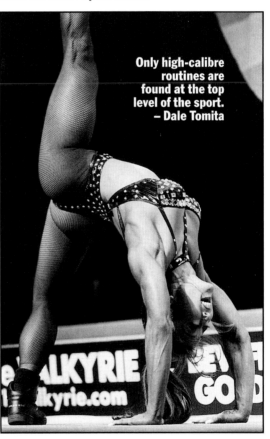

Only high-calibre routines are found at the top level of the sport. – Dale Tomita

EVENING GOWN

In this round the judges are looking for a radiant personality – a woman who carries herself with poise and dignity. In many cases you will be asked to give a brief biography of yourself and comment on some aspect of your life. With regards to your attire, choose something that is tasteful and elegant. You want something that will highlight your physique but at the same time can be used for a charming night out to dinner.

There were enough handstands, flysprings, walk ons, somersaults, star jumps, and physical contortions to raise the temperature and satisfy any fan of enthusiastically performed gymnastics. Those who marveled at what a fit body can do to a tight swimsuit were not disappointed either.

Johnny Fitness, *MuscleMag* **editor**

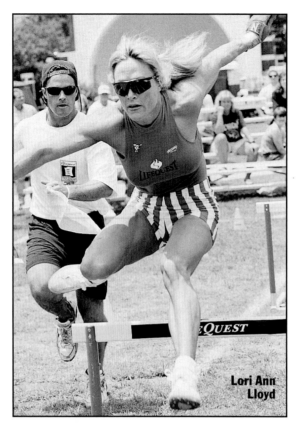

Lori Ann Lloyd

OBSTACLE COURSE

If your fitness event includes an obstacle course, there are a number of different "obstacles" you may be up against: a wall, cargo net, tires, horizontal bars, balance beam, cones, hurdles, long jump, sprint, underbar and overbar. It is best to run a clean round than to make mistakes by going too fast. You don't want to set yourself up for injury. Run the course with less speed until you are a better judge of where your body is in relation to the obstacles. Then you will be able to run the course as error-free as possible, increasing your speed as you become more accustomed to this type of competition.

Don't use a bodybuilding workout to train for the course because it will shorten your muscles. Any training you do needs to contain elongating or compound-type movements geared toward readying you for explosive movement. Try pliometrics, paced repetitions, quick burst work and sprinting.

Lori Ann Lloyd, winner of the '96 and '97 LifeQuest Triple Crown obstacle course events and the '97 Galaxy obstacle course round

STRENGTH AND STAMINA ROUND

This round will test your strength and endurance to the limit. It may also test your flexibility. A rower, Versa Climber, or other piece of cardio equipment may be used. You may have to perform dips or chins for reps. The 1997 Ms. Fitness Olympia chose a rower as its weapon of choice, while the 1997 Jan Tana Fitness Classic had the competitors cover as much distance in one minute as their muscles could bear on a Versa Climber.

This round varies from competition to competition, as well as within the same competition year to year. In 1998, the Ms. Fitness Olympia replaced the rowing segment with a one-minute mandatory moves routine (combining five strength moves, like one-arm pushups and a straddle-hold, with three feats of flexibility, such as full front splits and a high kick).

SHAVING DOWN

The purpose of shaving down is to remove any body hair that distracts from the body's muscularity. It doesn't make sense to spend years building a great physique only to have it obscured by long strands of hair. This is one area, however, where females have an advantage over their male counterparts. Most males limit their shaving to facial hair, and their first bodybuilding show introduces them to the art of removing unwanted body hair. Females on the other hand are used to shaving, and have less hair, so the precontest shave down is not that big a deal. For those who've never had to

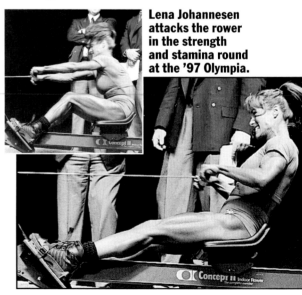

Lena Johannesen attacks the rower in the strength and stamina round at the '97 Olympia.

remove much body hair, the following suggestions should make things go smoother.

There are basically four ways to remove body hair – shaving with a razor, chemical, waxing, and electrolysis. Each has its advantages and disadvantages. Shaving can take two forms, electrical and straight edge. The advantage of a straight edge is the quality of the shave produced. Double-bladed shavers don't just cut the hair off at the surface, they actually cut below the surface. They do this by having the first blade lift the hair and the second cutting it before it snaps back into position. The result is a skin surface that appears like it never had hair to begin with. If such shaving has a disadvantage it's the close cutting often irritates the skin producing a rash. If you decide to go this route we suggest doing it a week before the show to allow any rash to clear up; however, by this time, stubble may start to appear.

The second type of shaving involves the use of an electrical razor. While the shave produced is not quite as close, it does have the advantages of not producing a rash, and taking a fraction of the time of straight-edge shaving. If you don't have a razor yourself, perhaps a boyfriend or husband can loan you theirs. As you know your better half better than we do, you may or may not want to tell them what you're using it for!

The second method to remove body hair is by chemical means. Most drug stores sell lotions that contain hair-removing agents. Such brands as Nair work by breaking down the hair's protein. Simply smear it on, wait 20 to 30 minutes (depending on the brand) and wash off. You may have to touch up with a razor but most of the hair will fall out. If this form of hair removal has a disadvantage it's that it may cause an allergic reaction. Our advice is to test a small area of skin before coating other areas of the body. If you develop a rash, you can try a different brand, but odds are you'll be allergic to every brand because most use the same active ingredients.

Many women prefer waxing because it lasts from three to six weeks. The only prob-

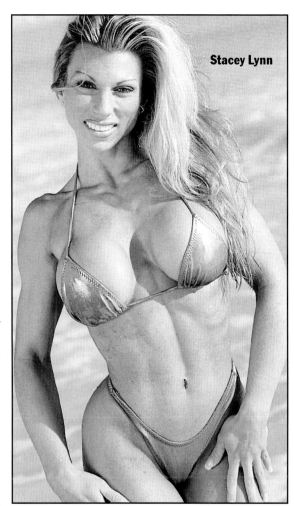

Stacey Lynn

lem is that the hair should be at least 1/2 an inch long before you wax, and some people don't like waiting. If it's going to be a problem you can bleach the hairs until they're long enough to remove.

Once the skin is exposed, warm wax is spread across the area, allowing the wax to penetrate the pores. A cloth is laid atop the wax, and firmly pressed against the skin. A short delay is given to allow the wax to dry, and then the strip is pulled off in a quick motion. A quick press of the hand over the stripped area will reduce any pain. Stray hairs that refused to give up the ghost can be pulled out with tweezers. Ingrown hairs present a special problem. Using a sharp-pointed tweezer (they're expensive but worth the cost), gently press the point on the skin to pop-out the hair. Once exposed you can tweeze. It is always better to have this done at a salon by a professional. The results and the experience are much more pleasant. Besides, imagine the expressions among the waiting clients when you let loose a blood-curdling scream. It's therapeutic, and you won't have to wait as long for an appointment the next time!

DO I HAVE TO SHAVE "EVERYTHING"?

Clearly from pictures of fitness and bodybuilder contestants, the genitals are clean shaven. How else do you wear a dental floss bikini? If you are not competing, it is a matter of personal preference. The bikini zone is easily waxed, and pubic hair can be trimmed into a Mohawk. But to completely remove the remaining hair, shave slowly and carefully.

While the first three techniques are temporary – the hair will grow back – the fourth category of hair removal is permanent.

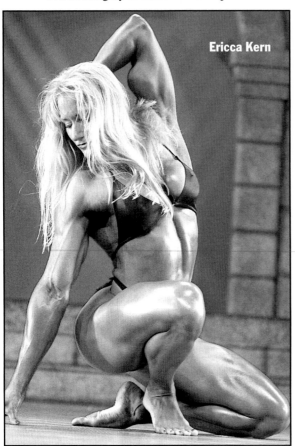

Ericca Kern

Called electrolysis it involves destroying the hair-generating follicles by electricity. The primary advantage of this technique is that it's a one shot deal. The hair won't grow back. The main disadvantage is cost. Depending on the amount of hair removed, electrolysis can cost thousands of dollars. You have to ask yourself if it's worth it for a local contest. Granted you won't have to shave again, but when weighed against the cheaper alternatives, most give electrolysis a pass.

GLASSES

This may seem like a trivial topic, but for those who depend on corrected vision, it does have some relevance. While there's nothing in the rule book about wearing glasses, some judges may see eye wear as a distraction to an otherwise great physique. This may seem petty but it happens; two competitors with similar physiques and presentations may not be scored evenly because one is wearing glasses.

To prevent such foolishness from happening either remove the glasses before stepping onstage or invest in contact lenses. Even if your vision is extremely weak, there's little to worry about onstage. Simply follow the other competitors as they exit and enter the stage and go through the compulsories.

Besides the appearance of glasses, there's a practical reason for not wearing them. A couple of minutes under the posing lights will have you sweating like the hardest of workouts. It won't be long before your glasses start sliding down your nose requiring readjustment.

CHOOSING A POSING SUIT

Bodybuilding and fitness competitions allow you to select two-piece swimwear from a broad range of colors. For specific regulations concerning posing suits it is best to check with the respective organization, as rules may differ from one competition to another.

Recent issues of *MuscleMag International*, *Oxygen*, or other bodybuilding/fitness publications can give you an idea of the scope of colors bodybuilders and fitness competitors are wearing. Everything from black and white, to red, blue, and purple can be seen. As a word of advice, choose your color based on your skin color and tone. For example, African-American bodybuilders should not wear black or brown trunks as they'll blend in with the skin. Conversely, light colors like yellow and white tend to draw attention to the midsection making it appear larger than it really is. Light colors also highlight stains more readily. Unless you live in a warm climate, you'll probably be using some form of artificial tanning lotion. Such lotions tend to streak and nothing looks as bad as a white posing suit cross-striated with brown stain.

With regards to style your physique also plays a role. Those with short legs should wear what's called a high-cut design as this will expose more of the thigh creating the illusion of leg length. Those with thigh cuts extending right up to the hip should also wear a high-cut design, to show off their great condition. On the other hand, those with long legs can get away with wearing a lower-cut design. Finally, there is a limit to how skimpy your posing attire can be. No thongs are permitted, despite how much the audience would love it!

If you live in a small town and none of the local stores carry posing suits, don't despair. Most of the top designers advertise in the pages of *MuscleMag International*, *Oxygen*, and other bodybuilding publications. Although the prices vary, $50 to $70 will get you a decent suit delivered to your door in two to three weeks.

STEPPING OUT

For those competing in fitness competitions there's one more piece of attire needed – footwear. During the comparison round, contestants are required to wear high-heeled shoes. As with posing suits, selecting the best footwear can be a chore. Some competitors match

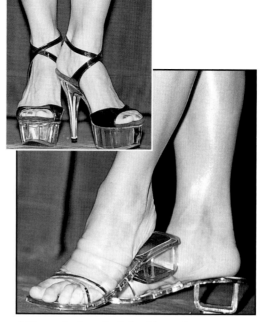

A three- to four-inch heel is preferable during a fitness competition.

the color of their footwear with their posing suits. If the right color can't be bought you have the option of dyeing. You can also play it safe and wear black or white shoes. Both colors match just about anything. Another option and one used by fitness champion and *Oxygen* columnist, Mia Finnegan, is to wear clear shoes.

In terms of heel size, stay around the three- to four-inch mark. Even this will be high for some. If you're not used to wearing high heel shoes we suggest practicing in the weeks leading up to the contest. The last thing you want to do is walk onstage and turn out an ankle.

TANNING

Although it's not a rule, for practical purposes you must darken the skin before competing. You may have the best physique onstage but if your genetics dictate light skin, chances are you won't crack the winner's circle. Tanning is one of those things that evolved over the years to the point that it's now a must for any serious competitor.

There are many reasons for tanning. The most practical is protection from the contest venue lights. The bright lights that flood the stage will wash out or diminish your physique's muscularity if you happen to have light skin. All things being equal, the darker-skinned competitor will look more muscular and in "better shape" than a lighter-skinned opponent.

Another reason for tanning is that the tanning process tightens the skin making it hug the muscles better. It also helps shed those few extra pounds of water under the skin that may blur muscularity. It's for these reasons that African-American bodybuilders also tan before contests.

HOW TO TAN

The cheapest and most natural way to tan is with sunlight. Rent the movie *Pumping Iron* with Arnold Schwarzenegger, and you'll see the competitors spending as much time lying on the beach as working out in the gym. If sunlight tanning has one disadvantage it's the risk to the skin. The thinning ozone layer means more harmful radiation is getting through. Such radiation causes skin cancer and a host of other problems. If you decide to go this route always wear a sunblock lotion to help filter out such harmful radiation. For most people nothing less than a sunblock 15 is recommended. And apply it frequently if you're playing games on the beach or swimming.

If you live in a northern climate or are fearful of the sun, you have the option of artificial tanning light. Tanning beds use an artificial light source that will also cause the body's skin pigment to darken, but they can be just as harmful to your skin as the real thing. (Some of the newer models have the harmful light rays filtered out.) Check out the sun solariums near you. Most have package deals that are ideal for precontest preparation.

Besides light, you can darken the skin with tanning lotions. This technique can be subdivided into two categories – overnight and instant. Overnight lotions mean just that. Apply the lotion all over the body before bed and hit the sack. In the morning your skin will

Although accelerators are likely ineffective they are also harmless – except to your pocket book. One important fact to remember, however, is that neither of these tanning aids or bronzers offer any protection against the rays of the sun. You'll still have to use an effective sunscreen to prevent sunburn and decrease skin damage.

Dr. Mauro DiPasquale, *MuscleMag* **columnist**

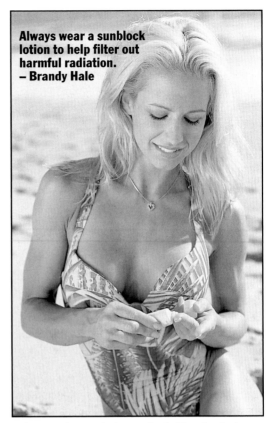

Always wear a sunblock lotion to help filter out harmful radiation.
– Brandy Hale

be sporting a whole new look. Tanning lotions work by reacting with enzymes in the skin. You might want to try different brands as the color produced can range from yellow to orange to brown.

If such lotions have a disadvantage it's that they'll darken everything your skin makes contact with. Your bed sheets are at the top of the list. Make sure to use an old set of sheets during the application process, or better yet, invest a few dollars in a set that can be put away strictly for contest preparation.

The other type of tanning lotions are something Picasso would be proud off. Instant tanning lotions are nothing more than coloring dyes that darken the skin then and there. Whether lotion or spray, they can turn the lightest of competitors into chocolate monu-

The average white male or female needs about four or five coats of skin dye over a good natural base tan to achieve the desired look come contest day. Have a trusted friend paint you, and leave enough time that the job can be done correctly.

Robert Kennedy, *MuscleMag* **founder and best-selling author**

ments! As with hair-removal products, try putting a small amount of lotion on the skin before covering the whole body. You may be allergic to the product. Compared to sunlight tanning, artificial tanning from a bottle is a safe, quick, year-round alternative.

The last category of tanning involves pharmacology. Taken in pill form, the "tan" is produced by one or the combination of two dyes: beta carotene found in fruits and vegetables, and canthaxanthin, a pigment found in some marine life. The tan is produced when the pigment accumulates in the skin, and can last for weeks, and in some cases months. Tanning pills are not considered toxic, but one side effect reported is anemia.

WHAT'S BEST FOR ME?

For those living in northern climates and competing during the winter, you have little option but to rely on tanning beds or tanning lotions. For those lucky enough to live down south, the choice is yours. Our advice is to rely on moderate sunlight or artificial light to get a good base tan, and then touch up just before the contest with artificial dyes and lotions. Those with sensitive skin, or Nordic genetics, may want to rely solely on lotions and dyes. A few degrees of skin darkening is not worth the risk of skin damage from solar radiation.

AFTER THE SHOW

Once the results have been announced and closing speeches made, the audience and competitors may head their separate ways, or they may take part in the post-contest festivities that are becoming popular these days. The best promoters often rent a club or large auditorium and invite all to a banquet. After months of dieting you've earned the right for a pig out! Enjoy yourself.

As a final comment please accept the contests results

After the show, always ask the judges how you could improve. Be able to accept criticism as well as praise. The criticism will help you if you learn and grow from it.

Marla Duncan, *Oxygen* **columnist**

no matter what your placing. There's nothing worse than a sore loser. Throwing a backstage tantrum ruins it for everyone. And you can be sure the episode will make its way to the judges' table. How do you think they'll view you next year? Bodybuilding and fitness contests have a habit of featuring the same judging panel year after year. A personal attack on one or more of the judges could stop your budding fitness career dead in its tracks. If you really were done an injustice the audience will let you know afterwards. We assure you their positive comments later will mean much more than any trophy ever could. Congratulate the winner, smile, and tell everyone how much fun you had. Many a great bodybuilding career started the moment an individual placed lower than deserved.

The bright lights onstage will wash out your muscularity (and set you back in the placings) if you don't present an evenly tanned physique.

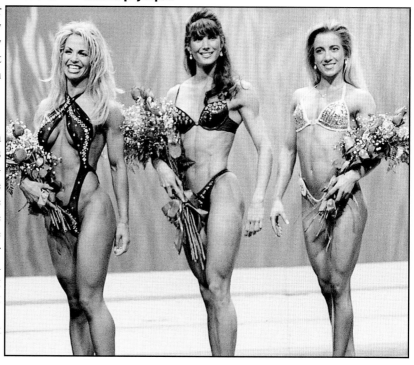

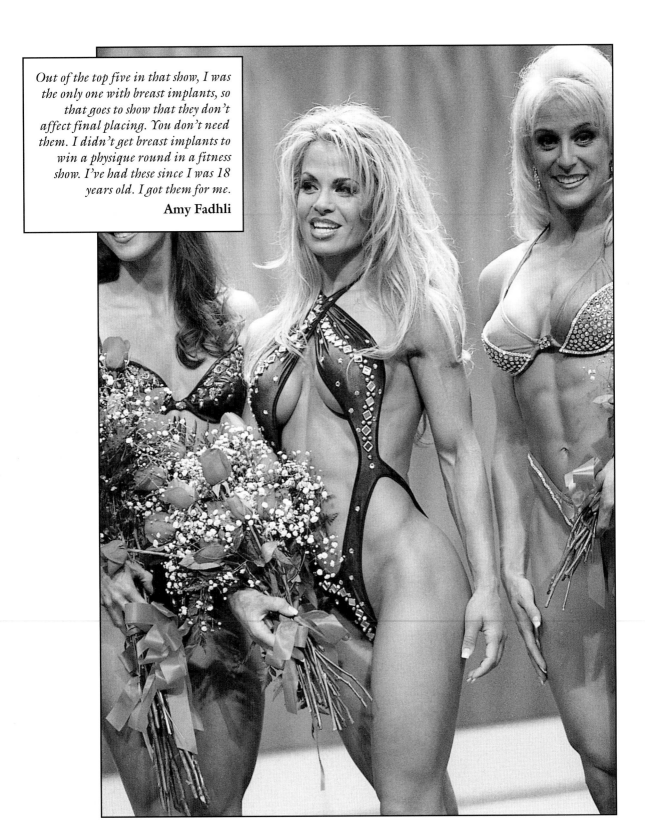

Out of the top five in that show, I was the only one with breast implants, so that goes to show that they don't affect final placing. You don't need them. I didn't get breast implants to win a physique round in a fitness show. I've had these since I was 18 years old. I got them for me.

Amy Fadhli

Chapter 21
Surgery

No! Take me for example. I won all my shows without breast implants. It isn't essential for success. I've never had them, I don't plan on getting them and it's just not part of my life.

Mia Finnegan, 1995 Ms. Fitness Olympia
and *Oxygen* columnist

PLASTIC SURGERY

Everyone wants an edge – that little advantage that helps one achieve success in work, love, and life. Genetics, disease and trauma may have left imperfections that can prevent you from achieving your goals. Modern medicine now has the tools to remove the scars that time has left. In this chapter we examine the procedures available, and what they're used for.

BREAST IMPLANTS

This is still one of the most controversial aspects of competition. The judges and the endorsement companies have a specific look in mind – a firm, lean body, girl-next-door to drop-dead-gorgeous face, and a bust that is prominent but not overly endowed. The problem is that the breasts are sweat glands (not two lumps of muscle). They are made up of bodyfat. Any dieting tends to cause weight loss in this area. Thus a biological conspiracy exists to prevent you, the reader, from having the breasts which are so happily paraded through the pages of fitness magazines, in combination with a low bodyfat level. It is a blatant contradiction, but to succeed at the higher levels of competition, surgical augmentation (or reduction), or

If you decide in favor of surgery, make sure you're doing it for the right reasons. As our fitness pros point out, larger breasts don't mean you'll win more medals on the fitness circuit.

Pamela Cottrell,
***Oxygen* editor-in-chief**

I would love to sit down with you and discuss just one issue – your boyfriend. The mere fact you mention his enthusiasm for breast-implant surgery worries me. Do it for yourself and not anyone else.

Amy Fadhli, top fitness competitor
and *Oxygen* columnist

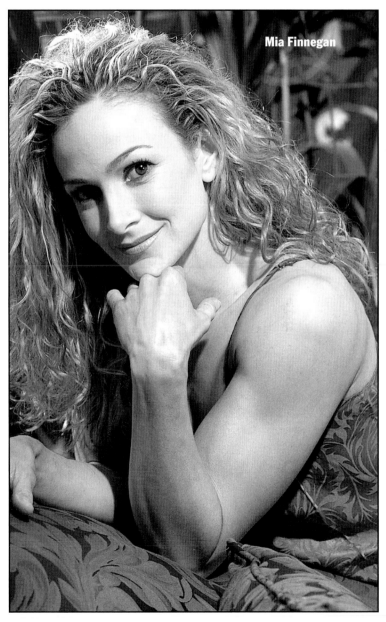

Mia Finnegan

CHAPTER TWENTY-ONE – SURGERY **241**

reliable padding, must be used. We didn't make the rules, but we know how the game is played.

BREAST DEVELOPMENT

At puberty, the breast develops under the hormonal influence of the ovaries, the hypothalamus and the anterior pituitary. Two hormones that are also of importance to this growth phase are insulin (produced in the pancreas) and thyroxine (produced in the thyroid gland).

Throughout a woman's reproductive life, her menstrual cycle will cause her breasts to change size. Three to four days before menses, increasing levels of progesterone and estrogen cause cell proliferation and water retention, which leads to swelling. After menstruation, water is lost and cellular proliferation regresses, and the breasts return to their normal size.

During pregnancy, estrogen, progesterone, placental lactogen, prolactin and chorionic gonadotrophin cause cellular proliferation in the breasts, resulting in a dramatic increase in size. At delivery, progesterone and estrogen levels drop, and milk production is chiefly under the influence of prolactin.

Menopause is the time when a woman's ovaries stop releasing eggs, and she is no longer fertile. Because the ovaries are no longer releasing estrogen and progesterone, there is a progressive loss of glandular tissue in the breasts. This leads to a loss in volume and firmness, and ultimately sagging.

SURGICAL PROCEDURE

Breast enlargement (or augmentation) is one choice available to fitness competitors. Women with underdeveloped breasts, who have lost breast size through dieting, drug use, or who have lost breast tissue because of disease or trauma, can have the breasts they desire. The operation consists of making an incision in three possible places: under the breast, within the armpit or around or within the areola (the pigmented tissue surrounding the nipple). The implant is placed either behind the breast tissue and in front of the chest muscle, or under the muscle. If the implant is placed under the breast tissue, the pain is minimal and recovery time tends to be faster. Placing the implant under the pectorals is more involved. The pectoral muscle must be stretched out in order to fit the implant. This usually results in severe post-operative pain, and a longer recovery period. As the following quote illustrates, mistakes in the operating room can be costly.

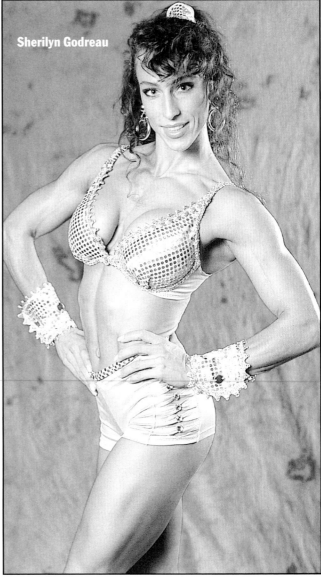

Sherilyn Godreau

"During the procedure the doctor noticed that my left pectoral was longer than my right, and in attempting to correct the problem he took it upon himself to actually cut the left one to match the right, and ended up cutting off half of my pectoral! That affected me in competition for about two years because originally he had put the implants up about half a foot too high. People were always talking about what a long torso I had. It made my waist look a lot longer. Having the implants under the muscle caused infections and a very long recovery process. I had to go to the emergency room twice to have the infections drained, so it was a real problem."

**Kim Chizevsky,
1996, 1997, and
1998 Ms. Olympia**

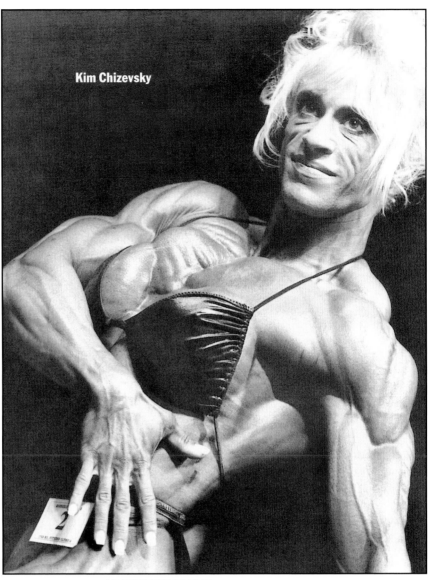

Kim Chizevsky

There is a great variety of implants to choose from. Almost all are made from a silicone rubber sack, which is filled with either saline or silicone gel. Your surgeon will help you decide which is right for you.

Scars are almost invisible because of their location. Scars are hidden in the armpit or under the breast, and placing the incision where the skin changes color at the border of the dark-colored areola makes very effective camouflage. Unfortunately, there is the risk of nerve damage, with the nipple becoming permanently numb. Implanted breasts are more firm and round than natural breasts of the same size. But implanted breasts, like larger breasts, will respond to gravity and sag with age.

ARE THEY SAFE?

There is considerable controversy surrounding the use of silicone implants. Despite numerous anecdotal reports of health problems attributed to implants, respected scientific journals have printed studies that demonstrate no relationship between silicone and autoimmune disease.[1] Sufferers claim that silicone is toxic, while scientists say that silicone is inert. Groups suing Dow Chemical (an implant manufacturer) say that up to 70 percent of implants rupture, but Dow claims

It comes down to which side has the most personal experts and puts on the best show.

Marcia Angel, executive editor of the *New England Journal of Medicine*

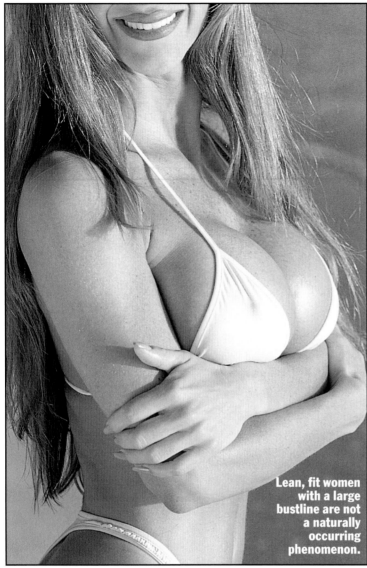

Lean, fit women with a large bustline are not a naturally occurring phenomenon.

There's no history in my family, no reason for me to be ill. There has to be something else.

Uneeda Laitinen, who went from a 34B to a 36C using silicone breast implants. Over the past 25 years since, she has suffered from memory loss, aching joints, severe migraines and nerves so badly damaged that she did not realize she was being burned by a hot skillet until she smelled her own flesh burning. She blames her health problems on her implants.

on your own, and check things out with a number of plastic surgeons. Then cool off for a couple of months and think very hard about this. Be sure to make an appointment with a breast cancer specialist. Some types of implants can obscure cancer in the early stages. Are you high risk for this disease? Perhaps padding or silicone supports that are worn in the bra might be safer. This is not a decision that should be taken lightly. You are thinking about having someone knock you out (and there is always a risk with any surgical procedure), open your body, and put foreign objects into it. There is the risk of infection and scarring. And there's going to be some post-operative pain. Is it worth it?

Some women say that it has enhanced their self-esteem, and thus helped them to achieve their goals. Others claim that it is a form of surgical abuse, designed to force women into an unnatural form that feeds our culture's fantasy of "Barbie-doll" women. You decide.

Perhaps the dumbest form of breast implants is using your own bodyfat. Basically, the surgeon removes fat from an area that you don't want it (your belly) and moves it to somewhere you want it (your breasts). Bad move. Fat naturally moves about the body, and surgically implanted fat tends to calcify,

only six percent break. Critics argue that Dow knew their implants were unsafe, Dow says their implants are safe. At any rate, going to court hasn't solved the controversy. Of 20 cases brought against Dow, 14 were settled in the company's favor. But in one class-action suit, a Louisiana jury found that Dow knowingly deceived the plaintiffs by hiding negative information about silicone. In numerous medical studies, there was found to be no connection between implants and illness. So what do you do? Discuss the issue with your doctor, your family, your friends, do some research forming bony granules. You don't want breasts that feel like bean bags. More seriously, a mammogram will identify the granule as a shadowy figure, requiring a biopsy. Any woman who has found a lump, and then experienced the terror of waiting to find out if it's breast cancer, will tell you to avoid this particular procedure at all costs!

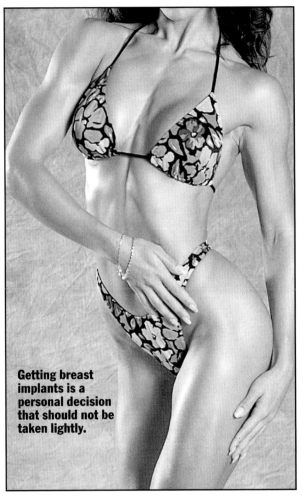

Getting breast implants is a personal decision that should not be taken lightly.

BREAST REDUCTION

For a number of women, this is a serious problem. Large breasts put a severe strain on the neck, shoulders and back. This can lead to joint problems such as arthritis and severe neck pain. Bras become uncomfortable as the straps cut into the skin. As well, constant chafing can lead to chronic skin irritation under the breasts. Mobility can be limited, and the

operation of a computer keyboard can become next to impossible. There are also social problems, usually in the form of unwanted comments and attention. Since the judges are looking at proportion in a fitness contest, overly endowed competitors are usually marked down. Clearly, while this is a type of plastic surgery, it is also an essential medical procedure that can drastically improve quality of life. Liposuction can also reduce the breasts, but the loss of volume results in sagging.

Breast reduction involves removing excess breast tissue while reshaping and lifting the breast. The reduction in weight means immediate relief for the upper body. There is less pain with this procedure than with breast augmentation. Because the nerves to the skin have been stretched out by the weight of the breasts, the skin is less sensitive. Recovery time is quicker and post-operative pain easily controlled. While the breasts are now smaller, they can become larger again through weight gain or pregnancy.

There is considerable scarring with breast reduction. The scars are placed so that they are only visible if you are topless. The scars are brown or pink, but may fade over the years. They are also long, and may thicken and widen over time.

BREAST LIFT

This procedure, also a called mastopexy, is done to correct sagging breasts. Breasts may sag because of weight gain or pregnancy (as skin stretches); because breast tissue shrinks (as you achieve a lower bodyfat level); or due to gravity over time. By decreasing the size of the skin or increasing breast volume, the surgeon can raise or lift the breast. That is why implants are often used with this procedure.

In a mastopexy, excess skin is removed from around the areola and sometimes the bottom of the breast. The remaining skin is surgically tightened. Volume in the form of an implant can be added to help further smooth the skin, as well as elevating the nipple and areola to a more youthful position.

It sounds simple, but it is an involved operation. It can take anywhere from two to five hours in surgery, but normal activities can be resumed in a matter of days. A support bra should be worn until the healing process is complete. The scars are minimal, but they are visible if you are topless.

LIPOSUCTION

This procedure is also called body sculpting, liposculpture, suction lipectomy and lipoplasty. It is a surgical way of removing bodyfat from the body. When it first became common in the 1980s, large suction tubes called canulas resulted in serious blood loss and the surgeon could not remove more than 1.5 litres of fat. The patient also required a blood transfusion, along with all the risks it entails. In the first few years, of the thousands that had this operation, 11 deaths were recorded, mostly the result of blood clots.

Thanks to smaller cannulas and the use of adrenaline to constrict blood vessels, blood loss is now minimized. The operation can be done under a local anaesthetic, which again lowers the risk. Through a tiny incision, the cannula (which can be as small as 1.8 milli-metres in diameter) is inserted into a problem area. A saline/adrenaline solution is injected. The saline distends the area and the adrenaline restricts blood flow. This type of procedure is called tumescent liposuction. The cannula is then connected to a machine or syringe that creates a vacuum, which sucks out the fatty deposits. The skin, nerves, blood vessels and muscles are left intact. Because of the use of adrenaline, the surgery becomes almost bloodless, making liposuction to the face possible. Less blood loss means less bruising and a quicker recovery time.

In abdominal liposculpture, the incision is made near the pubis or in the umbilicus (the belly button). With the arms, the incision is made near the elbow

crease or in the armpit. In the buttocks or thighs, the incision is made in the buttock crease. The neck can be liposculpted through incisions under the chin and behind the ear lobes. The knees and lower legs are incised from behind the knee. And the pad of fat under the chin can be removed at the source. Facial fat can be removed by syringe, using only a local anaesthetic.

Since fat cells do not regenerate, this is a permanent solution. But if you don't watch your diet, the remaining fat cells will get bigger. More than one Hollywood star has had

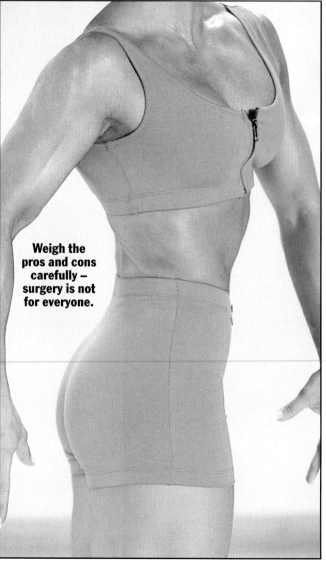

Weigh the pros and cons carefully – surgery is not for everyone.

the same area done more than once (one country singer had his abs done three times!).

This is still serious surgery and you can expect to have some postoperative soreness from a few days to a few weeks. Rest, limiting activities, and wearing restrictive bandages and clothing over the suctioned area are all mandatory.

TUMMY TUCK

Also called abdominoplasty, this refers to a procedure to correct the loss of elasticity to the skin over the gut and weakened abdominal muscles. Multiple pregnancies, weight fluctuation, and even liposuction can result in this problem. Excess fat and skin are removed from the umbilicus to the pubic hairline. The muscles are brought together and sutured to tighten the abdomen. More fatty tissue and skin are removed, and the umbilicus is restored to it's normal anatomic location. This is performed under general anaesthetic, and requires several weeks for complete recovery.

EYELID SURGERY

Also called blepharoplasty, this procedure improves the appearance of the eyes. Puffiness under the eyes can be caused by fat that protrudes under the eyelid skin. A heavy fold of skin that obscures the normal crease of the upper lid (and may even interfere with vision), is caused by excess skin. Removal of the fat by liposuction, and surgical removal of the excess skin can improve both appearance and vision. This type of surgery is normally done with a facelift. A local anaesthetic is used for blepharoplasty, and the suture can be removed after five days.

FACE LIFT

Age, gravity, genetics, and exposure to the sun lead to changes in the face. The skin on the neck and under the jaw becomes loose, fat builds up under the chin, wrinkles become more abundant and the crease between the nose and the mouth deepens. Abuse of drugs, tobacco and alcohol can also accelerate the aging process.

The incision is lengthy, beginning in the hair near the temple, continuing down the front of the ear, around the ear lobe and into the hair. This makes it easier to hide the scar. Excess skin is cut away, muscles and sagging tissues are tightened, and the skin is reposi-

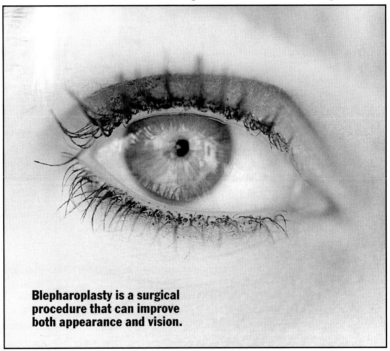

Blepharoplasty is a surgical procedure that can improve both appearance and vision.

tioned to give a smooth, youthful look. A double chin can be removed by liposuction. A variation of this, the deep plane lift, is a layered approach that permits tightening of the interlacing network of connective tissues that join the facial muscles beneath the skin. This procedure is said to provide a better and longer-lasting result.

The operation can take three or more hours, and the patient will look like she has been beaten with an ugly stick for the first few side effects should subside after several weeks. The scars remain pink for a few months, then change to a whiter color. Makeup is generally applied to help hide the scars. Because the face continues to age, some patients opt to have the procedure repeated every few years. Usually, once a lifetime is enough.

FACIAL IMPLANTS

These implants are used to enhance facial contours. Chin implants are used to correct a weak chin. A small incision is made inside the mouth, through which the implant is inserted, positioned and secured. Cheek implants are inserted through an incision inside the lower eyelid or upper lip. Jaw implants are inserted through an incision in the lower lip, and lip implants are inserted through an incision on the inside of both lips. Normal activities can usually be resumed after a week.

NOSE JOB

Also called rhinoplasty, this nasal reconstruction immediately brings Michael Jackson to mind. Most people are not interested in such a dramatic change in appearance. Whether genetics or trauma are at the root of the problem, the nose may develop in such a way that does not fit the face. A nose job can involve straightening of the nose and septum (which can improve breathing), reduction of a nasal "hump" in the bridge of the nose, and refinement of the tip. There are no visible scars because the surgeon operates from within the nostrils.

The operation is performed under general anaesthetic and takes about one hour. The nose is bandaged and splinted for protection, and the patient can expect bruising and two black eyes. The nasal protection is usually removed after a week, although the bruising may take longer to heal.

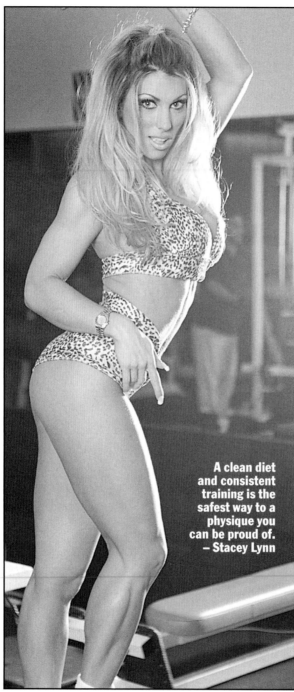

A clean diet and consistent training is the safest way to a physique you can be proud of.
— Stacey Lynn

days. After the swelling and bruising reduce, the beautiful results become apparent, and within two weeks the face regains its normal appearance. There can be postoperative feelings of pain, tightness and numbness. These

BROW LIFT

Aging and genetics can lead to a furrowed brow, giving a very serious or angry expression. To correct this, the brow can be lifted. This is done by endoscopic surgery under general anaesthetic. Adrenaline is injected locally to control bleeding. Parallel to the hair's center part, six, 1.5 centimetre incisions are made. A tiny scope on the end of a tube is put into one incision to locate the muscles. Surgical instruments are put into the forehead through other incisions. Nerves can be separated from muscles that are to be cut, and small pieces of fat can also be removed. Titanium screws are drilled into the skull, and the skin is sewn up, tightened and held in place by the screws. The screws are removed about ten days later. Recovery time takes about a week, and bruising should subside shortly thereafter.

DERMABRASION AND DERMAPLANING

Trauma, disease and genetics can all lead to alterations to the surface of the face. By surgically scraping the top layers of skin, the face can be refinished to appear more uniform. Dermabrasion is used to reduce facial scars, remove tattoos or to smooth out wrinkles. The surgeon sands off the outermost layer of skin until a safe level is reached that reduces the visibility of the wrinkle or scar. Dermaplaning is used to treat deep, or "ice-pick" acne scars. A hand-held planer is used to skim off layers of skin until the lowest point of the scar is even, or at least closer, to the level of the surrounding skin.

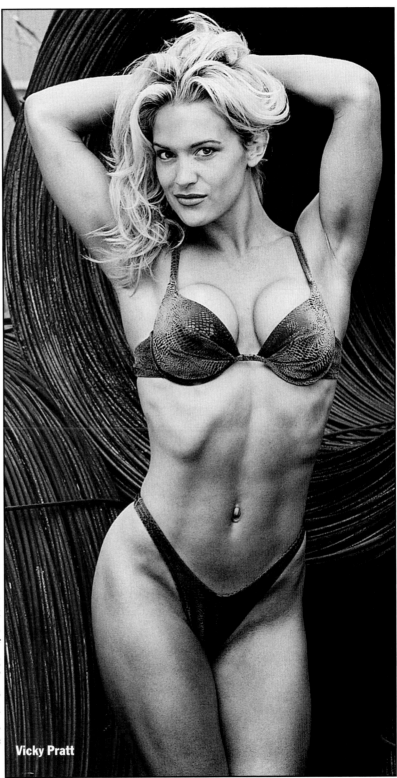

Vicky Pratt

Recovery time is variable, and depends on the amount of surface area involved. Dermabrasion produces considerable postoperative pain, and the scabs can take two weeks to heal.

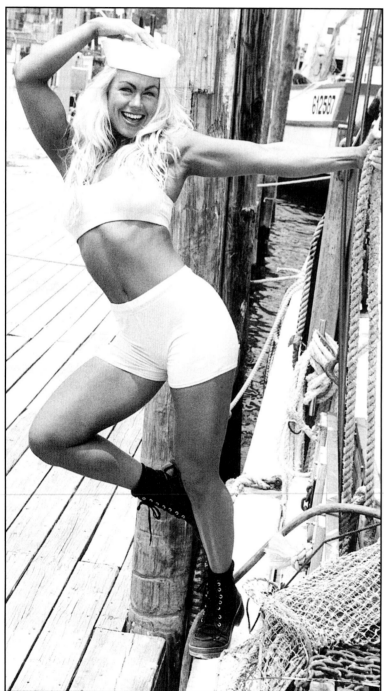

CHEMICAL PEEL

During World War I, it was discovered that ammunition workers who were exposed to the caustic chemical phenol had rejuvenated skin in the affected areas. After some study and practice, doctors began to use chemicals to peel away the damaged outer layers of the skin. Once it had healed, a youthful appearance resulted. Skin that has been damaged by acne, exposure to the sun, or has uneven pigmentation, precancerous growths or wrinkles can be treated with a chemical peel. Alphahydroxy acids (AHAs) are used in minor cases to produce a light peel. Trichloroacetic acid (TCA) produces a medium-depth peel. Both usually take 10 to 15 minutes to apply. Phenol is used for deep peeling. To do the entire face can take up to two hours. The use of phenol poses the risk of damaging pigment-producing melanocytes, leading to permanent depigmentation of the skin.

Because the face has been given a controlled chemical burn, appearance in the days immediately after treatment can be disturbing. But this is only temporary, and after about two months one can expect a full recovery.

A less drastic option is the mini peel. The face is given a deep steam cleansing, followed by a mask. Glycolic acid is then applied to the face, left on for a few minutes, and removed. This mild acid not only causes the outerlayer of dead cells to come off, it also affects the inner layers. Because it is the mildest peel, one application every two months for the first year, followed by one application every four months is the

Skin that has been damaged by the sun can be treated with a chemical peel.

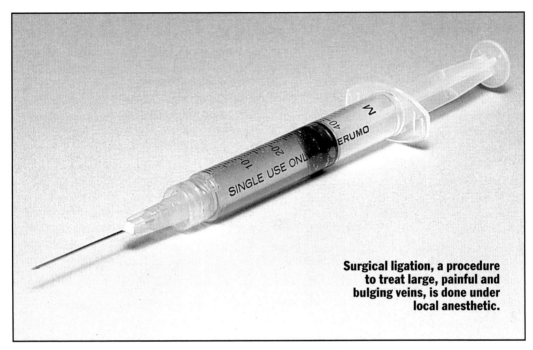

Surgical ligation, a procedure
to treat large, painful and
bulging veins, is done under
local anesthetic.

recommended regimen to maintain youthful skin.

LASER SURGERY

Laser light (light amplification by stimulated emission of radiation) is the ultimate scalpel. Because it seals blood vessels as it cuts them, little blood is lost, and blood-vessel constricting drugs do not have to be administered and the surgeon has a clear view of the operating area. Laser surgery is used for the same conditions as dermabrasion and the chemical peel. CO_2 lasers vaporize water in the epidermal cells, which results in a controlled burn. Because the surgeon can control the energy emitted by the laser, the doctor can precisely penetrate the skin to a consistent depth over the entire face. The burned skin is shed, and new skin regenerates. The risk of scarring is less than one percent. Since the laser light seals nerves as it cuts them, there is virtually no postoperative pain. There will be redness for at least ten days, and then a pinkish complexion for up to three months. Foundation can be used to correct this problem. This technique can also be used to remove varicose veins, stretch marks and unwanted tattoos.

SCLEROTHERAPY

This is the removal of varicose veins with the use of a sclerosing, or hardening agent (saline, dextrose or iodine). This irritates the lining of the vein, causing the walls to thicken and stick together. It eventually becomes scar tissue and is absorbed by the body. Circulation continues through healthy veins.

Sclerotherapy works best on veins smaller than three millimeters. Patients undergo an average of six sessions of sclerotherapy, comprised of 10 to 30 injections per session. Temporary side effects can include a burning or cramping sensation upon injection, swelling and bruising.

SURGICAL LIGATION

Also called stripping, this procedure is done under local anesthetic, primarily to treat large, painful and bulging veins. The abnormal vein is cut at both ends, then removed. The remaining veins are grafted onto other healthy veins. After surgery, patients are advised to rest at home for two weeks. Scars from the small incisions will eventually fade. They can be camouflaged with foundation.

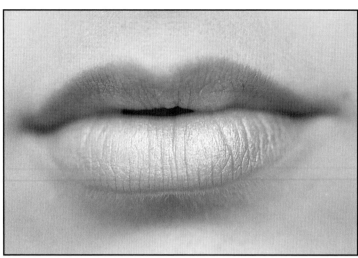

Lips can be enhanced with collagen injections, but the results will only last about six months.

COLLAGEN INJECTIONS

Collagen is a protein that is the principal component of connective tissue. It is also found in the skin. Collagen molecules are structured like three-strand ropes. Many of the processes of aging are possibly due to derangement of this structure. When the skin's own collagen wears down, wrinkles, depressions and gouges can appear. By injecting collagen directly into the affected area, the surgeon can fill in acne scars, reduce or eliminate wrinkles, or enhance the cheeks and lips. The body will absorb this injected collagen, so this procedure must be repeated every six months. Those with a history of autoimmune disease should not have this procedure.

FAT INJECTIONS

This is an option for those who cannot use collagen. The individual's own bodyfat is removed from where it's not wanted, and injected into an acne scar or wrinkle. Sounds safe since you're using your own tissue, but there are potential problems. Fat does not take kindly to being pushed around the body, and can calcify. Then you're stuck with a bony lump in your face. If the fat doesn't calcify, the body will reabsorb it over time, so the procedure will need to be repeated.

BOTOX INJECTIONS

Botulism is a potentially lethal form of food poisoning caused by the toxin that is produced by the bacteria clostridium botulinum. It thrives on badly preserved food, but only in the complete absence of air. Botox, a purified toxin produced by the same bacteria can paralyze the nervous system. This paralysis of muscles and nerves makes it a useful cosmetic tool. Injecting diluted doses of botox can cause local paralysis. No muscle movement, no creases, no wrinkles and no furrows. Having trouble maintaining that smile for the judges while you somersault across the stage? One treatment can keep you smiling for up to six months, even while you're sleeping! While Botox freezes features, there is the risk that the botox can spread and weaken surrounding muscles.

HAIR TRANSPLANT

Genetics, disease, trauma and drug use can all cause hair loss in women. Hair transplantation moves small grafts of scalp that contain hair follicles to areas that are thinning or bald. Normally, small plugs bearing two to 15 hairs are transplanted. Usually about six weeks after the transplant, the hairs begin to fall out, but they will grow back. There can be postoperative pain, swelling and bruising. Scabbing will heal within ten days, and numbness in the operated areas will disappear within two to three months. The scars are small and hidden under the hair.

SYNTHOL (PUMP 'n POSE)

For many years, bodybuilders have experimented with a variety of drugs that could either increase muscle mass, or give the illusion of mass. In the latter category, a number of competitors attempted to capitalize on the swelling effects of snake venom. In recent years, Esiclene, a weak anabolic steroid, has become a fashionable injectable among competitors. It causes a swelling that lasts about three days. It is also very painful, so an analgesic is usually taken as well. The latest product in this pharmaceutical arms race is Synthol. Though we refer to it by its original name Synthol (the name was dropped after it was discovered that the pharmaceutical company, Bristol-Myers, owned the name), it was renamed Synthosizze and is sold as Pump 'n Pose. There is a British product, which claims similar qualities, called Muscle Sheen.

Synthol is a German-manufactured oil believed to contain medical-grade MCT (medium chain triglyceride) oil, a painkiller and other secret ingredients. The owner, Chris Clark, will not divulge the exact contents. Sold as a posing oil and topical analgesic, it is being used by bodybuilders as an injectable to swell the muscles. If we are to believe the hype, you can make two years of gains in three weeks! Remember, there is no corresponding increase in strength. In fact, workouts are said to become painful after injection. The oil blends with the muscle fibers, which makes the entire muscle swell. Synthol increases both size and definition. This could also be of value for fitness contestants, who might have a weak bodypart that ruins their overall proportions.

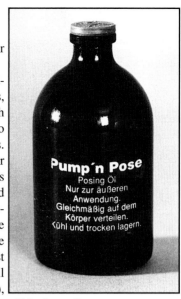

Because these products are sold as posing oils, they are not classified, which means they are not subject to legal or medical controls. Therefore, the manufacturer doesn't have to state what is in the oil, yet the oil is used as a body-modification substance. This could be the future of plastic surgery. Face lifts will be a thing of the past (sagging face muscles will suddenly get pumped up), and breasts will bounce up. This is really scary, because you know some idiot is going to inject every chest muscle! We don't know what happens to the injected muscle over the long term, or what happens if this stuff gets into the circulatory or lymphatic systems. Could it be carcinogenic? Will it calcify? There have been no medical studies done. Until it has been proven to be safe, avoid this treatment.

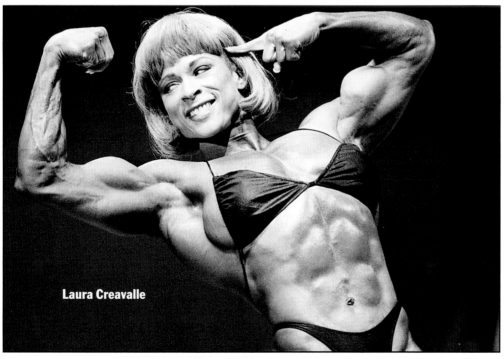

Laura Creavalle

NONSURGICAL OPTIONS

PADDING

One highly recommended form of padding is the IGIA WONDER FORM (TM). These figure-enhancing forms can increase the bust-line up to two full cup sizes, yet are made of light-weight silicone gel, so you barely notice them. The pads just slip into the bra and mould to your form. No mess, no fuss. And they look very natural, even in a swimsuit! Or you can go the supermodel route, and place duct tape under the breasts to lift them up. A lot cheaper, but definitely not as comfortable!

When you turn to the side, your glutes look so well developed that they make your chest appear even smaller than it is. What I would recommend to you is get a suit that will push you up and give you the illusion of having a chest.

A piece of valuable advice given by Carla Dunlap to Mia Finnegan. According to Mia, it worked!

HOW TO BE TWO-FACED!

Despite dieting and intense exercise, some women possess a pad of fat beneath the chin that won't go away. Others, due to genetics, age, or overexposure to the sun, find that parts of the face are wrinkling and even sagging. Still others seek a dramatic change by lifting the eyebrows. Is there a way to correct all this without surgery? You bet! But it's only temporary (but long enough for a stage show, photoshoot, job interview, or a big date). The solution is called taping. You can purchase specially made adhesive tapes that have holes for pieces of string to be connected using hooks. If you can't find these, make your own. Go to a medical supply store and buy adhesives designed to stick directly to the skin. You can then cut and modify them to suit your needs. Since natural oils and makeup prevent effective bonding, clean the skin with an alcohol swab or other astringent before applying the tape. When attaching the tape:

– Do it symmetrically, so that the face has an even appearance.

– Apply the tape in places where hair or shadow will easily conceal it.

– To remove that double chin, apply tape under the chin, just inside the corners of the jaw.

– To raise the eyebrows apply tape to the forehead (use bangs to conceal the tape).

– To alter the shape of the eyebrows or eyelids, apply tape to the temples (pulling up, down or to the sides).

– To go for the overall face lift (particularly to enhance the cheekbones), apply tape to the skin in front of the ears, but parallel to the apple of the cheek.

Once the tape is attached, the rest is easy, though not necessarily comfortable. Hook the strings to the tapes, pull the strings firmly until the desired effect is obtained, and tie them together. Then you can secure the strings to the hair with fasteners. Hair, flowers, or a fashionable hat will cover the evidence, completing the illusion. This is the sort of thing that you have to practice, and we strongly recommend that you have a friend assist you.

Carla Dunlap

Reference
1. www.brobeck.com/sslitplg/63.htm

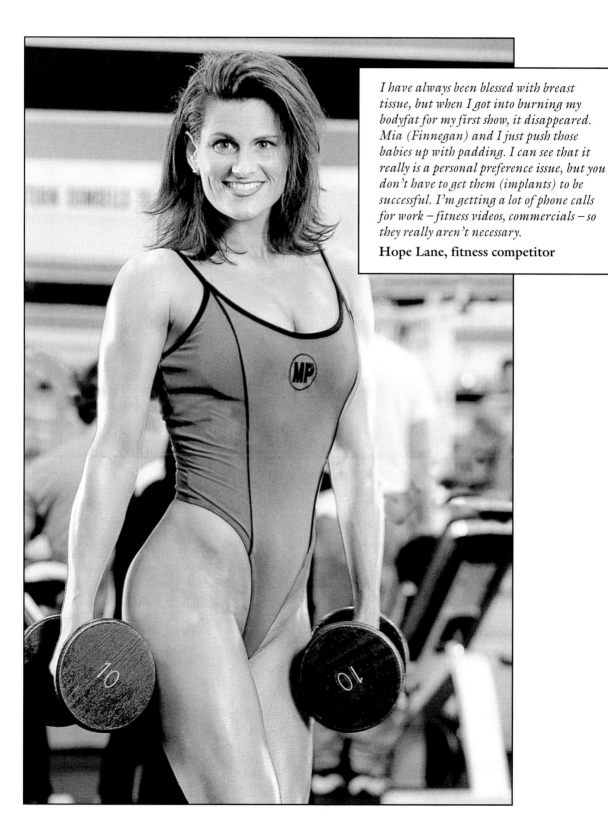

I have always been blessed with breast tissue, but when I got into burning my bodyfat for my first show, it disappeared. Mia (Finnegan) and I just push those babies up with padding. I can see that it really is a personal preference issue, but you don't have to get them (implants) to be successful. I'm getting a lot of phone calls for work – fitness videos, commercials – so they really aren't necessary.

Hope Lane, fitness competitor

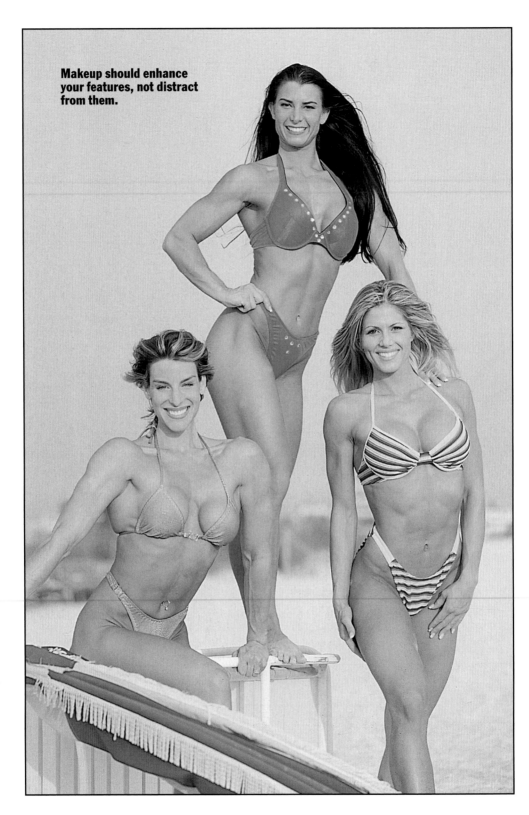

Makeup should enhance
your features, not distract
from them.

Beauty Tips

You can have a body to die for, and still lose a contest because of your complexion. The judges are looking for the complete package, and a mottled face just doesn't sell products. This chapter explains what cosmetics to use, and how to use them.

CONCEALER

Little imperfections like pimples and discoloration can distract from a beautiful face. The idea of concealer is to use as little as possible. Find a shade to match your skin type. If you're having trouble finding the right color, you can mix a small amount of concealer with a similar amount of eyeshadow in the shade you desire. Golden-toned concealers are the best for covering blue and purplish discoloration. If you have dark circles under your eyes because you couldn't sleep the night before the fitness contest, try a concealer that is several shades lighter. An alternative is to use foundation first, and then apply a reflective concealer over the foundation.

If you are an older fitness contestant, congratulations! But you may have run into the problem of "liver spots," brown patches that appear on the skin with age. Over-the-counter skin bleaches can help and so can your dermatologist. Check with a professional. You can also apply concealer, just use a lighter shade. Always apply concealer with a concealer brush. Its small tip allows you to be precise in applying concealer to where it's

Exercising without makeup is definitely the way to go. Sweat and dirt mixed with foundation powders and blushes is a nasty combination. Talk about clogging your pores.

Amy Fadhli, *Oxygen* **columnist and top fitness competitor**

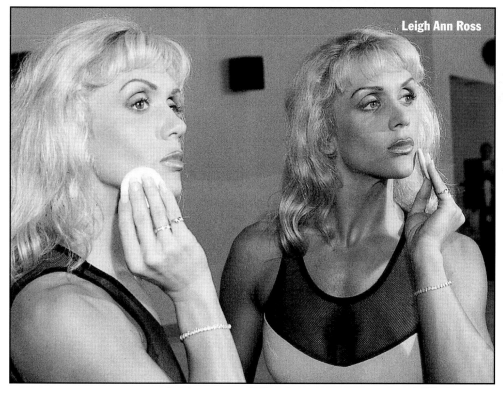

Leigh Ann Ross

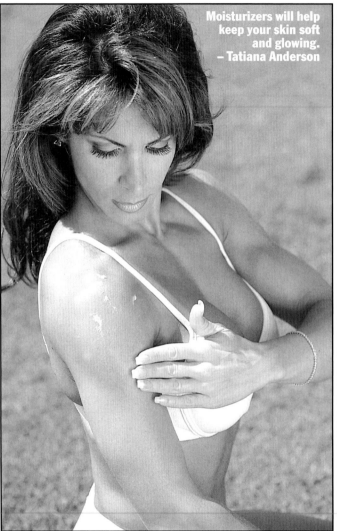

Moisturizers will help keep your skin soft and glowing.
– Tatiana Anderson

Cetaphil). A moisturizer will keep the skin soft and glowing, and help your makeup adhere to the skin. The only exception is for someone with skin irritation other than that caused by dryness. The skin needs to be dry to heal. For those of you with allergies, always use water-based moisturizers, not oil-based. See your dermatologist, and don't use a moisturizer until the doctor says it's okay.

First of all, always exfoliate and cleanse your entire body prior to applying bronzer. Use a scrub-brush or loufah with a scrubbing agent in the bath. This will eliminate dead skin cells which collect on your skin surface.

Amy Fadhli, *Oxygen* **columnist and top fitness competitor**

FOUNDATION

If you've applied the concealer properly, you might find that you don't need foundation. But the bright lights of the stage are harsh and unforgiving, so let's assume the worst and try the foundation anyway. First, find a color that matches your own. This is easier said than done. One option is to narrow it down to three shades. Apply one stroke of each down your cheek. The one that you can't see is the one for you. If you still find that your foundation is too dark for your skin tone, you can blend it with cornstarch. The more you add, the lighter the foundation will become. The cornstarch will hold. Just keep searching for that right tone for you. When applying foundation, use a makeup wedge. Make sure the wedge is lightly moistened, as this will aid in application and result in a more even tone. Begin at the center of the face and work outward. Use very little and sponge it out until the foundation disappears under the chin and at the hairline. Contestants of African ancestry sometimes find that foundation results in an ashen-look. They should always use foundations with yellow and red undertones.

needed. Remember, less is better! Concealer is not just for the face, you can also use it to cover stretch marks during a physique competition.

MOISTURIZER

No matter what type of skin you have, always apply a moisturizer before the rest of your cosmetics go on (though some will argue that those with oily skin should not, instead they should wash their skin first with a product like

Many women suffer from a condition called acnea roscacea. It is a skin condition in which the center of the face (primarily the nose and cheeks) becomes red and inflamed. People often cruelly assume that the sufferer has a drinking problem. Anyone with this condition should see a dermatologist. A foundation with yellow undertones is very good for restoring a normal pallor to the face.

If you're going onstage or are going to be photographed, continue applying foundation under the chin, over the throat and chest. A common mistake, still seen at contests, results in the contestant having a face that is light and a body that is dark. Foundation reflects the light but naked skin absorbs light, making it appear darker. Under the stress of competition and the bright lights, your face may begin to appear shiny. Powder-blotting papers will absorb excess oil while leaving the makeup. A quick powder touchup, and you'll look as good as new! And yes, you wouldn't be the first to apply foundation all over your body. After the foundation has been applied use powder to set and keep the foundation in place. Otherwise it may collect in the skin's creases. When applying powder use a large powder brush, knocking excess powder off the brush before you begin. Never rub or wipe across the face, rather use the brush in short blending motions.

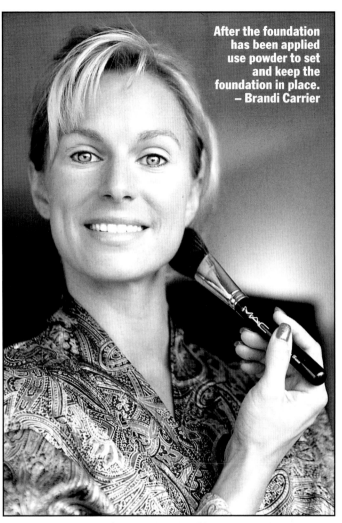

After the foundation has been applied use powder to set and keep the foundation in place.
– Brandi Carrier

CONTOURING

The goal here is to highlight what you like, and shade what you don't. Dark colors cause features to recede, while light colors make features stand out. Thus, you'll need highlighting powders and shading powders. To make the cheek bones prominent, apply dark shading beneath them. You don't need to apply light shade to the cheekbones themselves, as you'll be using blush shortly. To make the nose narrower and shorter, apply a dark shade across the front, and up the sides. Next apply a light shade to the bridge of the nose. A neat little trick for making the breasts pop out is to apply a light shade along the center of your cleavage, going up on both sides, following the natural contour of the breasts. A medium-sized blush brush works best for this task.

BLUSHING

This is the easiest part of doing makeup. To achieve that sun-kissed look, apply blush to the forehead, temples, chin and cheeks. To avoid the "clown" look when applying blush to the cheeks, begin at the hairline, and then gently swirl over the apple of the cheek. For white and Asian women, pink is a very good color. For women of African ancestry, mango powder is an ideal choice. If you are of a multi-racial background or tanned, you may find that bronzing powders hold the tone best suited for you. Use a blusher brush, shaking the powder off first, and then apply using quick, short strokes.

EYE SHADOW

The eyes are a region of personal choice. Go with the colors and styles that appeal to you. If you're trying to win a contest, read this section closely. You want the judges (and more importantly, the photographers), to love your face. Deep blue, green, glossy, or metallic eyeshadows are generally not seen among the winners. Endorsements depend on a natural look, not a look that's made up. Makeup must be used to enhance your features, not distract from them. Begin with an undereye concealer. This will hold your eye shadow in place. Dusting the eyelid with translucent powder will also help. When applying eye shadow, use either a disposable sponge applicator or an eye-shadow brush. You might need more than one brush to make sure you can comfortably cover the regions of the eye. Keep the eye open when applying eyeshadow to the crease. Though it is recommended that you remove your contacts before working on your eyes, a lack of time or simple inability to see may not make this the best choice. Just don't do this while driving! Apply the lightest shade to the lid, then do under the brow. Depending on the look you're going for, you can make the shade lighter, darker or the same.

A simple way to do the eyes is called "the sweep." Just one color is applied from lash to brow. This method has been around for years in Eastern Europe. Provided that soft, dark colors are used and they match your eye color, the effect is very erotic!

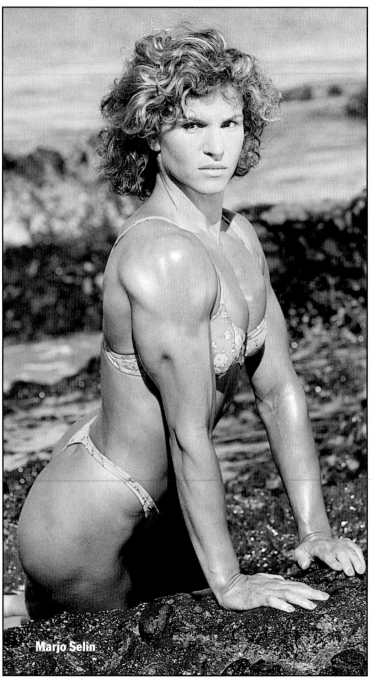

Marjo Selin

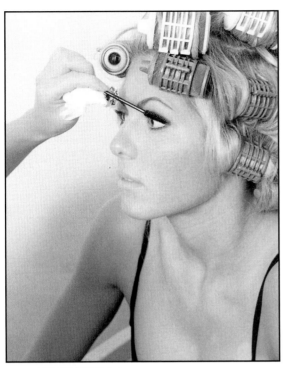

EYELINER

When applying eyeliner, try to stick to dark colors. A very popular look seen in many fashion magazines and contests is the "Kohl." By applying a dark line along the outer rims of the eyelid with an eyeliner pencil, you can outline the eye. Never put eyeliner on the inside rim, as this can lead to infection. Use a darker shade for the upper lid. With an eyeliner brush, you can smudge along this line, creating a seductive "smoky" frame that brings out the whiteness of the eye. In turn, the now intense white of the eye contrasts more strongly with the pupil.

EYELASHES (FALSE AND NATURAL)

If you have sparse lashes, or short ones, false eyelashes are a remedy. When attaching lashes, it is normal to work from the outer corner of the eye inward. If you want to apply individual ones, dip them in eyelash glue and attach them to the eyelid, between your natural lashes. If applying full lashes, apply glue to the lash-band. Let it dry a bit, and then apply next to the natural lashes. Careful snipping with a pair of scissors will give the lashes a more natural look.

To make your eyes appear wider and livelier, an eyelash curler is the ideal choice. By curling the lashes out from the eye, the eye is better defined and the lashes seem longer. Apply the curler as close to the base of the lashes as you can get and squeeze without pulling. After a few seconds, move outward and repeat. You should have the lashes completely curled after three or four repetitions.

The alternative is to have your eyelashes permed at a salon. This permanent curl will last for three months, but it is expensive.

MASCARA

When applying mascara, the goal is to create length and thickness. Begin by adding a tiny amount of translucent powder over the lashes, and then use the mascara. Beginning at the base of the lash, move the mascara brush upward and outward. Now you have the illusion of longer, darker lashes that are well defined and separated. Stick with dark, neutral colors (not blue) to create a more natural effect. Maybeline Volume is an excellent line of mascara, as well as any products made by

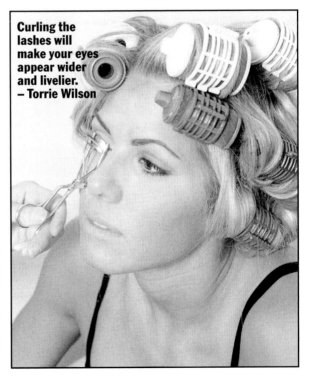

Curling the lashes will make your eyes appear wider and livelier.
– Torrie Wilson

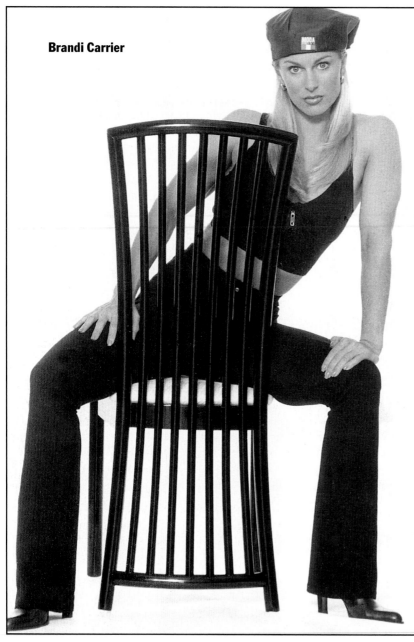

Brandi Carrier

until the eraser makes contact with the nose. Mark with concealer where the tip of the pencil is on your eyebrow. This is the outside boundary of the brow. Hold the pencil the same way, but against the side of the nose. The tip of the pencil now marks where the eyebrow should begin. To create a graceful arch, pluck stray hairs from the bottom of the brow. The top hairs usually form a natural bend in the brow. Be sure to clear the area between the brows. If you find that your brows are too sparse, you can fill in the gaps with an eyebrow pencil. To try out different colors, apply mascara with a mascara brush. To make the brows more prominent use a dark color throughout. If you want to minimize the brows, only color the center of the brows. If you want to create a gentler look, you can bleach the eyebrows. This will make the entire face look softer. If you have delinquent hairs that won't stay in place, a bit of hairspray will hold them down.

For your stage presentation, you and your choreographer may have cooked up a presentation that requires a drastically different look. The eyebrows you have may be suitable for daily activities, but you need something with more pizzazz for the big night. Here's a trick from the pros. Coat the entire brow in sealing wax. When that has dried add a coat of sealer, and let dry. Now apply your foundation, and voila! Your eyebrows have disappeared! Now you can paint on any style, any thickness you want.

"Did you always have the one eyebrow?"

"No. Not until I plucked the top one."

The Carol Burnett Show

Pupa. If you don't like using mascara and thickness isn't an issue, you can have your lashes tinted. This is not a cheap proposal. It should only be done at a salon and will have to be repeated every four weeks.

EYEBROWS

A variety of styles exist for the brows, but the styles all begin with a basic set of instructions. Take a standard-sized pencil, hold it vertically with the eraser end down, and place it at the center of the eye. Now lean the pencil over

Tweezing is still one of the few legal forms of torture that remains politically correct. What if you just can't stand the pain? Simple, just numb the area. Topically apply a toothache or teething remedy (Anbesol is really good) to the eyebrows, working it into the skin. Wait a minute, and then tweeze. You've really got to try it to believe it.

Many women prefer waxing. If done properly, it only has to be repeated once every three to six weeks. You should have this done at a salon.

LIPSTICK AND LIP LINER

Lipstick is made up of pigments, waxes and emollients. Pigments provide color, waxes provide a medium, and emollients move the pigment to the lips. While sheer (matt) lipstick gives a natural look by providing a hint of color, when onstage or out for the evening, the best choice is a shimmer (gloss) lipstick because it has microbeads that make the lips glimmer.

Getting the right shade of lipstick is an art form. It depends on your skin tones, your eyes, your hair and your choice of cosmetics. Once you have picked a shade, shaping the lips and getting the lipstick to stay is not all that hard. First, using a neutral-colored lip liner pencil (if the lipstick begins to wear off, it will still look natural), color the desired outline of your lips. Because of genetics, accidents, or age, the lips may lose their symmetry. To add on one side apply concealer over the new addition, or the area to be eliminated. Now color in the lips using the lip liner pencil. Using a lip liner brush, apply the lipstick to the lips. Stay inside the pencil barrier. Blot with a piece of soft tissue paper, and add a sprinkle of powder. This will help the second coat of lipstick stay put. Apply the second coat as you did the first, and blot again. If you want fuller lips, apply a slightly lighter shade of lipstick to the center of the lips using a lip liner brush. This will create the desired contour, making the lips more prominent. While the lip pencil will prevent bleeding, a lip sealer may also be used to extend the life of your lipstick. Just remember to carry your lipstick with you so you can touch it up as needed.

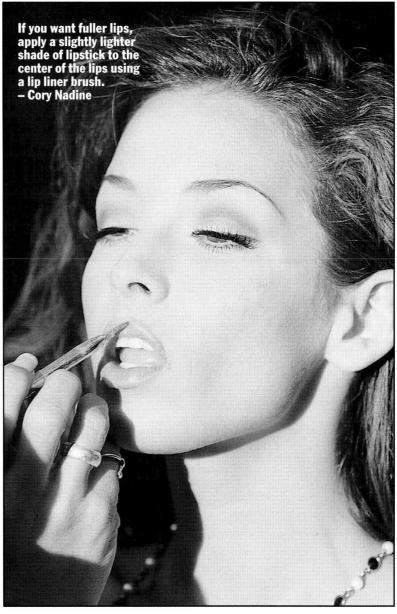

If you want fuller lips, apply a slightly lighter shade of lipstick to the center of the lips using a lip liner brush.
– Cory Nadine

REMOVING MAKEUP

To remove makeup, use Ponds face cream for oily skin. It removes the cosmetics, while gently cleansing your skin.

NOSE

You want to win a contest? Don't pierce your nose. It grosses people out. You may as well walk onstage and pick your nose to the third knuckle! Like we said before, we didn't make the rules.

ACNE AND RELATED PROBLEMS

Whether you have oily or dry skin, you can still have acne. It is believed that 95 percent of acne is hereditary, and despite what you were told in adolescence, it can persist throughout the adult years. Diet and personal hygiene are rarely factors. Aggravating factors are sleep deprivation, food excesses (bingeing), emotional stress and friction. Acne can also be a side effect of certain medications. While a sweat band might be fashionable, it can cause clogged pores and acne breakouts. Resting your chin on your hand or rubbing your face is another good way to get pimples. But you can only do so much. Acne is first and foremost a medical condition, so see a dermatologist. There are a variety of effective medications out there, but few that work overnight. If before a big contest you notice a huge, deep-seated pimple on your face, and you aren't allergic, a dermatologist can give you a corti-sone injection into the trouble spot, which will make it disappear.

Most acne medications are antibiotics. Minocin, a type of tetracycline, is particularly effective. It is also a photosensitive drug, which means that you will tan very quickly, so be careful! The result can be a severe burn! Benzoyl peroxide is a favorite among the medical establishment, but it's not the most effective. Vitamin A acid gels such as Retin-A are very effective in clearing up surface acne. They cause the outer layers to peel. At first this causes a flare-up, but three months into therapy the results are dramatic!

This treatment makes the skin much clearer. Another popular topical agent is Azelex. This cream is a mild emollient which contains azelic acid (from wheat). This acid not only keeps the skin cells shedding, it also acts as a mild bleach to prevent discoloration from healing skin. Because it's an emollient, the skin is kept moisturized, which minimizes the "flaky" appearance of the skin.

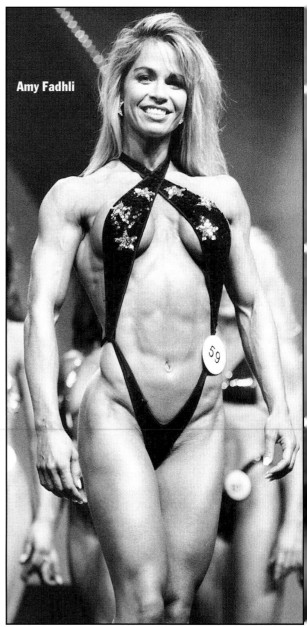

Amy Fadhli

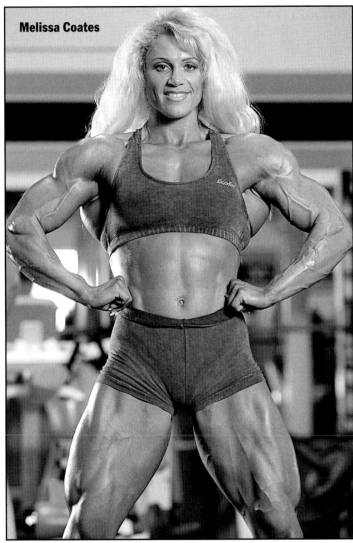

Melissa Coates

Deep-cysted acne, the type that leaves "ice-pick" scars, requires more aggressive treatment. If there has been no response to two or three courses of oral antibiotics, the next step is Accutane. It decreases the skin's oil production. Blackheads and pimples dry up and disappear. There may be an initial flare-up, but this quickly dies down. As the skin is dry, water-based moisturizers must be applied to the skin to stop itching, and balm to the lips to keep them from chapping. One course of Accutane lasts 16 to 20 weeks, and costs about $600 US, but after two courses most people are cured. There are a variety of side effects, so this drug is not for everyone. Some people have experienced depression, night blindness and rarely intra-cranial hypertension. You must not take this drug if you are pregnant or might become pregnant, as it can cause severe birth defects.

Some women may notice that their acne flares up at certain times during their cycle. The female hormone progesterone stimulates the oil-producing glands, as do androgens (male hormones), which women also produce (in smaller amounts than men do). When the ratio of female-to-male hormones in a woman's body changes, acne can flare up. Puberty, ovulation, menstruation and childbirth can all lead to acne outbreaks. A medical treatment for controlling these changing hormonal levels and also offer contraceptive protection is the birth control pill. (Ortho Tricylen is a low-dose pill that is effective against acne.)

If you have been on it, you should wait one month after discontinuing the drug before attempting to get pregnant.

Stay away from Clearasil and other so-called "acne treatments." They're actually sold as cosmetics! The way the advertisements are worded allow them to sound like a medical option. Maybe they help a little, but they certainly don't cure acne.

Since pimples are often three years old (seriously), many young women experience acnea cosmetica in their late twenties and early thirties. This condition is caused by the overuse of pore-clogging makeup over a long period of time. To prevent it, only use

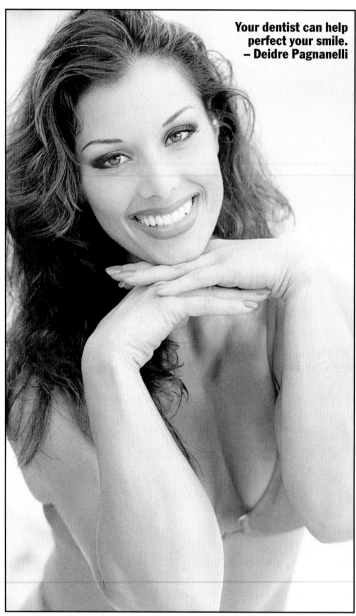

Your dentist can help perfect your smile.
– Deidre Pagnanelli

born pimples, as well as bleaching and loosening blackheads. To remove the blackheads and pimples, wipe the affected area with cotton swabs soaked in hydrogen peroxide. Let them sit on the skin for a minute. Rinse with water and repeat. Pat dry and with gentle pressure or using a Revlon blackhead remover, squeeze out the problem. If it comes out, wipe the area with hydrogen peroxide to disinfect. If it won't come out after a couple of tries, leave it alone and try again tomorrow. Patience is the key here. It didn't get there overnight, and it may take a little while to get it to leave. We often hear that you shouldn't squeeze blackheads and pimples because they'll leave scars. But if you leave them in, will they subside by themselves? Usually they just get bigger, cause social problems and leave a bigger scar when they finally pop. Discuss the technique with your dermatologist. Just be careful how you splash the hydrogen peroxide on, as you could end up bleaching your eyebrows and the hair around your face.

makeup that will not form comedones (the blockages that lead to blackheads and pimples). Get a regular facial at least once a month. By keeping the pores clean, you can prevent problems for years into the future!

Having seen your doctor, there are things you can do at home to help fight acne. Drink lots of water and get plenty of sleep. Hydrogen peroxide is an excellent topical agent for removing bacteria, clearing out stub-

Everybody goes to the dentist and has no compunction saying they go to the dentist. But people in the limelight want people to believe that whatever they have, they were born with.

Dr. Marc Lowenburg, who's clients are mostly celebrities, (and who shares a practice with Dr. Lituchy)

TEETH

To win a fitness contest you must present an image, one that includes a dazzling smile. Your dentist can not only correct medical problems, but also perform and recommend a number of techniques that deal with cosmetic issues. The most obvious are braces, which can be made out of clear materials. Bonding, which can be used to fill in gaps and build up teeth, can be done in the dentist's chair and produce dramatic results in half an hour. Capping and shaping are sculpting tools that the dentist can use to give you a million-dollar smile. Porcelain veneers can beautify every tooth visible to critical judges, prospective agents, and excited fans. But such smiles don't come cheap. They can cost as much as $20,000 US.

When you're watching TV and you see those incredible smiles, I would have to guess a lot of that is porcelain veneers. It's the Mercedes of smiles. It's predictable, it lasts, and it's an expensive luxury for yourself.

**Dr. Gregg Lituchy,
New York dentist to the stars**

Other approaches are not as expensive but they are not as permanent. One option is laser dentistry. Using a laser, a dentist bleaches your teeth white with a high-energy light beam. This can take an hour or more, and will definitely set you back a few hundred dollars, but the result is immediate. For thirty dollars, you can pick up home bleach-and-tray systems, but you won't get the same effect for at least eight weeks. For $2.50, you can pick up some cotton swabs and a bottle of hydrogen peroxide. Dilute with water and scrub your teeth with the peroxide-soaked swabs and rinse with water. You'll notice an instant whitening of your teeth. You can also brush with baking soda and water. Depending on your coffee and tea habits, you may have to repeat this procedure daily. At a cost of five cents for a daily treatment, this is the most affordable. But don't overdo it! You can wear the enamel off your teeth. Remember, check with your dentist before trying out any new system. It may not be right for you, and he or she may know of a better (and cheaper) way to go!

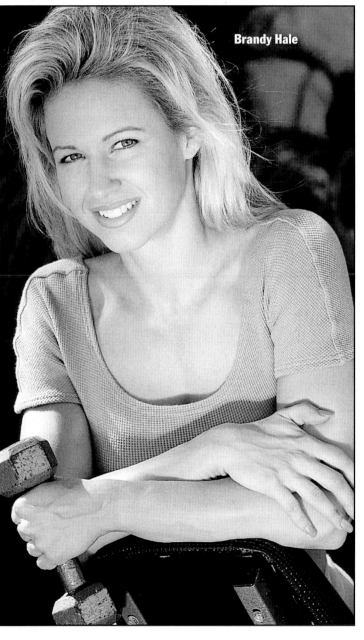

Brandy Hale

Other ways to improve your teeth's appearance include rinsing with PLAX, a liquid cleanser, and then brushing your teeth. The difference is amazing. Follow this with the previously mentioned peroxide procedure, and you'll have a Hollywood smile for sure! Of course, don't forget to see your dentist regularly, and floss and brush daily.

PERMANENT MAKEUP – THE ULTIMATE MISTAKE

Permanent makeup is trumpeted as being completely safe and of great convenience if you are visually disabled, old, or have arthritic hands. All this is true, but the pigments used in this form of tattooing all contain metallic compounds. These metals could prevent you from receiving the best medical care in the future. As we age our risk for stroke increases. One of the best diagnostic tools available is magnetic resonance imaging (MRI), which can provide the physician with an accurate picture of what is happening in the brain. If you have permanent eye liner, the metal oxides in your skin can fog the images, preventing the MRI from being of any use. And we're not just talking strokes, as brain cancer and trauma can occur at any age. Please, avoid this procedure at all costs. Your life could depend on it.

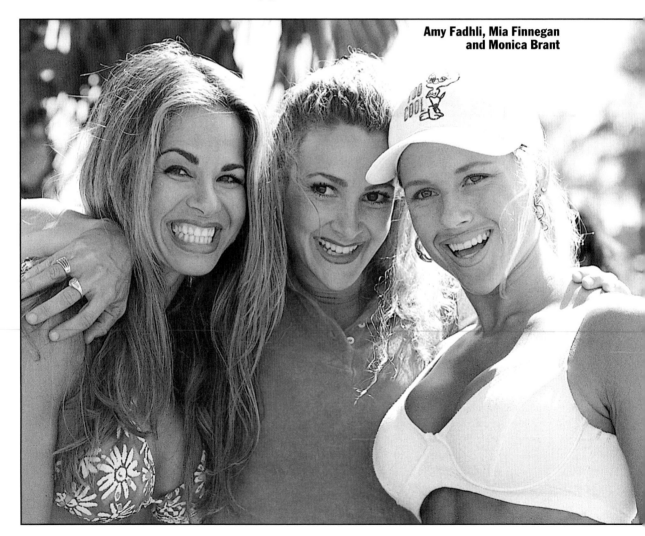

Amy Fadhli, Mia Finnegan and Monica Brant

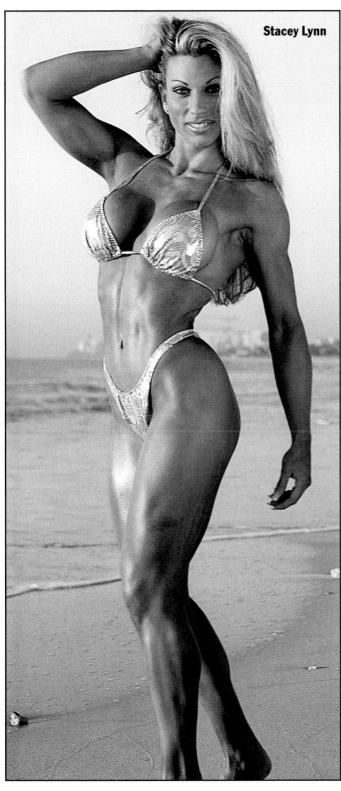

Stacey Lynn

HAIR

Hair is a cornified, thread-like outgrowth from the epidermis of mammals. It's length and texture varies according to ethnic background and body region. Hair follicles are found throughout the entire dermal layer, except on the palms, the soles and a few other regions. Individual hairs are formed in the follicles, which have their roots deep in the dermis layer. A papilla (a finger-like projection) of connective tissue projects into the follicle. Above the papilla are the epithelial cells, which constitute the hair root and the shaft of the hair. On the shaft, the hair cells secrete keratin (a protein which contains 21 amino acids), then die, leaving a compact mass that forms hair. The only living part of the hair is at the bottom of the follicle where growth occurs. That is why cutting the hair is painless, but tweezing the hair is painful. Attached to each hair follicle is a sebaceous gland. Its secretions make the hair more pliable. Each hair follicle is attached to a hair muscle, which pulls the hair up upon contraction (goosebumps).

The hair shaft consists of the medulla, the cortex and the cuticle. The medulla is the core of the shaft. The cortex, comprising three quarters of the hair shaft, forms the middle layer, which contains the pigment. This is called melanin, which can be broken down into two further types: pheomelanin – a yellow/red pigment and eumelanin – a black pigment. Together with the number of air bubbles present, these determine the color of the hair. As we get older the number of air bubbles in the hair increases, giving the hair its characteristic white color. The cuticle is the outermost layer and is made up of multiple layers of translucent cells that overlap each other like roof shingles. If the layers are flat and smooth on each other, more light is reflected and the hair looks shiny.

TOOLS OF THE TRADE

WIGS

Sometimes there is no time to prepare for a photoshoot, or you're just leaving the gym and there are fans outside. Actresses do it all the time. You're the one creating the illusion, so give people what they want. Besides, you're not going to sell posters with your hair glued to one side of your head. If you've lost your hair from chemotherapy, choose a wig made of synthetic hair, because it won't be affected by humidity and won't need to be set. Make sure that the wig is not overly tight. You'll probably be bald for a few weeks, and then your hair will start to grow back. Excessive pressure on the hair follicles will cause them to die, and then you will be permanently bald. Discuss this with your doctor, and see a hairstylist recommended by your hospital.

HAIRPIECES

Hairpieces are also called hair extensions. Make sure the color matches. Human hair tends to be more expensive, but it is easier to style and maintain. You can even color and perm your hairpiece with your own hair. Synthetic hair can't be restyled, but either straight or braided, it can have a magical effect. Hairpieces usually have clips, but your stylist can permanently attach some to your own hair. Mind you, the initial fee can be between $300 to $500, and expect to pay around $80 for a maintenance fee every six weeks.

JACQUIE'S PICKS FOR SHAMPOOS AND CONDITIONERS

Since Jacquie Molyneau-Petrie was our resident hair expert, we asked for her opinion on the best haircare products based on hair type. Here's what she said:

HAIR TYPE	SHAMPOOS	BRAND
Fine, limp hair	Complements Purifying Shampoo	Clairol
Fine, oily hair	Lavei	Joico
	CONDITIONERS	
Dry to normal hair	Osmose Daily Shampoo	L'Oreal
	Complements Daily Replenisher	Clairol
Coarse or chemically treated hair	Liquid Hair Moisturizing Shampoo then Wella Moisturizer Rinse, followed by Wella Restructurizer (which helps to reconnect protein bonds in the hair). Any chemical treatment needed would now be done.	Wella
Grey hair (to get rid of yellow tones) white, or heavily highlighted hair	Complements Revelation Brightening Shampoo	Clairol

HAIR COLOR

This is an easy question. You've found the right color if the first thing people notice are your eyes. Try it yourself, looking through pictures of fitness contestants. Some grab your view as if trying to establish a hypnotic trance! What they have done is found a hairstyle and color so matched to their own appearance that it does not distract from the person. Fine. And how did the person in the picture find the perfect match? Probably the same way you will, by trial and error. You can speed up the process by determining your skin tones. Those who have gray, blue or green eyes, and when tanning burn easily, have cool undertones. If your eyes are hazel or brown, and your skin doesn't burn easily, you have warm undertones. You can also do the T-shirt test: try on a white one and a beige one. If the beige one suits you best, you have warm undertones. If the white one looks better, you have cool undertones. If you have warm undertones, try the following hair colors: platinum blonde, golden blonde, auburn, and chestnut. If you have cool undertones, try: black, and different shades of red and dark blonde.

How do I get the shiny look I see in commercials and onstage? To achieve that illusion of a cascade of thick hair, different shades of the same color are weaved throughout. Fine lights and a color gloss is also added, providing the incredible shine you see onstage. If the style incorporates curls, butterfly tips on the ends make the curls light.

HOW TO MATCH YOUR HAIRSTYLE WITH YOUR FACE

You must be honest with yourself, and choose a hairstyle that compliments the shape of your face. The shape of your face provides a reference point to decide where you want to go with your hair. We will identify and examine the four types, using fitness contestants to illustrate what works (and what doesn't).

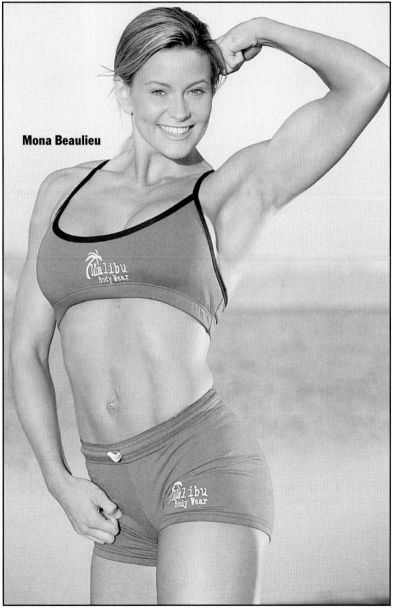

Mona Beaulieu

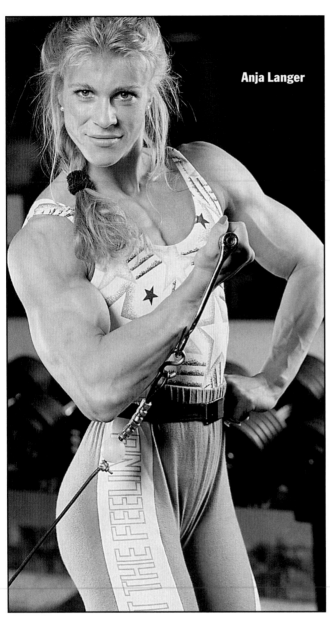

Anja Langer

braided hair or a long ponytail with the hair pulled away from the face creates a balance between the strength of the jaw and the femininity of the woman within. Always avoid jaw-length cuts as they make the jaw far too prominent.

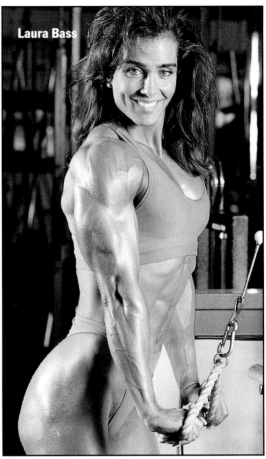

Laura Bass

THE SQUARE FACE

Square faces have strong, square jawlines with squared off hairlines and wide foreheads. The beautiful faces of Germany's Anja Langer and Bermuda's Keetha Steele illustrate the instant allure this type of face creates. To best frame these faces, short hairstyles should include soft waves, bouncy curls and off-center parts. Soft, fringe bangs soften the overall appearance. If you want a long hairstyle,

THE LONG FACE

Beauties with long, narrow chins, prominent jaws and high foreheads belong to this type. One only has to gaze upon fitness goddesses like Laura Bass and Milamar Flores to see this face come to life. These faces are best framed with short hairstyles that are layered. Soft bangs and fullness at the sides will add to the effect of widening a narrow face. People with this face type should avoid long, straight hair, styles with height at the crown (the topmost part of the head), and center parts. They make the face look longer than it really is.

THE HEART FACE

High cheekbones that taper into pointy chins, topped off by wide foreheads depict the heart-shaped face. We don't have pictures of Helen of Troy, but no doubt Jennifer Goodwin and Cory Everson could each launch 1000 ships. Face-framing layered styles with exposed foreheads and flipped ends will send erotic shudders through anything nearby with a Y chromosome. A saucy touch is the addition of a "Bear Claw," or standing set of curls (upright bangs that fall in a clockwise direction). This look became so popular in one Newfoundland town that the girls from that area became known as the "Mount Pearl Curl Girls." Avoid lifeless straight hairstyles or bangs that cover the forehead.

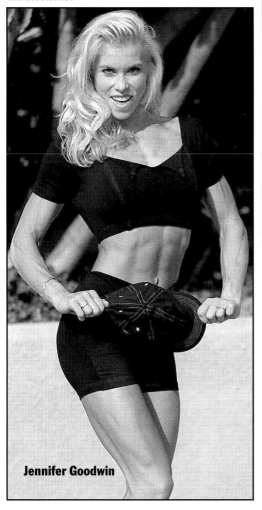

Jennifer Goodwin

THE ROUND FACE

Wide, full chins form the base for faces that have cheeks as wide as their foreheads and jaws. Lovely Dale Tomita and Marla Duncan show how incredibly attractive these faces can be. Long or short, always go for layered cuts that are parted at the side. This will slim the face. Avoid swept-back styles, as they make the face too round.

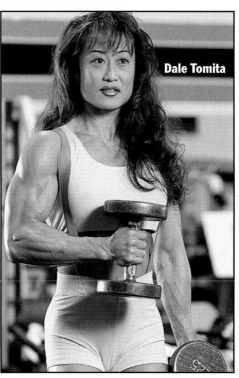

Dale Tomita

HAIR TYPES AND HOW TO CARE FOR THEM

If only life were so simple. These generalizations do not take into account the type of hair you may have. Hair type is determined by density (number of hairs per square inch) and diameter of the hair shaft. Density is classified, from least to most, as thin (usually those of Scandinavian descent), medium (Mediterranean descent) and coarse (Asian and African descent). Having said that, all three types can appear in just about any racial group. Humans are more alike than they are different. The diameter is classified, from smallest to widest, as fine, normal and coarse.

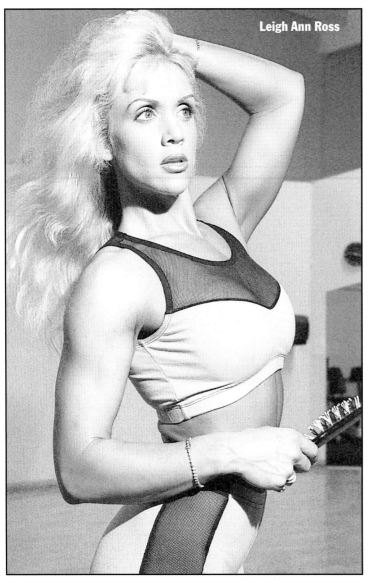

Leigh Ann Ross

THIN, FINE AND JUST PLAIN ANNOYING

Fine hair has the problem of being limp. To cope with this you can use body-building conditioners to add fullness. By coating the hair with layers of polymers and protein, the hair appears thicker. But once a week you should use a clarifying shampoo to remove the build-up. Another option is a short, blunt cut or bob. This will make the hair look thicker. To soften the style, try light layers around the face. Be careful when layering fine hair,

because you can end up making your hair look thinner. Remember that short hairstyles are more expensive in the long run because they require more maintenance. You should have a trim at least once every month to keep your new dynamite look. On the plus side, short hair is easy to maintain.

Another way to add volume to your hair is to grab your hairdryer. Begin by dampening the hair with water. Collect a dollop (not a very specific measurement, enough to fill one third of the palm, half an inch thick) of mousse, and work it into the roots of your hair. Be careful not to use too much mousse, as it can actually weigh your hair down. Scrunch your hair by lifting the curls at the base and continue lifting while the hair dries. Keep lifting as the weight of the water will push the hair down. By lifting the curl close to the roots you get the scrunched look. While scrunching, aim the air at the roots. This will not only add volume and body, but curl and texture as well. Another trick is to curl small sections of your hair on the crown with a curling iron. This will make your hair appear fuller. Volumizing spray can be used when the hair is dry. Lift the hair and spray at the roots. Sit back and glow in the difference! Another way to deal with fine hair is to go for the wet-look. Fine hair, when cut short, can sometimes decide to become spiked on its own, particularly if there's a lot of static electricity around. A simple and sexy way of correcting this problem is to slick back your hair with gel. Wet your hair, then comb gel through it using your fingers to shape the hair into waves, or whatever style flatters your face. This sleek style is great for the office, gym, or evening out.

MEDIUM HAIR, LUCK BE A LADY TONIGHT!

If you have medium hair, you are blessed! It is perhaps the ideal hair to work with because it is so versatile. On the negative side, other contestants will hate you and pray that you go bald. Oh well, you can't please everyone. But there is a problem that you may encounter. Perms can sometimes leave the hair brittle and damaged. The environment can also play havoc with your hair. Therefore a protein treatment should be used. Similar to conditioners (which only act on the cuticle), protein treatments add protein to the cortex, building strength into the shaft and helping the hair to retain moisture. Begin by using once a week, and after the first month use it bi-monthly. You should notice a drastic improvement in your hair. Since heat helps any conditioner or protein treatment penetrate the hair, your local gym or spa is a great place to go. After washing your hair, add the desired treatment, and luxuriate in the warmth of the sauna while your hair gets treated. Another place you should always bring conditioner is the beach. After coating your body in sunblock, coat your hair with conditioner. The sun will bake it into the shafts, and do wonders for split ends.

COARSE HAIR, THE HALLMARK OF NUBIAN BEAUTY

The luscious curly hair of African women has been celebrated from the temples of the Nile in ancient Egyptian times to the modern supermodel runways of Paris. Layered, excess curl can be controlled and the hair styled in the direction desired. Braided, it can frame the face in the style popularized in the mainstream by Bo Derek in the movie, *10*. Many African-American and Canadian women choose to relax (straighten) their hair, and this is commonly seen at fitness competitions. So we will focus for the most part on relaxed hair. With coarse hair, it is normal to have dry ends with an oily scalp. Coarse hair generally has less follicles, resulting in less oil and

drier hair. Thus the relaxation process and after-treatment are critical in maintaining healthy hair. To begin, a barrier cream protects the scalp. Then the relaxer chemical (the active ingredient is calcium hydroxide, milder and good for sensitive scalps; or sodium hydroxide, a lye relaxer that does not leave hair as dry) is applied to a section of dry hair for a specific time, depending on the strength of the relaxer. Various strengths are on the market. This is not surprising, as 70 percent of African Americans have white ancestry, therefore a considerable variety in hair types will be

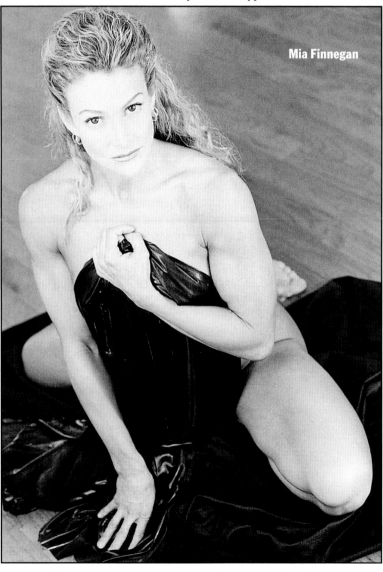

Mia Finnegan

found. There are three types of relaxer available: mild for fine hair, regular for medium hair, and super for very coarse hair. This is followed by a rinse and neutralizing shampoo. Now that the relaxing process has been stopped, the procedure is repeated. Once the entire head is done, a deep-penetrating protein treatment is applied to help the hair recover from its weakened condition. As new hair grows in, it should be retouched in the same way. It is not necessary to retreat relaxed hair.

Because coarse hair produces so little oil, it does not need to be washed as often. Once a week is usually sufficient. Obviously, if you work out heavily, work in a hot environment or wear a wig, you will need to wash your hair more often. Always wash with a conditioning shampoo followed by a leave-in conditioner. A good way of periodically adding moisture to your hair and scalp is to comb in castor oil. Remember to have weekly hot conditioning treatments. Relaxing the hair seriously weakens it, and many women complain of hair breakage. These treatments will restore your hair's health.

Your enemy is dryness. Whenever possible, air dry your hair. If you must use a hairdryer, use it on a low setting, but only after you've combed a moisturizer through. As well, if you're heading out into the sun, apply a leave-in conditioner. A good way to protect your straightened hair is to use gel for the sleek look. This also minimizes the chance of damage that can occur with other hairstyles. To get extra shine, use a color-enhancing conditioner or a super shiny hair color. But unlike fine or medium hair, never use Henna on coarse hair. Henna can act as a drying agent. Here's the simplest tip for outside protection – wear a hat.

NAILS

Nails are essentially flattened horny plates, formed from the epidermis, that are found at the ends of the fingers and toes. The nail grows from a tuck in the skin. The small patch of skin covered by the tuck forms the matrix. This is the site from which the nail originates.

The rest of the nail bed does not contribute to nail growth. This is why it is so important to be gentle with the matrix, because if it is damaged, the entire nail can be lost.

Like hair, nails are made of keratin. Nails are also dead. Except for the matrix, nails are made of dead skin cells. Good nail care will result in healthy-looking nails, and provide a nice finish to your professional look. In looking at pictures of fitness stars, it is quite common to see them hiding their nails by making fists, holding the hands behind the back, or sinking them into a vibrant head of hair. Working out heavy and having good-looking nails is not an easy task. Weight training often results in calluses and broken nails. Make it a little easier on yourself. Wear a pair of workout gloves. Just make sure to wash and dry your gloves regularly.

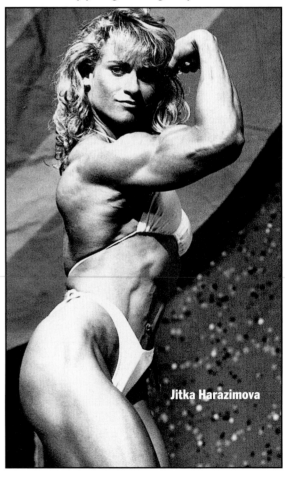

Jitka Harazimova

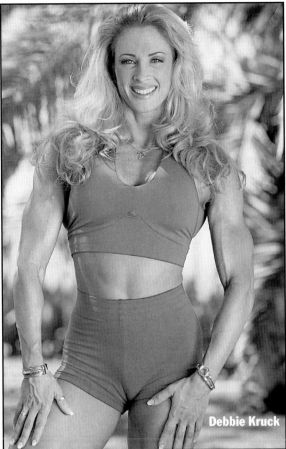
Debbie Kruck

THE X-FILES ON
NAIL FILING AND CARE

The best shape for your nails depends on personal taste and whatever is fashionable at the moment. The easiest shape is one that is natural and not long. Long nails are the look seen at contest time, and you can bet your last dollar that they're all artificial. But when you're onstage you have to be bigger than life to get noticed.

Once you've decided on a shape, pick up a shaper. This tool looks like a popsicle stick with a very coarse texture. They are routinely brown or black. Gently file the tips of the nails (always in one direction), using the flat edge of the file. Do this too aggressively and you'll damage your nails in the long run. If you've been taking good care of your nails all along, you are better off using a smoother. It is a nail file that is medium-coarse in texture, and is usually blue.

To round any sharp corners on the nails, use a disk file. This circular-shaped file is also great for buffing the tops of the nails without scratching the skin. If the nail is brittle you might want to shape your nails with a finisher. This nail file is less abrasive than the previous, and is usually light pink. Once the nail is shaped, rough edges or ridges can be smoothed away with a buffer. These rectangular-shaped tools are the least abrasive and are usually white or light-toned. For convenience, nothing beats a four-sided file. Everything you need to file your nails is on the same tool. You can shape, smooth, finish and buff. But most find the traditional files easiest to use.

Since the nails highlight the hands, we better take care of them too. Remove dead skin cells by cleaning them with an exfoliating cream of your choice. Rinse this off and then soak your hands in a bowl of lemon juice and water. This softens the cuticle, making it easy to gently push back with a cloth after you've dried the hands. Now, using nail-polish remover and a cotton ball, remove any remaining nail polish. At this point, nail ridges may pose a problem. Consistent use of a nail buffer, and application of a ridge filler should correct this. To help the nail polish adhere, apply a basecoat. It contains resins, which add strength to the nail.

Having chosen the color that's right for you, apply a thin coat of polish. Once the nails are dry, repeat. Next apply a top coat to produce a durable finish. It protects the nail polish from daily wear and tear. Some women opt for wraps, which are cappings made from silk, linen, fibreglass, glue or powders. See a professional for this one.

All that's left is a cuticle cream to nourish the living part of your nails, and a moisturising cream for your hands. If you want to add nail extensions, follow the manufacturer's directions, and if you can afford it, see a professional.

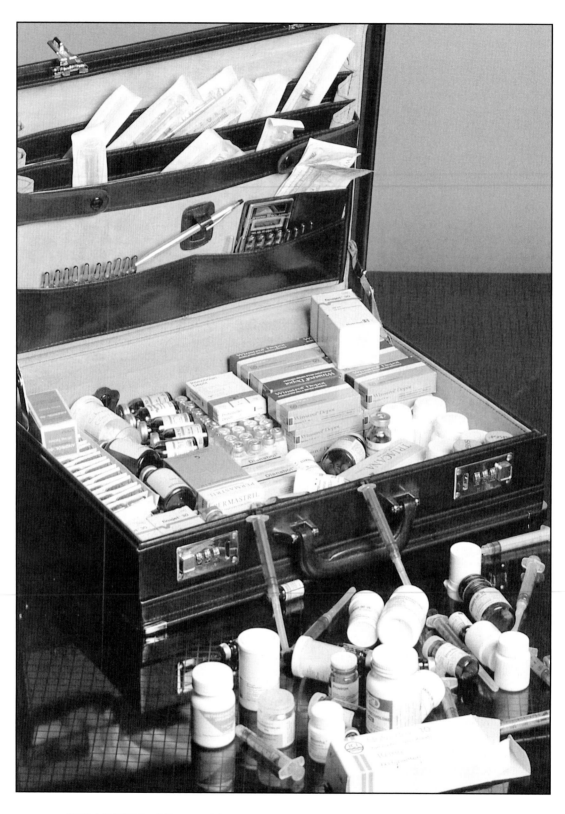

Chapter 23
Athletic Drugs

It didn't start with Canadian sprinter Ben Johnson in 1988, but the most famous drug test in athletic history helped expose the extent of drug use in sports. As long as humans have been competing in athletic events, a few have taken the extra step in their desires to be number one. And it's not just bodybuilding either. Such sports as football and track and field have just as much drug use as bodybuilding. Unfortunately the media tends to focus more on the fringe sports like bodybuilding rather the big "money sports."

Performance-enhancing drugs are simply defined as any substance that boosts an individual's athletic ability. The problem with such a definition is that food could be considered an athletic drug! Let's face it, if one athlete is eating nutritious food and the other is not, all things being equal, the former will most certainly outperform the latter. Another problem concerns the latest so-called natural supplements like creatine and HMB. The evidence does prove that these substances increase athletic performance, so are they not drugs? For the purposes of this text we are only going to discuss a few of the substances that are universally regarded as performance-enhancing drugs. For a full treatment of this topic please see *MuscleMag International's Anabolic Primer.*

ANABOLIC STEROIDS

Anabolic steroids are probably the most well-known performance-enhancing drugs. They are derivatives of the hormone testosterone, designed to emphasize the hormone's anabolic properties while minimizing its androgenic properties. Anabolic is a biochemical term defined as the synthesis of more complex substances from simpler ones. For example, amino acids join to form protein strands which in turn link to form muscle tissue. Androgenic is defined as any substance that promotes masculine characteristics such as a deep voice, facial hair, and masculinized genitalia. While testosterone is found in a woman's body, it's far more concentrated in a man, hence the physical differences between the sexes. Anabolic steroids were initially developed to treat concentration camp victims and patients suffering from wasting diseases.

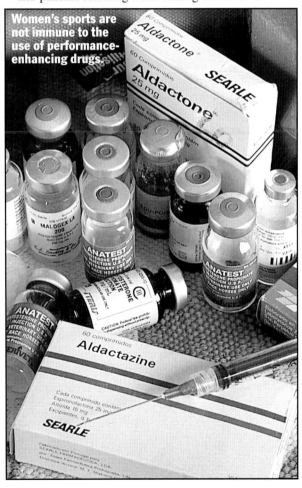

Women's sports are not immune to the use of performance-enhancing drugs.

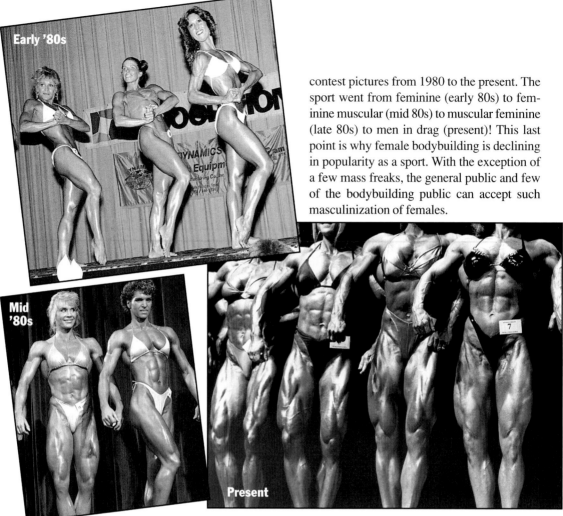

Early '80s

Mid '80s

Present

contest pictures from 1980 to the present. The sport went from feminine (early 80s) to feminine muscular (mid 80s) to muscular feminine (late 80s) to men in drag (present)! This last point is why female bodybuilding is declining in popularity as a sport. With the exception of a few mass freaks, the general public and few of the bodybuilding public can accept such masculinization of females.

Once athletes heard of their "muscle building" qualities, it wasn't long before they made their debut in sports. The first confirmed use was at the 1952 Olympics, but it's probably safe to say they've been used since their first synthesis in the late 1930s, early 1940s.

Despite their long history in men's sports, it probably wasn't until the 1970s that female athletics became tarnished. Although suspicions were strong about East German and Russian females, it wasn't until the fall of the Berlin Wall and breakup of the Soviet Union, that the evidence was found on paper.

With one or two exceptions female bodybuilding was probably clean until the mid 1980s. At first the drugs were only used to harden up for a contest, but now women are taking as much as their male counterparts. Anyone with a full collection of *MuscleMag International* can see the change. Look at the

Women's bodybuilding has gone from feminine (1980s) to masculine-feminine (present). Performance-enhancing drugs heavily influenced this transition.

SIDE EFFECTS

Most drugs cause side effects and steroids are no exception. Unfortunately the media have blown things way out of proportion. Yes, some users develop problems, but the vast majority do not. This is not so much our opinion as what the medical evidence says. As of this writing there are no large-sample, long-term studies that compare the health of users with nonusers. Everything negative you hear about steroids is based on a few case studies. A healthy individual dies of liver failure or heart disease and he or she just happened to be using steroids. Millions of people around the world die of such conditions and have never used steroids. In order to say a drug causes or contributes to a condition, you need to do long-term comparison studies. If the using group shows a higher incidence of a condition over the control nonusing group, you can start concluding the drugs played a role.

Having educated you on what won't occur, let's discuss what may occur. As steroids are derived from testosterone, they pose certain risks to females. Many women experience increased facial hair growth, and close ups of many female bodybuilders shows evidence of shaving.

Another common side effect is a deepening of the voice. Listen to some of the interviews on ESPN. Many of the ladies sound like James Earl Jones (the voice of *Star Wars'* Darth Vader). Biology is at the root of the problem as steroids cause the vocal chords to masculinize.

Perhaps the scariest side effect women may experience is a masculinizing of the genitalia. Both the male and female genitalia are derived from the same fetal tissue. In the presence of testosterone the tissue becomes male. In the absence of the hormone it becomes female. The interesting part is that the testosterone receptors are still there. If a female takes testosterone or its derivatives (anabolic steroids) later in life the receptors sort of "awaken" and start the masculinizing process – whereby the clitoris enlarges. Occasionally medical treatment in the form of drugs or surgery is needed to reverse the condition.

The choice to use steroids is yours. But you have to ask yourself if a few notches up the competitive ladder is worth the risk of developing side effects.

THYROID MEDICATIONS

The thyroid gland is a small organ located in the upper-neck region. Although it has many functions, its primary role is metabolic regulation. It does this by releasing two hormones: triiodothyronine (T3) and thyroxine (T4). Although T4 accounts for about 90 percent of thyroid secretions, both hormones consist of the amino acid tyrosine and the element iodine.

Thyroid hormones are popular with athletes because they increase the oxidation rate of fat. In other words, they allow the body to burn fat deposits at a faster rate. One of the causes of severe obesity is a malfunctioning of the thyroid gland. In recent years the use of thyroid medications is reported to have increased dramatically – especially of female bodybuilding and fitness contestants.

The primary drawback to using thyroid medications is dependence. As with any hormone derivative, thyroid medications can interfere with the body's natural production. When the outside drug use is stopped, the body's own production resumes, but sometimes it doesn't. There are reports of numerous bodybuilders and fitness competitors who screwed up their systems to the point where they are committed to using thyroid drugs for the rest of their lives.

I don't particularly care for thyroid hormones as I feel that they are among the more dangerous pharmaceuticals.

Bruce Kneller,
MuscleMag **contributor**

Our advice is to stay clear of thyroid drugs. For the sake of a few less pounds of fat it's not worth the risk.

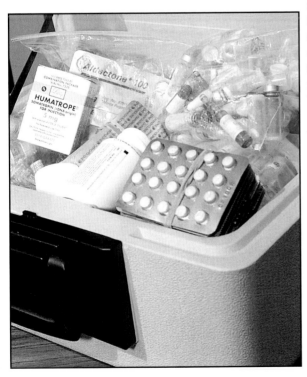

The metabolism is affected by more than one organ in the body, but is primarily associated with the thyroid gland in the throat. The thyroid dictates the health of your metabolism, but relies on other functions in the body to find information for it to make its decisions.

Nina Simone, *Oxygen* contributor

DIURETICS

Diuretics are substances that cause the body to lose water. With the emphasis on the "ripped" look these days, many bodybuilders and fitness competitors turn to diuretics to help shed those last few pounds of muscularity-blurring water. Despite a low bodyfat percentage, a thin layer of water under the skin can hide the competitor's muscularity.

Diuretics work in many different ways. The most common are those that interfere with the body's primary water-conserving hormone aldosterone. Unfortunately, besides shedding water the athlete also loses electrolytes. These electrically charged ions play a role in regulating most of the body's primary systems including muscle contraction. Lose too much and your skeletal muscles will cramp. Worse, you run the risk of interfering with proper heart contraction. A couple of bodybuilding's top stars, Hans Selemeyer and Mohammed Benaziza, have died from what was believed to be diuretic-induced electrolyte loss. Numerous others have collapsed onstage from dehydration. Only prompt medical attention saved their lives.

Water is essential for maintaining an electrolyte balance. The minerals potassium, sodium, and magnesium, and calcium are essential for conducting electrical currents from the brain to the nervous system to the muscles, signaling contractions.

Greg Merrit, *MuscleMag* contributor

As with thyroid medications, we strongly advise you to stay away from diuretic drugs. If normal dieting and exercise doesn't

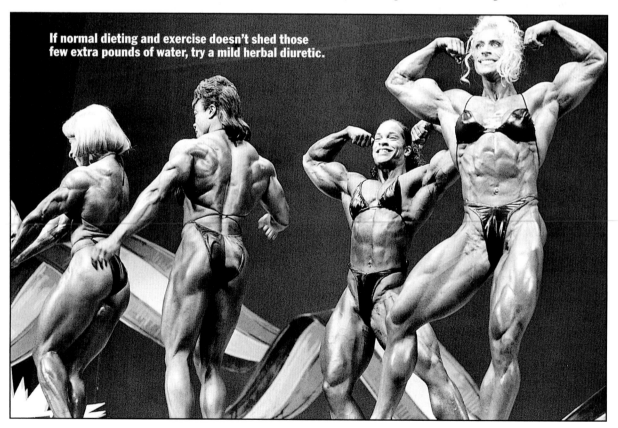

If normal dieting and exercise doesn't shed those few extra pounds of water, try a mild herbal diuretic.

If well-trained individuals are needed to monitor patients receiving diuretics because of potentially dangerous electrolyte changes, what makes bodybuilders think that self-medicating with diuretics is a risk-free proposition.

Scott Abel, top bodybuilding trainer

shed those few extra pounds of water, try a mild herbal diuretic. Even common caffeine-containing beverages like coffee and tea produce water loss. They are far safer and you won't have to worry about being hooked up to an electrolyte IV after the show.

INSULIN

Taking insulin is a perfect example of how far some athletes will go just to move a few notches up the competitive ladder. Insulin can be called the storage hormone of the body. Most are aware that it controls sugar, but few know it also influences protein synthesis by speeding amino-acid uptake. In effect, this makes insulin a powerful anabolic hormone and once word got around that some pros were using the stuff, use at all levels exploded.

Insulin is a particularly dangerous drug to fool around with. Like diuretics, insulin can kill you within a few hours if you abuse it. And if you use insulin when you're not a diabetic, you can become diabetic.

Greg Zulak, former *MuscleMag* **editor**

The dangerous thing about insulin is it's effects on glucose. Take too much and you run the risk of ending up in a diabetic coma. Even if you get the dosage right, your blood-sugar levels may be low to begin with. In either case you could be dead in a matter of hours. Unlike steroids where the risk of overdosing is practically nil, insulin abuse can and does lead to death. Please play it safe and avoid insulin.

CLENBUTEROL

Clenbuterol is another drug initially developed for medical purposes but is now being widely used by athletes. Biochemically it's a beta agonist, that among other things, stimulates the smooth muscles of the lungs and associated tissues. Initially used to treat asthma patients, studies with animals discovered it

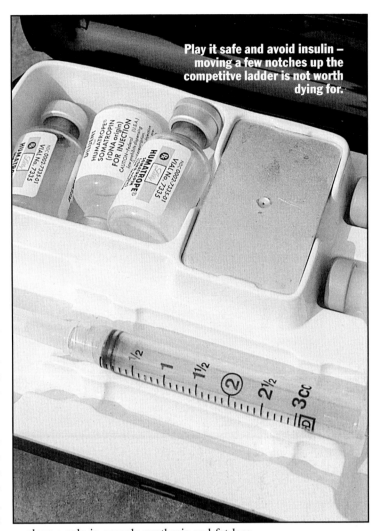

Play it safe and avoid insulin — moving a few notches up the competitve ladder is not worth dying for.

plays a role in muscle synthesis and fat loss. Despite the lack of scientific evidence involving human subjects, athletes were quick to give it a try. The anecdotal evidence suggests clenbuterol is more beneficial for fat loss than muscle gaining. Further, its effects seem to be limited to six to eight weeks. A combination of tolerance and receptor down loading seems to quickly reduce the drug's effectiveness.

Bodybuilders find that clenbuterol does cause reductions in bodyfat and noticeable increases in body leanness and definition but as with most drugs there is no free ride. Common side effects to clenbuterol use are shakiness, tremors, nervousness, headaches, and insomnia. The more you take the worse the negative side effects.

Greg Zulak, former *MuscleMag* **editor**

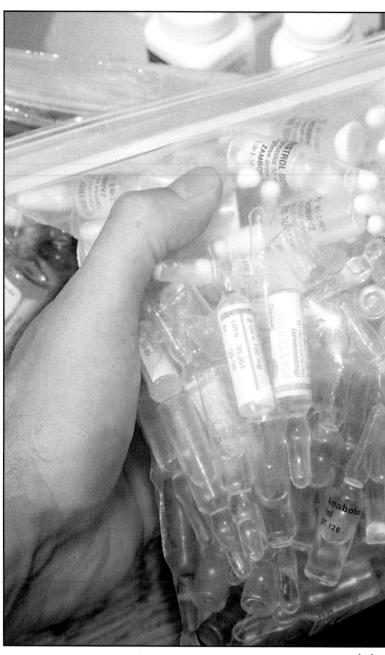

LEGAL ISSUES

Most sports federations ban many of the drugs discussed in this chapter. As a competitive athlete the onus is on you to know your sport's rules. Athletes are usually one step ahead of the testers and most don't get caught. As well, drugs like thyroid and insulin are difficult to test for because they're naturally occurring substances.

From a legal standpoint the water is far murkier depending on the country you live in. At one extreme you have the United States and Canada where drug laws are very harsh. In the US anabolic steroids fall into the same category as heroin and other street drugs, and possession will get you hard jail time. Other drugs like clenbuterol and thyroid fall under various prescription drug laws and while the sentence would not be as severe as anabolic steroids, the wrong combination of judge and prosecutor could get you convicted.

The drug laws in most other Western countries are not as archaic as North America but you should become familiar with them before engaging in any drug use. Despite the authors viewing drug use as a moral and health issue rather than a legal one, the bottom line is the law. As stated in *MuscleMag International's Anabolic Primer*, it's far more fun to pump iron in the gym than in the prison courtyard!

Since it's a beta agonist, clenbuterol can cause heart problems. For this reason the drug was never granted approval for use in the United States. Still, it's use as a bodybuilding and fitness contest drug is believed to be widespread. For those athletes in drug-tested sports, be warned as clenbuterol is one of the easiest drugs to detect.

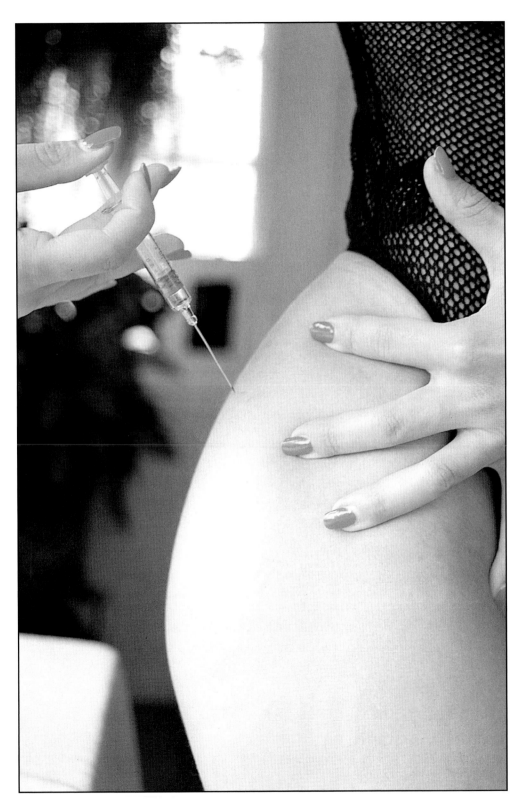

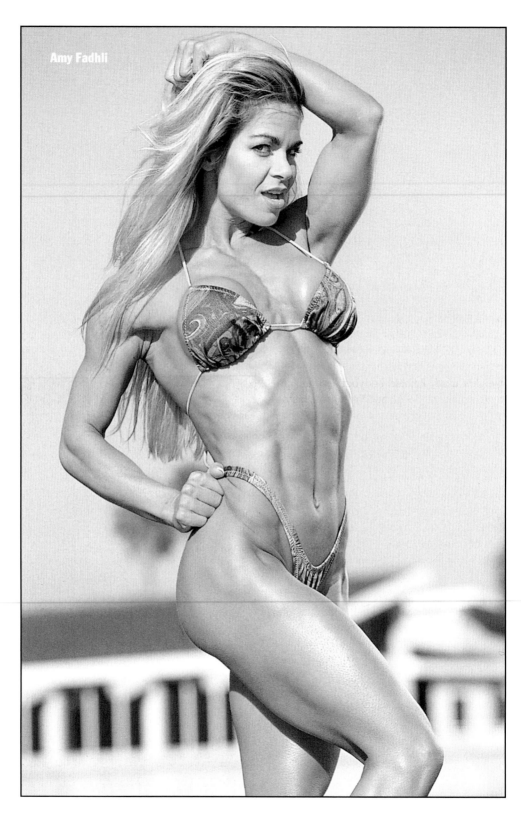

Amy Fadhli

Chapter 24
Routines of the Stars

Throughout MuscleMag International's twenty-five year history, virtually every physique star has been profiled. Readers constantly tell us they love reading about what such and such a star does for his or her training. When *Oxygen* was launched we knew one of its biggest selling points would be training tips from the top fitness and female bodybuilding personalities.

Recognizing that readers of this book come form all backgrounds, we have chosen a broad selection of training programs. As you'll see the exercises are identical. The primary difference is found with the rep ranges and weights used. Female bodybuilders are primarily concerned with building as much mass as possible and hence use lower rep ranges with heavier weights. Fitness contestants are more interested in overall muscle tone and proportions, and keep the reps in the 12 to 15 range. We should add that many of the female bodybuilders you see onstage are taking anabolic steroids and other performance-enhancing drugs. There's no way the average female can add 30 to 40 pounds of pure muscle tissue naturally. Female biochemistry won't allow it. We're saying this so the fitness contestants and general trainers out there won't be afraid to try some of the following bodybuilding routines. Trust us, you won't accidentally gain too much muscle mass!

CHEST TRAINING WITH TONYA KNIGHT

One of the more popular bodybuilding stars of the late 1980s and early 1990s was two-time Ms. International winner Tonya Knight. Besides her dynamic personality, Tonya was famous for combining good muscle quality with feminine proportions.

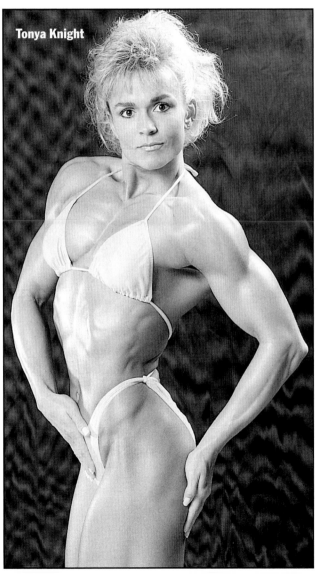

Tonya Knight

When I started – we all thought we knew what we were doing back then – it was always heavy, heavy, heavy. I have since learned to go only as heavy as I can do each repetition slowly, controlling the motion every inch of the way.

Tonya Knight, two-time Ms. International champion

Tonya attributes her great physique to variety, alternating between high-rep (20 reps) and low-rep (8-12) days. The following is a sample high-rep chest workout.

EXERCISE	SETS	REPS
Decline smith-machine presses	4	20
Flat dumbell flyes	4	20
Incline dumbell presses	4	20
Cable crossovers	4	20

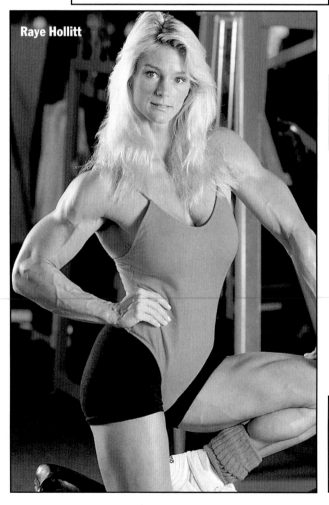

Raye Hollitt

SHOULDER TRAINING WITH RAYE HOLLITT

For those interested in the strength benefits of weight training look no further than Ms. Los Angeles winner Raye Hollitt. At a bodyweight of 150 pounds Raye has done what few females have even thought possible – lifting 300 pounds in the bench press! Yet there's no mistaking the fact that Raye is female. It wasn't long before Hollywood discovered Raye and featured her in the movie *Skin Deep* with John Ritter, and as "Zap" on *American Gladiators*. The following is a sample shoulder routine that Raye used to develop her amazing delts.

I like to train heavy even up to the show. I diet for detail and definition. During the off-season I train heavier, yet starting with light weight and working up in poundage to my maximum.

Raye Hollitt, bodybuilding champ and movie star

EXERCISE	SETS	REPS
Dumbell lateral raises	3	12
Dumbell front raises	3	12
Bent-over laterals	3	12

LEG TRAINING WITH LAURIE DONNELLY

Top fitness competitor Laurie Donnelly is one of the new wave of fitness superstars that are starting to surpass their bodybuilding colleagues in popularity. Like all fitness competitors, Laura uses weight training to enhance her physique. She trains her legs every third workout, performing 2 to 4 sets of four exercises. She often uses supersets and giant sets to keep the muscles guessing.

My routine is basic and simple enough that most women, even those who have never picked up a weight in their lives, are capable of doing it.

Laurie Donnelly, top fitness competitor

EXERCISE	SETS	REPS
Squats	2-4	10-20
Lunges	2-4	15-20
Stiff-leg deadlifts	2-4	15-20
Glute/leg raises	2-4	20-25

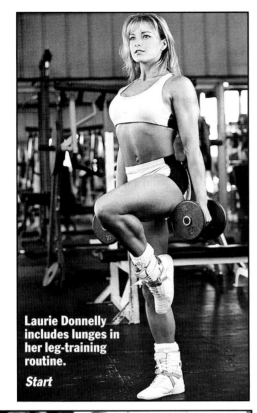

Laurie Donnelly includes lunges in her leg-training routine.

Start

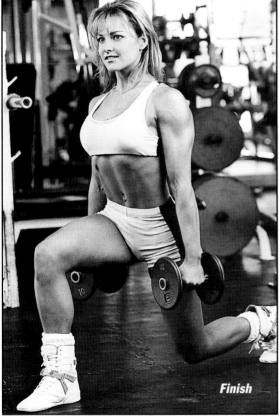

Finish

CHEST TRAINING WITH TRISH STRATUS

It seems every month brings forth a new face to the fitness scene, and one of the prettiest is Trish Stratus'. Trish is currently under the tutelage of Canadian trainer supreme Scott Abel. Scott first spotted Trish at World Gym and it wasn't long before his advice paid off as Trish is now a top fitness model. The following is a sample chest routine performed by Trish.

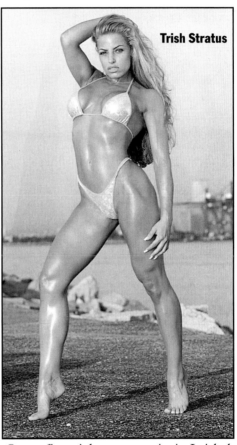

Trish Stratus

On my first night as a receptionist I picked up a copy of MuscleMag. *I saw this blonde (Marla Duncan) who looked like a million dollars, and I knew that I wanted to look as beautiful.*

Trish Stratus, fitness model

EXERCISE	SETS	REPS
Incline dumbell presses	3	8-10
Flat dumbell flyes	3	10-12
Pec-deks	3	15

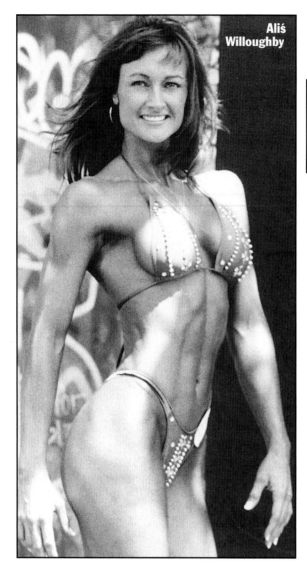
Aliś Willoughby

Instead she treats them like most other muscles and trains them two to three times a week.

EXERCISE	SETS	REPS
Hanging knee raises	3	15
Hanging side leg raises	3	6
Ab crunches (machine)	3	25
Ab crunches (free)	3	50

ARM TRAINING WITH DENISE RUTKOWSKI

When she competed back in the early to mid 1990s Denise Rutkowski was easily one of the most muscular women onstage. She's considered one of the originators of the all-out muscular look for female bodybuilders.

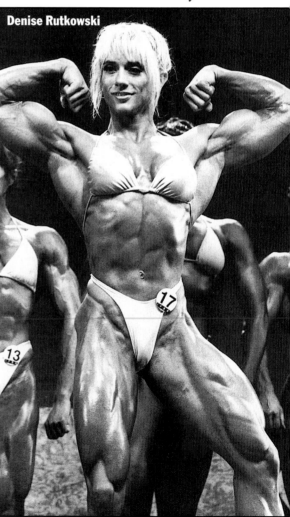
Denise Rutkowski

ABDOMINAL TRAINING WITH ALIŚ WILLOUGHBY

Most people who receive 270 stitches from a car accident at 17 would probably consider themselves lucky and play it safe for the rest of their lives, but not Aliś Willoughby. Just a few years later this native of New York City was winning the 1994 Sarasota Bodybuilding Championships. A year later she had switched to fitness and was competing in the Galaxy Fitness Competitions.

Like many trainers, Aliś doesn't believe in training the abdominals every day.

It all comes down to how much you want it. Without desire there's no commitment. Without commitment results are zero.

Aliś Willoughby, fitness competitor

Some people's form is so bad that you can't tell whether they're trying to work arms or back. I try to squeeze and contract on every rep.

Denise Rutkowski, champion bodybuilder

Picking a best bodypart on Denise is difficult as she's built from head to toe. Her arms received a lot of attention during her competitive days, so we have outlined one of her typical arm routines.

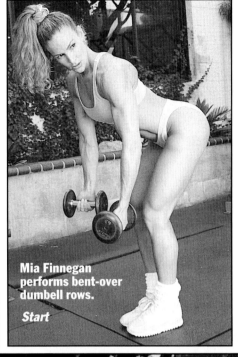

Mia Finnegan performs bent-over dumbell rows.
Start

BICEPS EXERCISE	SETS	REPS
Straight-bar curls	4	8-10
Hammer curls	4	8-10
Concentration curls	4	8-10
TRICEPS EXERCISE	SETS	REPS
Triceps pushdowns	4	8-10
Lying EZ-bar extensions	4	8-10
Behind-the-head dumbell extensions	4	8-10

DAZZLING DELTS WITH MIA FINNEGAN

The first-ever Ms. Fitness Olympia in 1995, Mia is the epitome of proportion and feminine grace. At the center of her physique are two of the most balanced delts in the business. Unlike some women who focus most of their energy on the side delts, Mia targets all three heads with equal ferocity.

Some people start out heavy and then go light, but I like to go light to heavy.

Mia Finnegan, 1995 Ms. Fitness Olympia

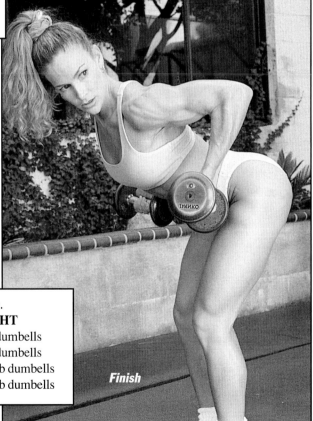

Finish

Warmup – 3 sets to failure with three-pound dumbells.

EXERCISE	SETS	REPS	WEIGHT
Dumbell lateral raises	3	to failure	5-8 lb dumbells
Single-arm lateral raises	3	to failure	5-8 lb dumbells
Bent-over dumbell rows	3	to failure	10-15 lb dumbells
Seated cable presses	3	to failure	10-15 lb dumbells

BICEPS TRAINING WITH SARYN MULDROW

With the ever-increasing muscularity of female bodybuilders, it was only a matter of time before a counter movement began for women not wishing to sacrifice femininity at the expense of muscle mass. In the past five years the fitness movement has exploded and in many respects, has surpassed female bodybuilding in popularity. The second Ms. Fitness Olympia was held in 1996, and Saryn Muldrow had the pleasure of being crowned the winner.

Realistically it takes much longer than four months for most women to make great strides and changes in their physiques. To take your time is not only natural, it is what creates a truly enduring, beautiful figure for years to come.

Saryn Muldrow, 1996 Ms. Fitness Olympia

With more than seven years training under her belt, Saryn displays a physique that is as close to perfection as genetically possible. Although her arms took longer to respond, they are now considered one of her best body-parts. A sample biceps routine follows.

EXERCISE	SETS	REPS
Alternate dumbell curls	3	10-15
EZ-Bar curls	4	8-12
Cable hammer curls	3	10-12
High-pulley cable curls	4	10-15

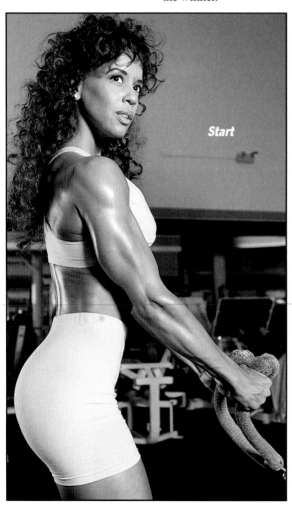

Start

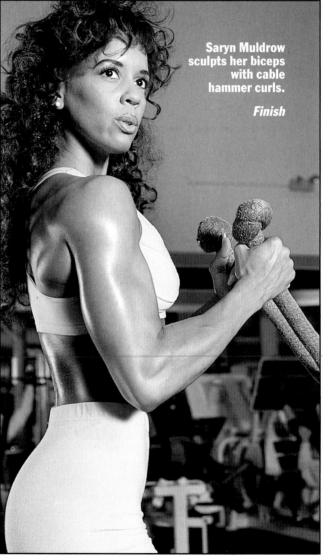

Saryn Muldrow sculpts her biceps with cable hammer curls.

Finish

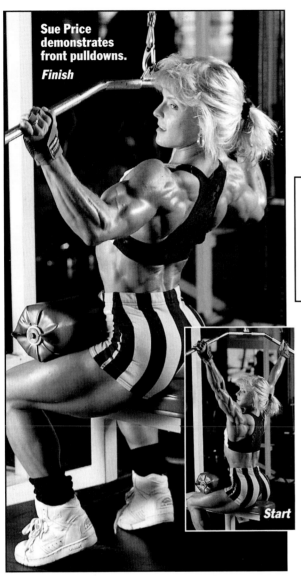

Sue Price demonstrates front pulldowns.

Finish

Start

A trim waist is a function of diet and aerobics, but a toned waist is more a function of ab exercises.

Cory Everson, Six-time Ms. Olympia

Like many weight trainers, Cory doesn't rely on one routine to work her abs. She alternates the exercises and reps to add variety to her training. No matter what the routine, she always tries to spend 15 to 20 minutes training her abs. Cory followed the routine below while on her record Ms. Olympia run in the late 1980s.

EXERCISE	SETS	REPS
Crunches	3	50
Rope crunches	3	50
Decline situps	3	50
Side crunches	3	50
* Note: Cory often performed the previous in 1 or 2 giant sets.		

BACK TRAINING WITH SUE PRICE

One of the top bodybuilding competitors in the early 1990s, Sue Price was known for her combination of muscularity and femininity. This is not surprising as one of her first idols was bodybuilding's first Ms. Olympia, Rachel McLish. A sample back-training routine follows.

I started seriously training at 19 years old when I attended Northern Illinois College. I ran cross-country in high school but I let myself get fat from too many pizzas. I joined an aerobics class that had Nautilus machines. I enjoyed the Nautilus training more than the aerobics because the weights changed the shape of my body while the aerobics only got rid of the fat but did little for my muscle tone.

Sue Price, 1994 Jan Tana Classic bodybuilding champion

ABDOMINAL TRAINING WITH CORY EVERSON

Although Rachel McLish was the first multi-winner of the Ms. Olympia contest, it was six-time winner Cory Everson who brought the benefits of weight training to millions of women. With her perfectly proportioned physique, Cory combined the best qualities of symmetry, muscularity, and most importantly, femininity. In short, she was the epitome of what weight training could do for the female form.

EXERCISE	SETS	REPS
Chins	4	8-10
Barbell rows	3	6-8
Pulldowns	4	8-10
T-Bar rows	3	8-10
One-arm rows	3	8-15

During one of my first photoshoots I was told that I would someday be a champion if I brought my shoulders up. So from then on, every time I went into the gym to train shoulders I started doing barbell presses to build mass.

Tonya Knight, former *MuscleMag* columnist and American Gladiator

SHOULDER TRAINING WITH TONYA KNIGHT

Considered to have one of the best balanced physiques in the late 1980s and early 1990s, Tonya Knight was no stranger to shoulder training. The following is one of the routines she used to bring up what was once a lagging muscle group.

EXERCISE	SETS	REPS
Barbell presses	4-5	15-20
Side lateral raises	4-5	8-12
Bent-over laterals	4-5	8-12
Shrugs or upright rows	4-5	12-15

LAURA BINETTI'S ARMS

If it's hardcore muscle you like, look no further than Canada's own, Laura Binetti. This 142-pound resident of Toronto won the Canadian Bodybuilding Championships, her class at the North American Championships, and the 1995 Canada Pro Cup. Laura is an example of a female body-builder who gives the hardcore element just what they want – lots and lots of eye-popping, striated muscle!

Laura is another bodybuilder who doesn't rely on one routine to train her physique. The following are three routines she uses to blast her triceps and biceps.

My people use moderate poundages but they're training much harder than the guy who puts five or six plates on the bar and does 3 reps with a lot of speed and momentum. Many bodybuilders who try to follow Laura through a routine go outside and throw up or have to stop from exhaustion.

Scott Abel, Canadian "trainer of champions," commenting on the training intensity of Laura Binetti

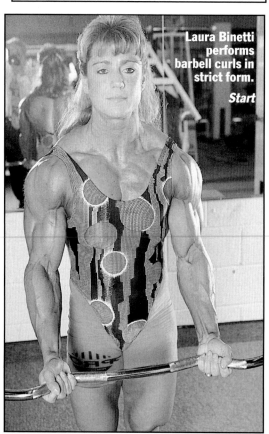

Laura Binetti performs barbell curls in strict form.

Start

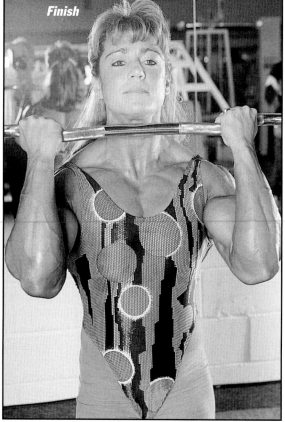

Finish

TRICEPS ROUTINE A

EXERCISE	SETS	REPS
Pushdowns	6	8-15
Overhead rope extensions	3	12-15
One-arm dumbell extensions	3	8-12
Kickbacks	3	15

TRICEPS ROUTINE B

EXERCISE	SETS	REPS
Close-grip bench presses	6	8-12
Pushdowns	3	12-15
Lying triceps extensions	3	10-12
Kickbacks	3	15-20

TRICEPS ROUTINE C

EXERCISE	SETS	REPS
Lying EZ-Bar extensions	6	10-12
One-arm dumbell extensions	3	10-12
Rope extensions	3	12-20
Kickbacks	3	15

BICEPS ROUTINE A

EXERCISE	SETS	REPS
Concentration curls	6	8-12
One-arm preacher curls	3	8-10
Barbell curls	3	15
Hammer curls	3	10-12

BICEPS ROUTINE B

EXERCISE	SETS	REPS
Alternate dumbell curls	6	6-10
One-arm preacher curls	3	10-12
Cable preacher curls	3	15-20
Hammer curls	3	10-12

BICEPS ROUTINE C

EXERCISE	SETS	REPS
Concentration curls	6	8-12
One-arm preacher curls	3	8-10
One-arm cable curls	3	12-15
Hammer curls	3	10-12

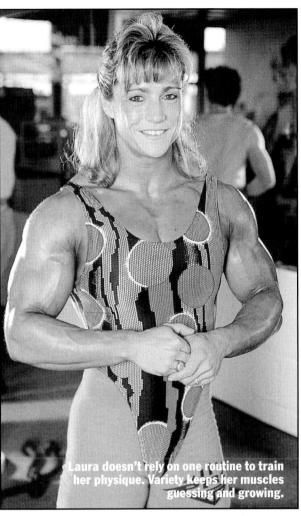

Laura doesn't rely on one routine to train her physique. Variety keeps her muscles guessing and growing.

LEG TRAINING WITH MONICA BRANT

It's difficult to pick up a bodybuilding or fitness magazine these days without being confronted with the lovely image of Monica Brant. Currently one of the most sought after personalities in the fitness field, Monica is another example of what weight training can do for the female form. Early in her career she realized her legs were growing proportionally faster than her upper body. Monica gave up training her legs for almost two years. Even now she uses light weight and high reps for overall conditioning rather than building mass.

I took about two full years off training my legs. Instead I ran sprints on a track and distance in the sand to work them and keep them conditioned.

Monica Brant, 1998 Ms. Fitness Olympia

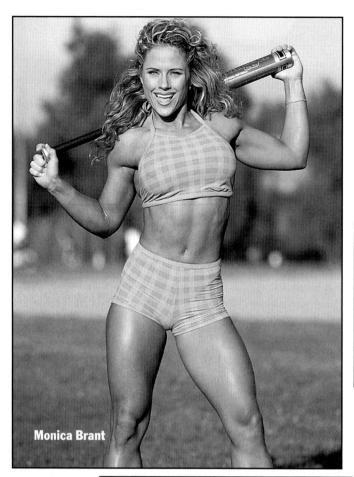

Monica Brant

I believe keeping active is at the heart of developing good calves. I feel that exposing calves to a tremendous amount of diversity in activity is when they really buckle down and respond.

Dale Tomita, fitness competitor

Great calves or not, Dale has good advice for those trying to build the "lowers." She's a firm believer in the old adage that variety is the spice of life. High reps, low reps, heavy weight, light weight, she recommends it all. In fact she utilizes all the previous in the following calf routines.

DAY 1		
EXERCISES	**SETS**	**REPS**
Seated calf raises	4	12-20
Standing calf raises	4	15-20
DAY 2		
EXERCISE	**SETS**	**REPS**
Seated calf raises	4	12-20
Dumbell calf raises	4	15

Warmup – 5 minutes plus light stretching		
EXERCISE	**SETS**	**REPS**
Leg presses	3	30-40
Leg extensions	4-6	25-40
Lunges	4-6	to failure
Squats	4-6	to failure
Leg curls	4-6	20

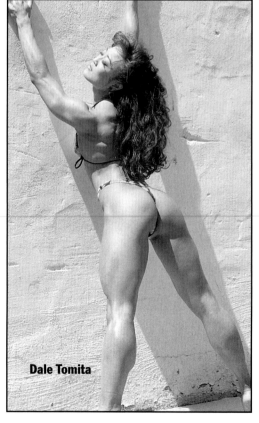

Dale Tomita

DALE TOMITA'S CALVES

Dale Tomita is a product of the mid 1980s approach to women's weight training. Being influenced by Cory Everson and Gladys Portuguese, she places heavy emphasis on symmetry, femininity, and shape. Unlike many individuals who have to slave thousands of hours for calf development, Dale was blessed with great calf-building genetics. She had to stop training them heavy to keep them in proportion with the rest of her physique.

GLUTE AND LEG TRAINING WITH VICKY PRATT

One of our great pleasures at MuscleMag headquarters is helping further the careers of young, up-and-coming fitness and bodybuilding competitors. One such sensation is Canada's own Vicky Pratt. With an honor's degree in kinesiology, this certified fitness appraiser knows her way around a fitness center. Like regular *MuscleMag* columnist Marla Duncan, Vicky has a set of legs and glutes most women would die for. There are those who blame good genetics, but these same people are nowhere to be seen when Vicky hits the gym for a workout. The following is one such workout.

I focus on keeping constant tension on the muscle and squeezing it throughout the entire set. I'm not concerned about how much weight I use. Instead, I want to work the muscle as much as possible.

Vicky Pratt, Canadian fitness model

EXERCISE	SETS	REPS
Lying leg curls	3	20-40
Barbell lunges	3	12
One-leg leg presses	3	20-25
Low kickbacks	3	30-40

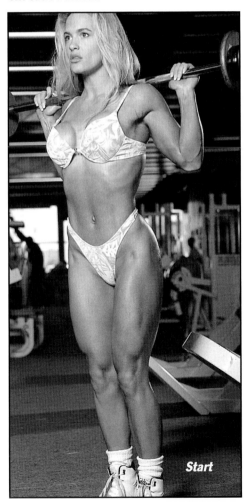

Start

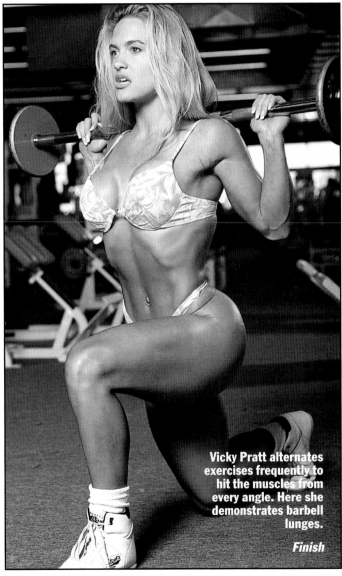

Vicky Pratt alternates exercises frequently to hit the muscles from every angle. Here she demonstrates barbell lunges.

Finish

BICEPS TRAINING WITH LAURA CREAVALLE

Laura used to do a lot of sets like 16 sets for biceps, and since she trains hard they were all-out sets. She used to like to superset them and drop set them. I thought she was overtraining so I suggested she cut back her sets to only 9 or 10, say 3 sets each of what she felt were her three favorite exercises.

Chris Aceto, top trainer and husband to Laura Creavalle

With three Ms. International titles and a Ms. Olympia runner-up placing to her credit, Laura Creavalle is easily one of the top female bodybuilders in the world. While famous for her complete physique, her biceps deserve special attention. Measuring a rockhard 15 inches in contest shape, Laura's biceps are the envy of many a competitor. The following is one of her favorite biceps routines.

EXERCISE	SETS	REPS
Dumbell curls	3	8-10
Cable preacher curls	3	10-12
Hammer curls	3	8-12

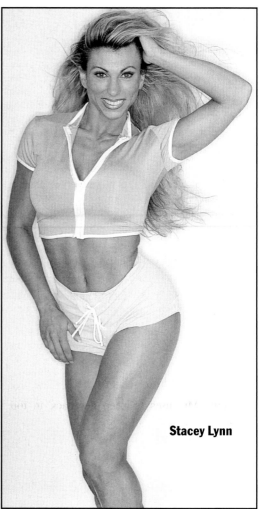

Stacey Lynn

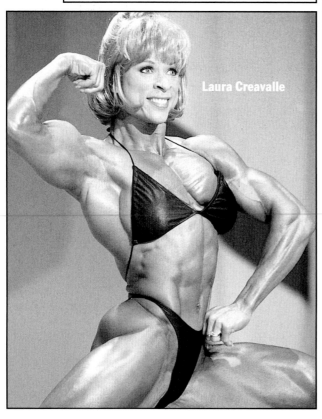

Laura Creavalle

LEG TRAINING WITH STACEY LYNN

It was only a matter of time before fitness sensation Stacey Lynn was bitten by the weightlifting bug. Working for MuscleMag International she was constantly surrounded by the top physiques in the world, and with the encouragement from *MuscleMag* founder, Robert Kennedy, Stacey took the weight-training plunge. The rest is history as Stacey is one of the most sought after fitness models. The following is a sample leg-training routine.

I was amazed at the results. I didn't have to lose or gain weight, but the firming and shaping effect from the weight workouts was awesome. Every part of my body got toned. I increased my base strength by 50 percent in only a few weeks and I felt fitter and healthier than ever before in my life.

Stacey Lynn, top fitness model

EXERCISE	SETS	REPS
Leg extensions	4	20
Squats	4	10
Leg presses	4	15-20
Lunges	3	15-20
Cable kickbacks	3	25-30
Stiff-leg deadlifts	3	10-15
Leg curls	3	10-15
Standing calf raises	3	15-20
Seated calf raises	3	15-20

BACK TRAINING WITH MIA FINNEGAN

Looking at Mia's well-balanced physique makes it hard to believe she was all legs and no upper body at one time. Yet this is the predicament she found herself in after 10 to 12 years of gymnastics. It took a combination of hard work and intelligent training to balance her symmetry. The following is a sample routine Mia uses to keep her back in top condition.

As an athlete I find I can't rely only on isolation movements. If I did I would be all show and no go.

Mia Finnegan, top fitness competitor and *Oxygen* columnist

EXERCISE	SETS	REPS
Wide-grip chins	3-4	12-17
Wide-grip pulldowns	4	8-12
Seated cable rows	4	8-12
Dumbell rows	3	12-15

LENDA MURRAY'S TRICEPS TRAINING

With her sixth Ms. Olympia win in 1995, Lenda Murray accomplished what few people thought possible, tying Cory Everson's record of six straight Ms. Olympia wins. It's not surprising given her almost unparalleled genetics. Besides her world famous delts, Lenda has two of the best triceps ever to grace the Ms. Olympia stage.

She has the ideal combination of triceps mass, length, and shape.

Greg Zulak, former *MuscleMag* editor

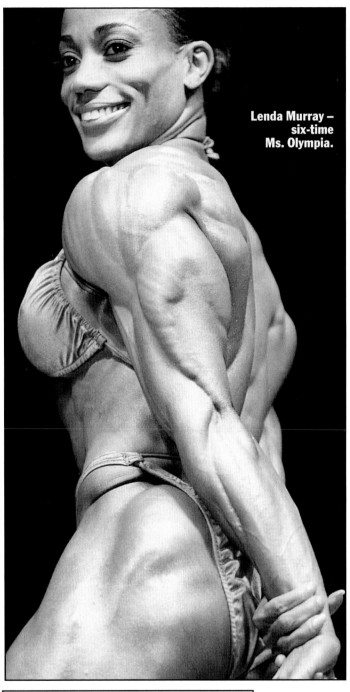

Lenda Murray – six-time Ms. Olympia.

EXERCISE	SETS	REPS
Narrow bench presses	4	12
Superset with:		
Bench dips	4	12-15
One-arm extensions	4	10-15

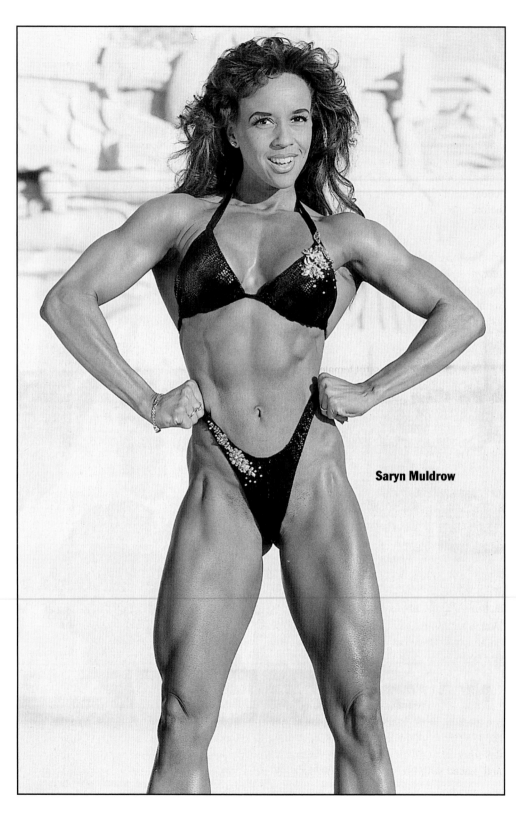

Saryn Muldrow

Chapter 25

MuscleMag's Gallery of Stars

Over the past twenty-five years *MuscleMag International* has interviewed and profiled virtually every top female bodybuilder and fitness superstar. In many cases the interviews were conducted before the individuals reached international status.

The following is a brief look at some of the women who have graced the pages of *MuscleMag International* and *Oxygen* magazines over the years. Our apologies to anyone we have inadvertently omitted.

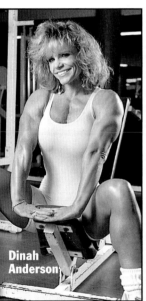

Dinah Anderson

DINAH ANDERSON – Dinah was one of the more successful female competitors of the mid 1980s. Her string of 10 consecutive firsts is among the longest in the sport's history. Included in this record run is the USA National Championships.

DORIS BARRILLEAUX – One of the true pioneers of women's bodybuilding, Doris has been promoting the benefits of weight training for over 35 years. With her boundless energy and youthful enthusiasm Doris is presently active as an IFBB representative.

LAURA BASS – Laura was born in Livingston, New Jersey, and among her titles are the New Jersey State Championships, and the 1991 Jr. USA Championships. She is now devoting her energy to fitness competitions, and placed seventh at the 1997 Jan Tana Pro Fitness Classic.

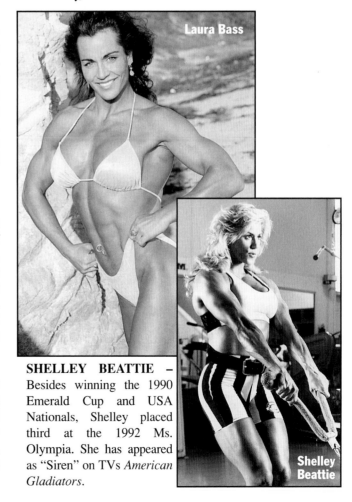

Laura Bass

Shelley Beattie

SHELLEY BEATTIE – Besides winning the 1990 Emerald Cup and USA Nationals, Shelley placed third at the 1992 Ms. Olympia. She has appeared as "Siren" on TVs *American Gladiators*.

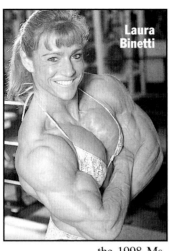
Laura Binetti

LAURA BINETTI – One of Canada's most successful pro bodybuilders, Laura has won the Canadian Championships, her class at the 1989 North American Championships, and the 1994 Canada Pro Cup.

MONICA BRANT – Always placing high in fitness contests since 1991, Monica finally received her dues by winning the 1998 Ms. Fitness Olympia, after placing seventh in 1995 and 1996, and sixth in 1997. She also placed third at the 1997 Pro World Fitness, second at the 1997 Ms. Fitness International, and second at the 1998 Fitness International.

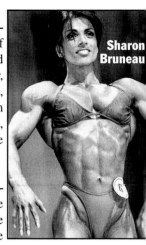
Sharon Bruneau

SHARON BRUNEAU – With her combination of muscularity, symmetry, and athleticism, this Vancouver, British Columbia native, won the 1991 North American Championships, and placed fourth at the 1992 Ms. International.

BRANDI CARRIER – This popular fitness athlete won Ms. Galaxy Physique in 1994 and 1995 and is the 1996 Ms. Galaxy champion. She has competed in the 1995 Jan Tana Pro Fitness Challenge, and the 1997 Fitness America Pageant. She is also the LifeQuest Triple Crown World champion for 1997 and 1998. Brandi has been featured in numerous magazines, is a personal trainer, and is a spokesperson for a nutritional company. She is currently going in the direction of hosting fitness events rather than competing.

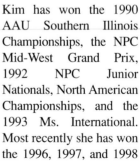
Brandi Carrier

KIM CHIZEVSKY – Kim has won the 1990 AAU Southern Illinois Championships, the NPC Mid-West Grand Prix, 1992 NPC Junior Nationals, North American Championships, and the 1993 Ms. International. Most recently she has won the 1996, 1997, and 1998 Ms. Olympia contests.

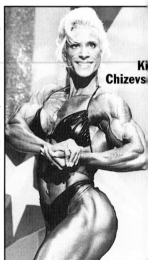
Kim Chizevsky

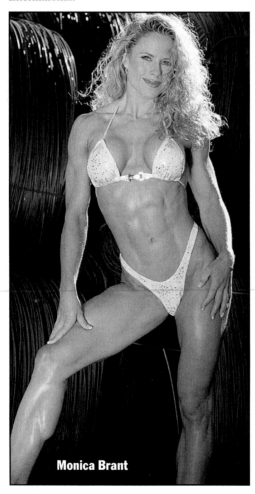
Monica Brant

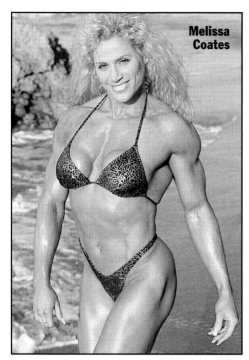

Melissa Coates

MELISSA COATES – A Canadian body-builder, Melissa won her first pro show, the 1996 Jan Tana Classic. She also placed fifth at the 1996 Ms. Olympia and sixth at the 1997 Ms. International.

LAURA COMBES – One of the pioneers of women's bodybuilding, Laura won the 1980 Ms. America. With a level of muscular development never seen before on a woman, Laura set the standard for things to come. Her physique was years ahead of its time. Her death in 1989 shocked and saddened the bodybuilding community.

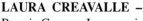

Laura Creavalle

LAURA CREAVALLE – Born in Guyana, Laura emigrated to Canada thirteen years later. With wins at the World Championships and Ms. International, Laura is considered one of the top female bodybuilders in the world. She placed a very controversial second behind Lenda Murray at the 1994 Ms. Olympia. She followed this up with the 1995 Ms. International win.

CANDY CSENCSITS – One of the true pioneers of women's bodybuilding, Candy lost her battle with breast cancer in January of 1989. In her short 33 years she accomplished more than what most accomplish in a lifetime. Besides being a pro bodybuilder, she was a model, school teacher, health-food store owner, and IFBB official. She also held degrees in nutrition and psychology. Her death was felt throughout the bodybuilding world.

SUSAN CURRY – Susan became a fitness pro in 1996, winning the NPC North Carolina Championships, the Junior USAs, the NPC Nationals and the IFBB World Amateur Fitness Championships. She followed her flawless 1996 season with a third at the 1997 Fitness Championships, a first at the IFBB World Pro Fitness Championships and a fourth at the Fitness Olympia. She also walked away with the 1998 Fitness International win, and moved up to second place at the 1998 Fitness Olympia. She currently co-owns a gym in Bremen, GA.

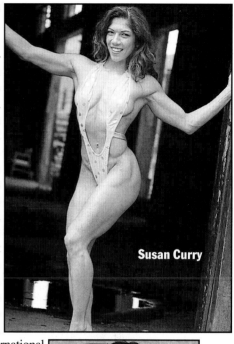

Susan Curry

DEBBIE DOBBINS – One of the saddest days in MuscleMag's history was the tragic death of Debbie Dobbins. With two *MuscleMag* covers to her name, and a growing popularity in the fitness world, Debbie's career was skyrocketing. Debbie was training for the Ms. Galaxy contest when she died in a house fire on New Year's Eve, 1993.

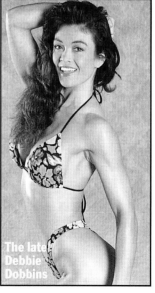

The late Debbie Dobbins

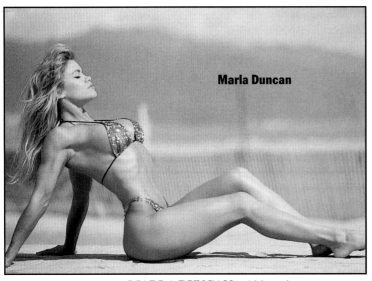
Marla Duncan

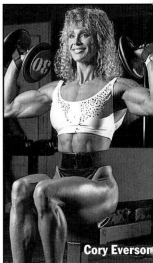
Cory Everson

was due to her combination of symmetry, muscularity, and presentation. In short, she combined the best features of bodybuilding without taking on a masculine appearance. When other competitors began looking like males, Cory retained her femininity and the bodybuilding public loved her for it. Since retiring she has appeared in a number of films, served as a TV color commentator, and most of all, still does her part for the promotion of women's bodybuilding.

MARLA DUNCAN – Although not competing any longer, Marla was one of the very first fitness athletes to grace a stage. She has won several fitness competitions, including the 1990 Ms. Fitness USA. She has also been on the cover of over 25 magazines. She is currently a columnist for *Oxygen*, and is kept busy with seminars, guest appearances, and personal training.

CARLA DUNLAP – Few women bodybuilders have accomplished as much as Carla Dunlap. Besides being one of the sport's pioneers, Carla won the 1983 Ms. Olympia and is an accomplished broadcaster and personal trainer. Although retired from competition, Carla is still devoted to the sport and trains regularly.

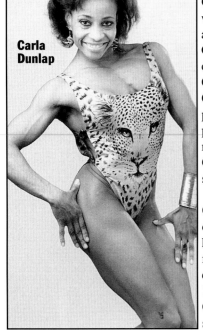
Carla Dunlap

CORY EVERSON – Without a doubt, Cory Everson has established herself as female bodybuilding's greatest star. Before she retired in 1990, Cory had won the Ms. Olympia contest no less than six times. Cory's domination

MIA FINNEGAN – Mia is aptly called the queen of fitness, winning the industry's most prestigious titles with her stunning physique and athletic prowess. A list of her competitive titles is as follows: 1992 Ms. Natural Universe, 1993 Ms. Fitness Western USA, 1994 Ms. Galaxy Fitness (first runner-up and obstacle course winner), 1994 Ms. Fitness California, 1994 Fitness America National Champion, 1995 Ms. Galaxy Fitness, 1995 Ms. Fitness Olympia (first ever), and 1996 Ms. Fitness Olympia runner-up. Mia has retired from competition, but still plays an active role in the fitness world, hosting fitness contests for ESPN, and running her own fitness show titled *Fitting It In*.

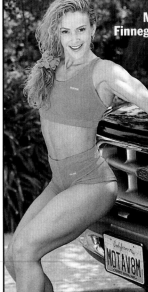
Mia Finnegan

BEV FRANCIS – Hailing from Australia, Bev dominated powerlifting in the late '70s and '80s (winning six world championships back to back). She was also a pro bodybuilder,

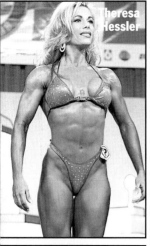

Theresa Hessler

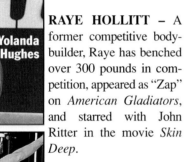

Yolanda Hughes

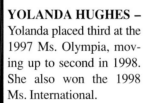

Lena Johannesen

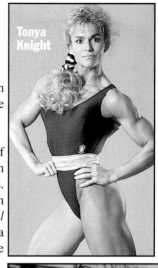

Tonya Knight

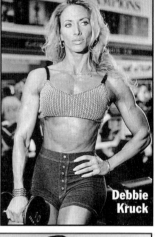

Debbie Kruck

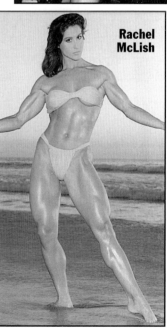

Rachel McLish

placing third at the Ms. Olympia in 1987, 1988 and 1989, and second in 1990 and 1991. She is now retired.

THERESA HESSLER – Theresa won the 1995 NPC Maryland Fitness Championships and was the runner-up at the NPC Nationals the same year. She went on to win the 1996 Florida Pro Fitness and the Italian Pro Fitness Classic, as well as the 1996 and 1997 Jan Tana Pro Fitness Classic.

RAYE HOLLITT – A former competitive body-builder, Raye has benched over 300 pounds in competition, appeared as "Zap" on *American Gladiators*, and starred with John Ritter in the movie *Skin Deep*.

YOLANDA HUGHES – Yolanda placed third at the 1997 Ms. Olympia, moving up to second in 1998. She also won the 1998 Ms. International.

NEGRITA JAYDE – Negrita has been a multi-Canadian women's champion, and has placed as high as third in the World Championships.

LENA JOHANNESEN – Lena was a heavyweight runner-up at the 1992 Nordic Bodybuilding Championships. Turning to fitness, she placed third in the 1997 Ms. Fitness Olympia, fourth at the 1998 Fitness International, second at the 1998 Jan Tana Pro Fitness Classic and fifth at the 1998 Ms. Fitness Olympia.

TONYA KNIGHT – Tonya was one of the most popular female bodybuilders on the pro scene, winning the Ms. International title. Tonya had her own column in *MuscleMag International* called "KnightTime." She was also a regular on *American Gladiators* in the early '90s.

DEBBIE KRUCK – Debbie began her string of wins with the 1992 Fitness America Regional Championships, becomming the first ever Ms. Fitness USA. She also won the 1993 and 1994 Strong and Shapely Pro Fitness Championships, and was 1994 Fitness Model of the Year. Today she is the promoter of the "Debbie Kruck Fitness Classic," emcee of the NPC Wheelchair Nationals, and is busy guest posing in both the US and Europe.

ANJA LANGER – Often called the "Katerina Witt" of women's bodybuilding, Anja was one of the sport's top stars in the late '80s and early '90s. Her combination of muscularity, femininity, and creative posing earned her second place at the 1988 Ms. Olympia.

RACHEL MCLISH – Another of women's bodybuilding pioneers, Rachel was the sport's first Ms. Olympia, (1980 and 1981).

SARYN MULDROW – Saryn is well known for her 1996 Ms. Fitness Olympia win, following a third-place finish at the 1995 Fitness Olympia. She placed second in 1997 and fourth in 1998. She also placed first at the 1998 Czech Republic Pro Fitness Classic and 1998 Panatta Pro Fitness Classic of France.

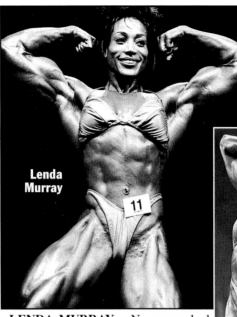

Lenda Murray

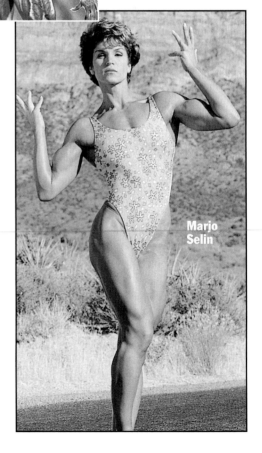

Sandy Riddell

SANDY RIDDELL – This former fire fighter from Arizona first came to bodybuilding prominence in the fall of 1989 when she placed a close second to Cory Everson at the Ms. Olympia contest. In recent years she has shown her athletic ability by competing in the Ms. Galaxy contest.

ANJA SCHREINER – Born and raised in Bad Wimpen, West Germany (now Germany), Anja is considered to be the epitome of what a female bodybuilder should look like. After winning the WABBA Ms. World Championship, Anja joined the IFBB, where she has placed as high as third at the Ms. Olympia, and second at the Ms. International.

LENDA MURRAY – No sooner had the reign of six-time Ms. Olympia Cory Everson ended, when women's bodybuilding found a new queen – Lenda Murray. Her first major win was the 1989 North American Championships, which earned Lenda her pro card. Not being one to waste an opportunity, Lenda won six Ms. Olympias in succession from 1990 to 1995.

GLADYS PORTUGUES – A top female bodybuilder in the early to mid '80s, Gladys became more famous after marrying actor/martial arts champion, Jean-Claude Van Damme.

SUE PRICE – This Chicago native won the 1994 Jan Tana Invitational and placed sixth in her first Ms. Olympia appearance. She also won her weight class at the 1987 Collegiate Illinois and 1990 Midwest Grand Prix.

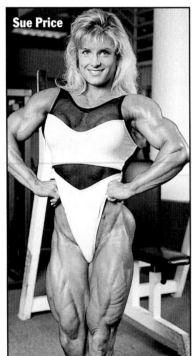

Sue Price

Marjo Selin

MARJO SELIN – Marjo has been one of the world's top female bodybuilders for over a decade. She was also a regular member of the *MuscleMag International* family with her monthly "Repping With Marjo" column.

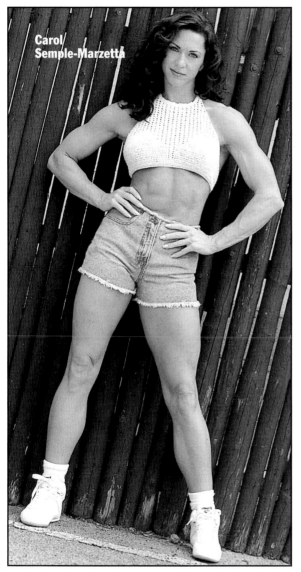

Carol
Semple-Marzetta

CAROL SEMPLE-MARZETTA – Carol is a true fitness champion. A list of her overall wins follows: 1991 Ms. Fitness Colorado, 1992 and 1993 Ms. National Fitness, 1994 and 1995 Ms. Fitness USA, 1994 and 1995 Ms. Fitness World, 1997 Fitness International and the 1997 Ms. Fitness Olympia.

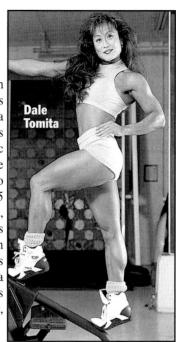

Dale
Tomita

DALE TOMITA – Dale has won the 1995 NPC National Fitness Championships, the 1997 Florida International Pro Championships and the 1997 Czech Republic European Championships. She also placed second at the 1997 Pro World Fitness, fourth at the 1995 and 1996 Ms. Fitness Olympias, and fifth at the 1997 Ms. Fitness Olympia. Dale holds a BA in Speech Communications. She is currently a spokesperson for a nutrition company, and gives seminars on healthy eating, fitness and motivation.

BETTY WEIDER – Betty is the wife of bodybuilding publisher supreme, Joe Weider. Betty has been involved with women's fitness for decades and was promoting the benefits of weight training for females long before the current generation of stars was born. She is truly a pioneer of women's fitness and is a regular contributor to *Muscle and Fitness*, and *Shape* magazines.

MARY YOCKEY – Stunningly proportioned and strong to boot, Mary is making her move in the fitness arena. Placing second at the 1997 NPC National Fitness Championships, she went on to place seventh at the 1998 Fitness International, but regained herself, placing second at the 1998 Panatta Pro Fitness Cup in Italy. A superb showing at the 1998 Ms. Fitness Olympia brought her into third-place standings.

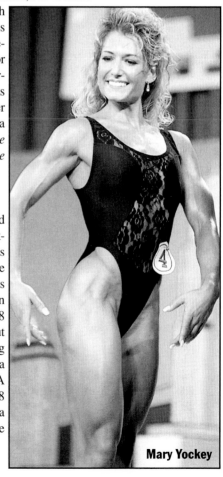

Mary Yockey

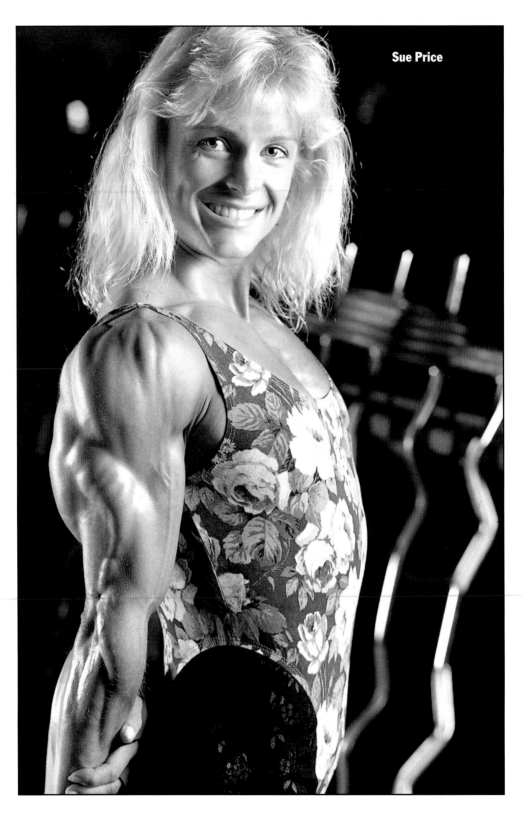

Sue Price

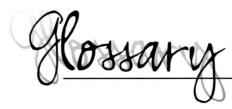

Glossary

Abdominals – The series of muscles located on the lower midsection of the torso. They are used to contract the body forward through a range of six to eight inches.

Acupuncture – The ancient Chinese practice whereby the body's well-being is controlled by pressure points. Acupuncture involves stimulating these points with long needles.

Aerobic Exercise – Any long-lasting exercise that can be carried on within the body's ability to replenish oxygen in working muscles.

AFWB – The American Federation of Women Bodybuilders. This organization is an affiliate of the IFBB, and is responsible for organizing and running women's bodybuilding contests in America.

AIDS – Short for Acquired Immune Deficiency Syndrome. AIDS is caused by a virus and is contracted by the exchange of bodily fluids. There have been some cases of bodybuilders contracting AIDS from the sharing of needles (used for anabolic steroid injections).

Amenorrhea – Absence of menstrual periods due to a low bodyfat percentage.

Amino Acids – Called the "building blocks of life," amino acids are biochemical subunits linked together by chemical bonds to form polypeptide chains. Hundreds of polypeptides, in turn, linked together from a protein molecule.

Anabolic – Metabolic process whereby smaller units are assembled into larger units. For example, the combining of amino acids into protein strands is a form of anabolism.

Anaerobic Exercise – Any high-intensity exercise that outstrips the body's aerobic capacity and leads to an oxygen debt. Because of its intensity, anaerobic exercise can only be maintained for short periods of time.

APC – The American Physique Committee. This federation is responsible for organizing and running men's amateur bodybuilding contests in America. It is also an affiliate of the IFBB.

Arm Blaster – Short, curved metal training apparatus used for bracing the arms when performing exercises such as biceps curls.

Arthritis – Chronic condition marked by an inflammation of the tissue surrounding the joints.

Asymmetric Training – Any exercise that targets only one side of the body. One-arm dumbell curls, lateral raises, or triceps extensions, are all examples of asymmetric training.

Back – The series of muscles located on the dorsal region of the body. The back muscle complex includes the latissimus dorsi, spinal erectors, trapezius, rhomboids and teres minor and major.

Barbell – One of the most basic pieces of bodybuilding equipment. Barbells consist of a long bar, collars, sleeves, and associated plates made of steel or iron. They may be either adjustable (allowing the changing of plates) or fixed (the plates are kept in place by welded collars). Barbells average between five and seven feet in length, and usually weigh between 25 and 45 pounds.

Basic Exercises – Exercises that work more than one muscle group simultaneously. Basic exercises form the mainstay of a bodybuilder's mass-gaining routine. Examples include: bench presses, shoulder presses, squats, deadlifts, and bent-over rows.

Belt – Large leather support worn around the waist by bodybuilders. Weightlifting belts are usually four to six inches in width and provide support to the lower-back muscles and spine.

Biceps – Flexor muscles located on the upper arm. The biceps are composed of two "heads," and are responsible for bending the lower arm towards the upper arm.

Biofeedback – Any physiological or psychological symptom given off by the body. The best bodybuilders are those who recognize such biofeedback signals and use them to improve their training, eating, and competitive preparation.

BMR – Short for Basil Metabolic Rate, the BMR is the speed at which the resting body consumes energy (calories).

Bodybuilding – Competitive or noncompetitive subdivision of weight training in which the primary goal is the improvement of one's physique. For most, the objective is not competition. For those who do compete the final placings are determined by a panel of judges who look at such physical qualities as muscle size, shape, symmetry, bodyfat percentage, and presentation (posing).

Bodyfat Percentage – The ratio of fat to bodyweight. For most bodybuilders, eight to 12 percent is the competitive goal.

Breathing Pullovers – Specialized exercise important to a bodybuilder as it stretches the rib cartilage, producing a large rib cage and, therefore, a larger chest measurement.

Bulking Up – Bodybuilding term which refers to the gaining of 30 to 40 pounds of bodyweight over a short period of time. This practice has become less common given the increased number of competitions, and the demand for guest posers on a year-round basis.

Burn – Unique term to the sport of bodybuilding describing the feeling a muscle gets as it's exercised. Burns are partial reps done at the end of a set when performing full reps is impossible.

Bursae – Flat sacks filled with fluid. They support and protect joints.

Buttocks – Another term referring to the gluteus maximus, medius and minimus, extensors and abductors of the thigh at the hip joint.

Cables – Long wire cords attached to weight stacks at one end and a hand grip at the other. Cable exercises keep tension on the working muscle throughout a full range of motion.

Calves – Also called "lowers" and "bodybuilding's diamonds," the calves consist of the soleus and gastrocnemius muscles located on the backs of the lower leg bones. The calves are similar to the forearms in that they are composed of extremely dense muscle tissue. Their function is to flex the feet.

Carbohydrate Loading – The practice of depleting and replenishing the body's glycogen levels in the weeks leading up to a bodybuilding contest. This technique allows bodybuilders to saturate their muscles with stored water, thus making the muscles fuller and harder.

Cartilage – Connective tissue that acts as a shock absorber between bones. It's found wherever two bones articulate over one another.

Chalk – White, fine-grained powder, used to improve the grip on a barbell or dumbell. Chalk is formed from the shells of dead marine microorganisms.

Cheating – An advanced training technique that consists of utilizing fresh muscles to assist in the completion of an exercise, when the muscle being trained is nearing fatigue.

Chelation – The process by which protein molecules are bonded to inorganic minerals, making them easier to assimilate by the human body.

Chest – The large pectoral muscles located on the front of the upper torso, responsible for drawing the arms toward the center of the body.

Cholesterol – Naturally-occurring steroid molecule involved in the formation of hormones, vitamins, bile salts and the transport of fats in the bloodstream to tissues throughout the body. Excessive cholesterol in the diet can lead to cardiovascular disease.

Circuit Training – A specialized form of weight training which combines strength training and aerobic conditioning. Circuit training consists of performing 10 to 20 different exercises, one after the other, with little rest between sets.

Clean – Weightlifting technique whereby the barbell is hoisted to shoulder level using the arms, legs, hips, and lower back. The competitive version is called the "clean and jerk."

Collar – Small, round, iron or plastic clamp, used to anchor plates on a barbell or dumbell. In most cases collars are screwed on but some versions are held in a spring-like manner.

Compound Exercises – Any exercise that works more than one muscle group. Popular compound movements include: bench presses, squats, shoulder presses, and bent-over rows.

Compulsory Poses – Seven poses that are used to compare contestants in a bodybuilding contest. They include: side chest, rear lat spread, front lat spread, front double biceps, rear double biceps, side triceps, abdominal and front thigh.

Cortisol – Catabolic hormone released by the body in response to stress (of which exercise is one form). Cortisol speeds up the rate at which large units are broken down into smaller units (catabolism).

Cut – Competitive term used to describe the physical appearance of a bodybuilder. To be "cut," implies that you are in great competitive shape, with extremely low bodyfat levels.

Cycle Training – Form of training where high-intensity workouts are alternated with those of low intensity. The technique can be applied weekly or yearly.

Decline Bench – Bench used to work the lower and outer pectorals. Decline benches require the user to place their head at the low end and their feet at the upper end of the bench.

Definition – Another term to describe the percentage of bodyfat carried by a competitive bodybuilder. A bodybuilder with good definition shows a great deal of vascularity and muscular separation.

Dehydration – Biological state where the body has insufficient water levels for proper functioning. As the human body is over 90 percent water, athletes must continuously replenish the water lost during intense exercise.

Density – Term used to describe the amount of muscle mass carried by a bodybuilder. It generally refers to muscle thickness and hardness.

Descending Sets – An advanced training technique involving the removal of weight at the completion of a set, and then performing additional reps with the lighter weight.

Diet – A term that refers to a fixed eating pattern. In general usage it usually means to try and lose weight.

Dislocation – Type of injury where the end of one bone (called a "ball") slips out of a hollow indentation (called the "socket") of another bone. It is usually accompanied by tearing of the joint ligaments, which makes the injury extremely painful.

Diuretics – Some bodybuilders use diuretics before a contest as it improves their muscularity. Diuretics are any natural or synthetic chemical that causes the body to excrete water. In most cases the drug interacts with aldosterone, the hormone responsible for water retention. Diuretics also flush electrolytes from the body. One of the functions of electrolytes is to control heart rate, so using diuretics to get "cut" is a dangerous practice. A few pro bodybuilders have died of diuretic-induced heart attacks.

Down the Rack – An advanced training technique involving the use of two or three successively lighter dumbells during the performance of one set.

Dumbell – Short bars on which plates are secured. Dumbells can be considered the one-arm version of a barbell. In most gyms, the weight plates are welded on, and the poundage is written on the dumbell.

Ectomorphs – Body type characterized by long thin bones, low bodyfat levels, and difficulty in gaining muscle mass.

Endomorphs – Body type characterized by large bones and an excess of bodyfat.

Endorphins – Chemicals released by the brain in response to pain. Often called "natural opiates," endorphins decrease the individual's sensitivity to pain.

Epiphysis – Locations on bones at which growth takes place. They fuse by the late teens or early twenties, but they can prematurely close in young teens by anabolic steroid use.

Exercise – In general terms, any form of physical activity that increases the heart and respiratory rate. In bodybuilding terms, an exercise is one specific movement for one or more muscle groups.

Flexibility – The degree of muscle and connective tissue suppleness at a joint. The greater the flexibility, the greater the range of movement by an individual's limbs and torso.

EZ-curl Bar – Short, S-shaped bar used for such exercises as biceps curls and lying triceps extensions. The bar's unique shape puts less stress on the wrists and forearms than a straight bar.

Fast-twitch Muscle Fiber – Type of muscle fiber that is adapted for rapid but short duration contractions.

Fluid Retention – Bodybuilding term referring to the amount of water held between the skin and muscles. A bodybuilder "holding water" appears smooth, and his muscularity is blurred.

Forced Reps – An advanced training technique where a training partner helps you complete extra reps after the exercised muscles reach the point of fatigue.

Fractures – Complete or partial break of one of the body's bones.

Free Posing – Held in round three of a bodybuilding contest, free posing consists of individual poses set to the bodybuilder's personal choice of music.

Free Weights – Term given to barbells and dumbells. Free-weight exercises are the most popular types performed by bodybuilders.

Genetics – The study of how biological traits or characteristics are passed from one generation to the next. In bodybuilding terms it refers to the potential each individual has for developing his or her physique.

Giant Sets – An advanced training technique where four or more exercises are performed consecutively. In most cases the term refers to exercises for one muscle group, but bodybuilders have been known to use exercises for four different muscle groups.

Gloves – Specialized hand apparel worn while working out. Gloves help prevent blisters and calluses.

Glycogen – Primary fuel source used by exercising muscles. Glycogen is one of the stored forms of carbohydrate.

Golgi Tendon Organ (GTI) – Stretch receptors located at the ends of muscles. They terminate muscular contractions when too much stress is placed on the muscle.

Gym – Although this can apply to almost any exercising venue (e.g. high school gym), for bodybuilders the term refers to a weight-training club.

Hamstrings – The leg biceps located on the back of the upper legs, responsible for curling the lower leg to the upper leg. The hamstrings are analogous to the biceps in the upper arm.

Head Straps – Leather or nylon harness that is placed over the head allowing the user to attach weight and train the neck muscles.

Hypertrophy – Biological term that means muscle growth. Muscles do not grow by increasing the number of cells, but by increasing the size of existing muscle fibers.

IFBB – International Federation of Bodybuilders. First founded in 1946 by Joe Weider, the IFBB is the largest bodybuilding federation in the world and the fifth largest sporting federation.

Injuries – Physical injuries include any damage to bone, muscle, or connective tissue. The most common bodybuilding injuries are muscle strains.

Instinctive Training – An advanced training technique, whereby you train according to how you "feel." In short, you deviate from the normal routine and train according to intuition. It takes many years of experience to become fine-tuned with your body to train instinctively.

Intercostals – Small, finger-like muscles located along the sides of the lower abdomen, between the rib cage and obliques.

Isolation Exercises – Any exercise aimed at working only one muscle. In most cases, it's virtually impossible to totally isolate a muscle. Some common examples are: preacher curls, lateral raises, and triceps pushdowns.

Isometric – Type of muscle contraction where there is no shortening of the muscle's length. Isometric exercises were popularized by Charles Atlas.

Isotension – Exercising technique where continuous stress is placed on a given muscle. Extending the leg by contracting the quadriceps, and holding the position for 10 to 20 seconds or more, is an example of isotension. Bodybuilders make use of the technique during the precompetition phase as it improves muscle separation.

Isotonic – Type of muscle contraction where the contracting muscle shortens. The muscle may also be lengthening, as when doing a "negative." Most bodybuilding exercises are examples of isotonic contraction.

Joint – The point at which two bones meet. Most joints have a hinge-type structure which allows the bones to articulate (bend) over one another.

Lactic Acid – A product given off during aerobic respiration. Lactic acid was once thought to be strictly a waste product, however recent evidence suggests that a version of lactic acid called lactate is used by the liver to replenish glycogen supplies.

Latissimus Dorsi – Called the lats, these large fan-shaped muscles are located on the back of the torso, and when properly developed give the bodybuilder the characteristic V-shape. The lats function to pull the arms down and back.

Layoff – Any time spent away from the gym is called a layoff. It can be referred to as a training vacation.

Ligament – Fibrous connective tissue that joins one bone to another.

Lymph System – Parallel system to the cardiovascular system, responsible for collecting and removing waste products from the body. The system's fluid is called lymph, and collects at nodes found in the neck, armpits, and groin.

Massage – Recovery technique that involves a forceful rubbing, pinching, or kneading, of the body's muscles. Massage speeds up the removal rate of exercise byproducts, helps athletes relax, and improves performance. The most popular forms of massage are Soviet and Swedish.

Mesomorphs – Body type characterized by large bones, low bodyfat levels, and a greater than average rate of muscle growth.

Muscularity – Another term used to describe the degree of muscular definition. The lower the bodyfat percentage the greater the degree of muscularity.

Muscle – The series of tissue bellies located on the skeleton that serve to move and stabilize the body's various appendages.

Nautilus – Type of exercise equipment invented by Dr. Arthur Jones. Nautilus machines employ a wide assortment of cams, pulleys, and weight stacks, to work the muscles over a wide range of movement.

Negatives – A portion of the rep movement which goes in the same direction as gravity, but the user concentrates on resisting it.

Neuromuscular System – The combination of nerves and muscles that interact to control body movement.

Nutrition – The art of combining foods in the right amounts so the human body receives all of the required nutrients. In bodybuilding terms, eating to gain muscle size and reduce bodyfat levels is considered proper nutrition.

Nutrients – The various minerals, vitamins, proteins, fats, and carbohydrates, needed by the body for proper maintenance, health, and growth.

Off-season – Competitive bodybuilding term used to describe the period of the year primarily devoted to gaining muscle mass.

Oil – Mineral or water-based liquid used by bodybuilders to highlight the muscles while onstage. Most bodybuilders use vegetable oils as they are absorbed by the skin and give it a better texture.

Olympia, Ms. (and Ms. Fitness Olympia) – The top professional contest in women's bodybuilding. The first Ms. Olympia was held in 1980 (won by Rachel McLish). The first Ms. Fitness Olympia was held in 1995 (won by Mia Finnegan).

Olympic Barbell – The most specialized and refined barbell in weightlifting. Olympic barbells weigh 45 pounds and are made from spring-steel.

Overload – Term used to describe the degree of stress placed on a muscle. To overload means to continuously increase the amount of resistance that a muscle has to work against. For bodybuilders the stress is in the form of weight.

Overtraining – The physiological state whereby the individual's recovery system is taxed to the limit. In many cases, insufficient time is allowed for recovery between workouts. Among the more common symptoms are: muscle loss, lack of motivation, insomnia, and reduced energy.

Peak – This can mean the degree of sharpness or shape held by a particular muscle (usually the biceps), or it may refer to the shape a bodybuilder or fitness competitor holds on a given contest day. A woman who has "peaked" is in top condition.

Plateau – A state of training where no progress is being made. Plateaus usually occur after long periods of repetitious training. Breaking the condition involves shocking the muscles with new training techniques.

Plates – Small to large cast-iron weights that are placed on a barbell or dumbell. Plates range in size from 1-1/4 pounds to 100 pounds. The most common plates in bodybuilding gyms weigh 5, 10, 25, 35, and 45 pounds.

Posedown – Final round in a competitive bodybuilding contest, whereby the top three to six contestants match poses in a posing free-for-all.

Posing – The art of displaying the physique in a bodybuilding or fitness contest.

Positives – Part of the rep movement that goes against gravity. In barbell biceps curls, the positive phase would occur during the curling of the barbell. The lowering of the bar is the negative phase.

Poundage – Another term used to describe the weight of a barbell, dumbell, or machine weight stack.

Powerlifting – The competitive sport that utilizes three lifts – the squat, deadlift, and bench press. The objective is to lift more than your opponent both in the three individual events, and in total.

Precontest – Period of the year devoted primarily to refining muscle size and shape. Bodybuilders, on average, devote the last three months before a contest to this type of training.

Pre-exhaust – Advanced training technique first described by *MuscleMag's* Robert Kennedy. The technique involves fatiguing a desired muscle with an isolation movement, and then using a compound exercise to stress the muscle even further. Pre-exhaust is ideal for eliminating the "weakest link in the chain" effect, often encountered during compound exercises.

Prejudging – Section of a bodybuilding contest where most of the actual judging takes place. Although the competitors may go through their free-posing routines, most of the emphasis is placed on the compulsory rounds.

Priority Training – Training strategy where an individual devotes most of her energy to targeting weak muscle groups.

Proportion – Term used to describe the size of one muscle with respect to the whole body. A bodybuilder or fitness competitor with good "proportions" would have all her muscles in balance with regards to muscle size.

Protein – Nutrient composed of long chains of amino acids. Protein is primarily used in the production of muscle tissue, hormones, and enzymes.

Psychological Warfare – Any verbal or behavioral strategies employed by competitors to interfere with their opponents' preparation or competition.

Pump – Biological condition where an exercised muscle swells and becomes engorged with blood.

Pumping Up – The practice of performing light exercise just before walking onstage at a contest. Pumping up gives the muscles a temporary size increase.

Pyramiding – Training technique where weight is added for the first couple of sets, and then decreased for the remaining sets. A half-pyramid technique may also be performed where the weight is only added or decreased for the given number of sets.

Quadriceps – Commonly known as the "thighs," the quads are the large, four-headed muscles located on the front and sides of the upper legs. They are analogous to the triceps, and are the extensors of the legs. Their primary function is to extend the lower leg forward (bringing the upper and lower legs to a locked-out configuration).

Repetition – Abbreviated "rep," this simply refers to one full movement of a particular exercise.

Resistance – The amount of force being placed on a muscle. In bodybuilding circles it refers to the amount of weight being lifted.

Rest/Pause – A training technique where the user completes one set, and then rests about 10 seconds before starting the next set. The technique is based on the biological fact that a muscle recovers about 90 percent of its strength within 10 to 15 seconds.

Ripped – Another term to describe the percentage of bodyfat carried by a competitive bodybuilder. A ripped bodybuilder has a very low bodyfat percentage (eight to 12 percent).

Routine – Another word for program, schedule, agenda, etc. It refers to the complete number of sets, reps, and exercises performed for a given muscle or muscles on a particular day.

Set – Term referring to a given number of consecutive reps. For example, 10 nonstop reps would be called one set of 10.

Shocking – Training strategy that involves training the muscle with a new form of exercise. Shocking techniques are used to "kick start" muscles that have become accustomed to repetitious training routines.

Shoulders – The deltoid muscles – anterior, medial and posterior – located at the top of the torso. The deltoids are responsible for elevating and rotating the shoulder girdle.

Sleeve – Short, hollow, metal tube fitted over both ends of a barbell. The sleeve allows the plates to rotate on the bar, thus reducing the stress on the user's wrists.

Slow-twitch Muscle Fiber – Type of muscle fiber adapted for slow, long duration contraction. The spinal erectors of the lower back are primarily composed of slow-twitch muscle fibers.

Somatotype – Term referring to an individual's body characteristics including such things as muscle size, bone size, bodyfat level, and personality.

Soreness – The mild pain felt in muscles after a workout. It is primarily caused by lactic acid build-up, and usually appears 12 to 24 hours after exercising.

Spinal Erectors – Two long, snake-like muscles located at the center of the lower back. The spinal erectors help maintain posture by keeping the upper body perpendicular with the floor.

Split Routines – Any routine where different muscle groups are worked on separate days. The most common split routines are four- and six-day splits.

Sponges – Sponges are used to protect the hands from blisters and callouses. Many bodybuilders find sponges more convenient to work with than gloves.

Spot – In short, a helping hand when performing a particular exercise. A spot is provided by a training partner when you fail during an exercise. In most cases it involves providing a few pounds of upward pressure to keep the barbell, dumbell, or machine handle moving.

Staggered Sets – An advanced training technique where the user adds sets for a weak muscle group between their regular training exercises. For example, many bodybuilders with weak calves add extra calf training between other muscle groups. In many cases, the calf exercise is performed instead of taking a rest.

Steroids – Synthetic derivatives of the hormone testosterone that allow the user to gain muscle mass and strength more rapidly.

Sticking Point – The point during an exercise where the user is in the weakest biomechanical position. In other words, this is the most difficult part of the movement. The sticking point is usually close to the bottom of an exercise.

Straps – Long, narrow pieces of material used to increase one's gripping power on an exercise. Straps are wrapped around the lower forearm and bar in such a manner that as the user grips the bar, the straps get tighter. They are used on such exercises as deadlifts, shrugs, and chins.

Stretching – Form of exercise where the primary goal is to increase flexibility. Stretching is also an excellent way to warm up the body and prepare it for more stressful forms of exercise.

Stretch Marks – Red or purple lines caused by thinning and loss of elasticity in the skin.

Strict Form – Training technique which involves performing exercises in a slow, controlled manner, and through a full range of motion, without the aid of a partner or cheating techniques.

Stripping Method – An advanced training technique where the individual removes a few plates at the end of a set and forces out extra reps. The technique allows the user to force a muscle past the point of normal failure.

Supersets – Advanced training technique where two exercises are performed consecutively without any rest. Supersets may consist of exercises for the same muscle group (e.g. dumbell curls and barbell curls) or exercises for different muscle groups (e.g. triceps extensions and biceps curls). When performing supersets for different muscle groups, it is common to work opposing muscle groups (triceps/biceps, quads/hamstrings, chest/back, etc.).

Supination – Technique where the palms start off facing the body during a dumbell curl, and rotate outward as the dumbell is raised. At the top of the movement, the palms are facing upward. The technique takes advantage of the wrist-rotating properties of the biceps.

Supplements – Any form of vitamin, mineral, protein, or other nutrient, that is taken separately or in addition to, normal food. Supplements come in many forms including: tablet, capsule, powder, oil, or plant material.

Sweat Bands – Small pieces of material, usually cloth, wrapped around the forehead to absorb sweat.

Symmetry – In bodybuilding terms this refers to the overall balance of the body. Symmetry is closely related to proportion. A bodybuilder with good symmetry does not have any overdeveloped or underdeveloped muscle groups.

Tanning – Biochemical reaction where the skin releases pigment upon exposure to sunlight (or artificial tanning light). Competitors tan because a darker complexion improves skin appearance in a contest or photoshoot, highlighting muscularity.

Tendinitis – Form of inflammation involving tendons and the points where they attach to muscles and bones. Tendinitis is usually caused by overstressing a particular area. Bodybuilders often get tendinitis in the biceps-tendon region.

Tendon – Tough cord of connective tissue that joins a muscle to a bone.

Testosterone – Androgenic/anabolic hormone responsible for such physiological effects as: increasing muscle size and strength, facial hair growth, scalp hair loss, decreasing sperm production (males), and increasing aggression levels. Although both sexes have circulating testosterone, males have it in greater concentrations.

Training Diary – Daily journal, or record, useful for keeping track of such items as weight, exercises, sets, reps, calories and overall motivation levels.

Training Partner – Any individual who matches you set for set during your workout. Training partners allow you to go for that extra rep. They also serve as a sort of coach on days when you just don't feel like working out.

Training to Failure – Any form of exercise where you terminate a set only after the muscle cannot contract for additional reps. Most bodybuilders train to positive failure and then have a training partner help them perform a few extra reps.

Triceps – Extensor muscles of the upper arm. The triceps are composed of three "heads," and work opposite to the biceps in that they extend the lower arm to a locked-out position.

Trisets – Similar to supersets but involving the use of three different exercises for the same muscle group.

Twenty-one's – Advanced exercise technique where you perform 7 half reps at the bottom of the movement, 7 half reps at the top, and finish with 7 full reps.

Universal Machine – The most common type of training apparatus (not counting free weights) found in bodybuilding gyms. The machines may train one muscle group, or have numerous stations to train the whole body.

Vascularity – The degree of vein and artery visibility. In order to be "highly" vascular, a bodybuilder must have an extremely low bodyfat percentage.

Warmup – Any form of light, short duration exercise that prepares the body for more intense exercise. Warming up should involve increasing the heart and respiratory rate, and stretching. A good warmup helps prevent injury.

Weight – This term refers to the plates or weight stacks themselves, or it can be used to describe the actual poundage on the bar.

Weightlifting – A term used to describe weight training, or an Olympic event. The competitive version involves two lifts – the snatch, and clean and jerk.

Workout – The program or schedule of exercises performed on any given day.

Wraps – Long pieces of material (usually a first-aid bandage) that bodybuilders wrap around weak or injured bodyparts. Wraps keep the area warm and provide extra security. Many bodybuilders wrap the knees during squats, and the wrists during bench presses.

GLOSSARY **315**

INDEX